U0344559

༄༅། །ལུས་གསོའི་རིས་མོས་དོན་འགྲེལ། །

An Illustrated Guide to

HEALTH CULTIVATION IN TIBETAN MEDICINE

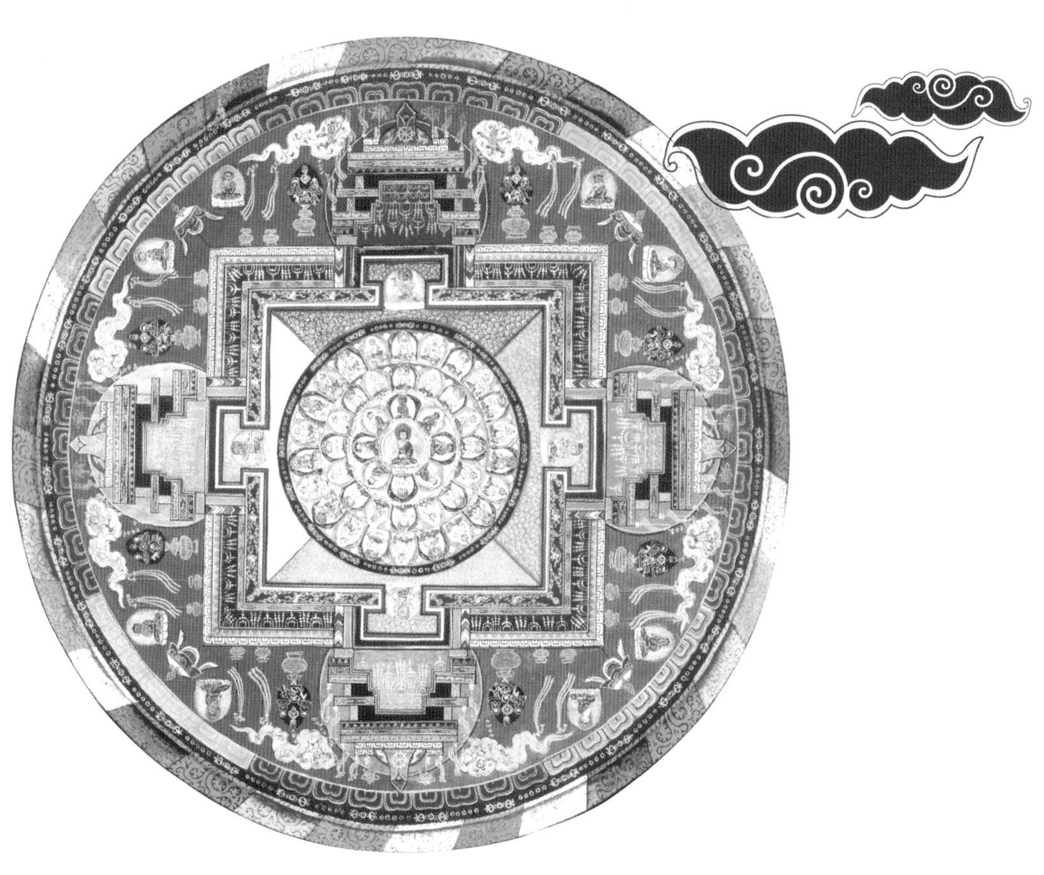

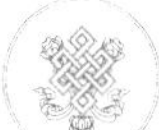 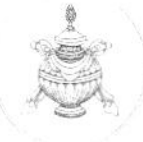 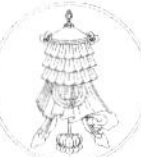 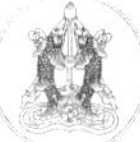 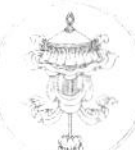 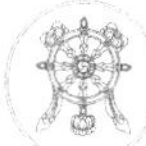 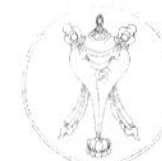 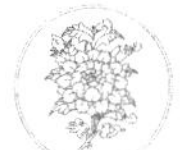

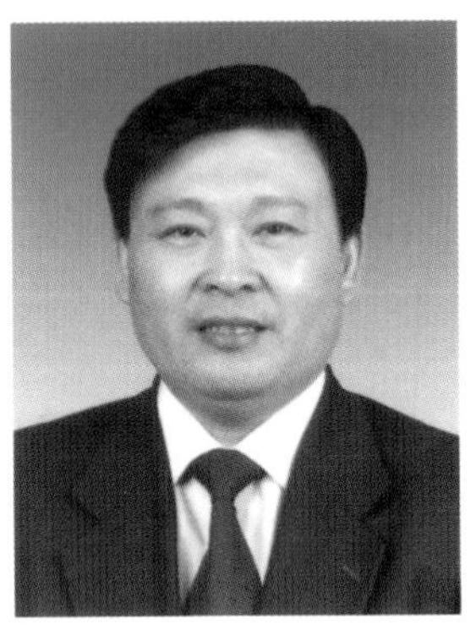

ABOUT THE AUTHOR

Professor Huang Fu-kai, born in 1958 in Huainan, Anhui province, is an associate chief-physician of Tibetan medicine. Presently he is the president of the Beijing Tibetan Medicine Hospital, professor of Tibetan medicine at the Central University for Nationalities, and the deputy secretary-general of the Chinese Association of Minority Medicine. His main interests are Tibetan medicine and the integration of traditional and Western medicine. He has published over twenty articles, including *Report on the Research of Development of Tibetan Medicine under the Situation of Development of Western China.* His monographs include *Chinese Tibetan Medicinal Bathing.* He is the chief editor of *Bibliography of Articles on Tibetan Medicine (1907-2001), Research Anthology of Tibetan Medicine, Chinese Epidemic Diseases, Guide to Chinese Minority Medicine,* and other titles. Professor Huang has also been in charge of several projects under the State Administration of Traditional Chinese Medicine, including *National key constructed specialties of priority - Department of cardiovascular and cerebrovascular diseases in Tibetan Medicine.*

Project & Managing Editor: Zhang Nai-ge & Carl Stimson
Book & Cover Designer: Hui Lin
Typesetter: Wei Hong-bo

༄༅། །ལུས་གསོའི་རིས་མོས་དོན་འགྲེལ། །

An Illustrated Guide to HEALTH CULTIVATION IN TIBETAN MEDICINE

Huang Fu-kai

President of Beijing Traditional Tibetan Hospital,
Professor of Tibetan Medicine, Central University for Nationalities

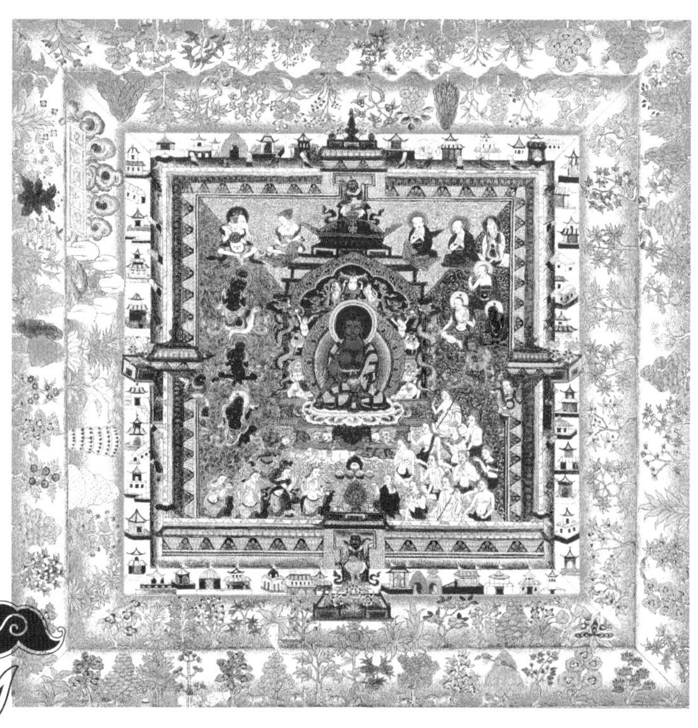

Translated by **Zhen Yan**, Ph.D. TCM
Edited by **Cai Jing-feng**, Professor of China Academy of Chinese Medical Sciences

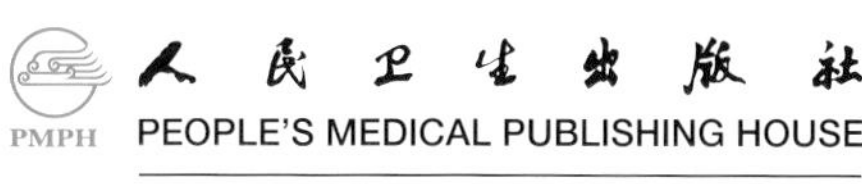

PMPH 人民卫生出版社
PEOPLE'S MEDICAL PUBLISHING HOUSE
BEIJING • LONDON • NEW YORK

人民卫生出版社
PMPH PEOPLE'S MEDICAL PUBLISHING HOUSE

Website: http://www.pmph.com
Book Title: An Illustrated Guide to Health Cultivation in Tibetan Medicine
图说藏医养生

Contact address: Bldg 3, 3 Qu, Fangqunyuan, Fangzhuang, Beijing 100078, P.R. China, phone/fax: 8610 6769 1034, E-mail: pmph@pmph.com

For text and trade sales, as well as review copy enquiries, please contact PMPH at pmphsales@gmail.com

Disclaimer

This book is for educational and reference purposes only. In view of the possibility of human error or changes in medical science, neither the author, editor, publisher, nor any other party who has been involved in the preparation or publication of this work guarantees that the information contained herein is in every respect accurate or complete. The medicinal therapy and treatment techniques presented in this book are provided for the purpose of reference only. If readers wish to attempt any of the techniques or utilize any of the medicinal therapies contained in this book, the publisher assumes no responsibility for any such actions.

It is the responsibility of the readers to understand and adhere to local laws and regulations concerning the practice of these techniques and methods. The authors, editors, and publishers disclaim all responsibility for any liability, loss, injury, or damage incurred as a consequence, directly or indirectly, of the use and application of any of the contents of this book.

First published: 2008
ISBN:978-7-117-09101-5/R・9102

Cataloguing in Publication Data:
A catalog record for this book is available from the CIP-Database China.

Printed in The People's Republic of China

PREFACE

Recently Tibetan medicine, one of the most ancient traditional medical systems in the world, has been gaining in popularity among people all over the world. Currently, there are institutions of Tibetan medicine worldwide, offering hospital, clinical, and educational services as well as performing research based on Tibetan medicine. In addition to presentations on Tibetan medicine in international academic conferences dealing with Tibetan studies, workshops and conferences exclusively on Tibetan medicine have been held in Tibet and abroad. Besides the institutions in the areas where the Tibetan people live (Tibet, Qinghai, Gansu, Sichuan, and Yunnan), traditional Tibetan hospitals, colleges, and research institutes have been established all over China. The Beijing Hospital of Tibetan Medicine (now promoted as a hospital that includes ethnic medicines of many other minority groups) is open to the public for outpatient visits, and has 200 beds for inpatient care. Here, patients can receive treatment that integrates Tibetan medicine, other minority medical techniques, modern biomedicine, or traditional medicine of the Han nationality (commonly known as traditional Chinese medicine).

People's awareness of Tibetan medicine has gradually increased. However, only those who have sought the help of Tibetan medicine to relieve health problems have some knowledge of its techniques and theories. Most people only have a superficial understanding or are even ignorant about Tibetan medicine. Furthermore, quite a large number of people even say that Tibetan medicine is "superstitious", "non scientific", "backward", "tainted with religion", and so on.

It is true that since the Tubo Dynasty was established in the 7th century, Buddhism has played an important role in Tibet, diffusing to all aspects of life in Tibetan society, including the medical world and people's habits and customs.

To remedy the wrong ideas about Tibetan medicine that exist in some people's brain, it is best if people can experience the benefits of Tibetan medicine in person. Unfortunately, it is practically impossible for everyone to have such an opportunity, especially in the West. An alternative approach is to learn Tibetan medicine through books. Popularization of common knowledge about Tibetan medicine is an effective approach to remedy incorrect ideas about Tibetan medicine. Among others, Dr. Huang Fu-kai's *An Illustrated Guide to Health Cultivation in Tibetan Medicine*, is a distinguished example of popular knowledge about Tibetan medicine made available to the general public.

The major part of this book is devoted to illustrations taken from the *Sman-thang*, a superb series of Tibetan medical paintings consisting of seventy-nine paintings unparalleled and unprecedented in the history of traditional medical systems. The author of this book extracts the essence of these paintings with numerous examples relevant to health.

All the illustrations in this book are full of the flavor of Tibetan culture, displaying vividly the daily life of the Tibetan people. It gives readers knowledge about Tibetan medicine and lets them enjoy the art at the same time.

Last but not least, this is not only a quality book giving valuable knowledge about health, but also outlines theories and concrete measures for implementing them in simple language that is readily acceptable.

As the Chinese economy flourishes and the living standard of the Chinese people rises, what the people demand is not only an elevation of material enjoyment, but also an increase in cultural accomplishments. Popularization of knowledge is essential for this. The demand for learning and access to Tibetan medicine is part of this process. And the publication of *An Illustrated Guide to Health Cultivation in Tibetan Medicine* should be recognized as an important step in a positive direction.

The publication of *An Illustrated Guide to Health Cultivation in Tibetan Medicine* is a welcome event.

Cai Jing-feng

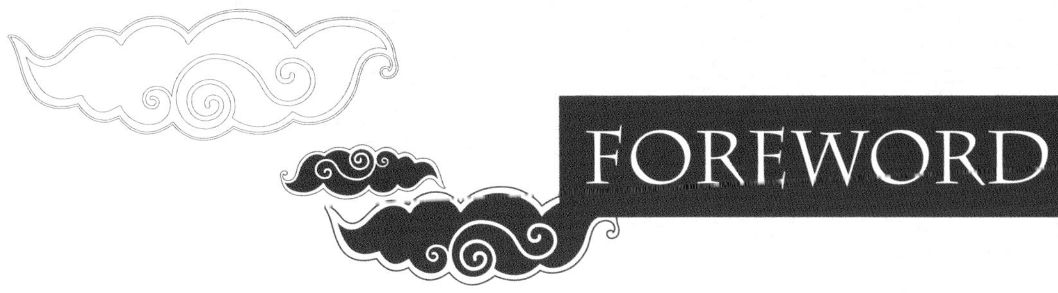

FOREWORD

Every civilization contributes her traditional medicine.

According to the archeologists, since 40,000 to 50,000 years ago there have been people living on the Qinghai-Tibetan plateau. Knowledge of health maintenance and the treatment of disease accumulated over this long period of time. As cultural relics and literature reveal, around 2,000 to 3,000 years ago the ancestors of the present Tibetan people had mastered a considerable amount of medical knowledge, which formed the basis for the maturation of Tibetan medicine in later centuries.

In the 7th century A.D., King Srong Btsan Sgam Po did all he could to make his kingdom prosperous. He is credited with not only opening a new era in the history of Tibetan civilization, but with raising the standard of medicine. He invited prominent doctors from all areas of the kingdom to help compile the early Tibetan medicine classic *Mi 'jigs pa mtshon cha (The Fearless Weapon)*. In the 8th century, the fundamental classic *Rgyud bzhi (The Four Medical Tantras)* was written by Gyuthog Yontan Gonpo. This book established Tibetan medicine as a complete system. Since it holds the fundamentals for the later development of Tibetan medicine, this book is often seen as the origin and core of Tibetan medicine and the author Gyuthog Yontan Gonpo is known as the father of Tibetan medicine. In the subsequent 1,200 years, numerous interpretations, elaborations, and commentaries on this book were published. As a result, Tibetan medicine was propelled from one peak to another.

From a contemporary medical perspective, traditional Tibetan medicine not only has a sound theoretical system, but also contributes important knowledge in the fields of internal medicine, surgery, gynecology, pediatrics, disease prevention and health maintenance. Tibetan medicine is extremely profound and comprehensive, especially in its understanding of embryology and urinary diagnostics, which are considered the most highly developed of all traditional medical systems. Knowledge from these fields are still of great academic and practical value.

Originating from the experiences of generations of Tibetan doctors, knowledge of health maintenance is abundant and unique. It forms an important segment of Tibetan medicine. As the opening of *The Four Medical Tantras* goes, "To prevent and treat disease, the people should read this book; to live longer, the people should read this book; to get the Dharma, wealth and health, the people should read this book; to help all sentient beings escape from the sufferings of disease, the people should read this book." At the end of *The Four Medical Tantras* it summarizes, "Lengthy though *The Four Medical Tantras* is, it talks about only two conditions:

health and disease." The 13th through 18th chapters of *Description Tantra* in *The Four Medical Tantras* discuss everyday principles of health maintenance and health maintenance through the use of proper diet. The 23rd chapter is on prevention of disease. The 71st chapter of the *Secret Tantra* in *The Four Medical Tantras* is on nursing, and the 90th is on preventing aging. There are numerous places in other chapters that offer insights into health cultivation and disease prevention. The present book is a refinement and summary of the chapters on health maintenance in *The Four Medical Tantras*, with wisdom on health maintenance from generations of prominent Tibetan doctors included.

This book is also illustrated with vivid pictures in the colorful style of the Tibetan people. In the 17th century, Sangs rgyas rgya mtsho sponsored and designed the now famous medicinal *Thangkha* series, which was then called *Sman thang*. *Sman* means medicine and *thang* is an abbreviation of *thangkha*, an art form unique to Tibetan culture. Simply stated, a *thangkha* is a kind of scroll. Thus *Sman thang* refers to a medical scroll, something we might compare to a teaching wall chart. The text portions of the *Sman thang* are mainly from the text *Baidurya sngon po (Blue Lapis Lazuli)*, complemented with information from *Sman dpyad zla ba'i rgyal po (Medical Investigations of the Lunar King)*. The dimensions of the original *Sman thang* are basically the same for each piece, about 30 - 43 cm × 90 - 100 cm. There are eighty *Sman thang* in all and are a perfect combination of Tibetan art and medical scholarship. These comprehensive charts interpreted the profound contents of *The Four Medical Tantras* with original images. Sangs rgyas rgya mtsho once said, "To make *The Four Medical Tantras* more accessible, and help those from beginning students to knowledgeable scholars understand medicine, we produced this *thangka* series. With these charts, the contents of *The Four Medical Tantras* will be as clear as an emblic flower on the palm, and a student can see it clearly at a glance."

In order to increase the dissemination value, we have selected a large number of images from *Sman thang* to help introduce the concepts of health cultivation in Tibetan medicine. In order to help readers learn more about the cultural background of the Tibetan concepts of health cultivation, other Tibetan art forms such as frescos, *Thangkha*, and folk decorations have been used in the book. We tried our best to achieve excellence both in the text and the illustrations, thus making the Tibetan concepts of health maintenance accessible and helpful to everybody.

When explaining the causes of disease *The Four Medical Tantras* says, "In the sky the birds fly, on the ground the shadows attend by; sentient beings live with seeming joy, for their ignorance disease goes by." With calmer hearts and easier access to Tibetan wisdom of health cultivation as described in this book, we eliminate our ignorance of illness bit by bit, and draw closer to eternal wellness and true joy.

EDITOR'S FOREWORD

Tibetan culture and the form of Buddhism practiced by the Tibetan people have become very popular in the West in the past few decades. As access to the Himalayan region has increased, so has travel to this amazing area. People from Western countries are attracted to the beauty and purity of the region and the kindness and open-heartedness of the people that live there. In recent years the artistic styles of Tibet have also become increasingly popular, with paintings and sculptures in high demand.

The aim of this book is to introduce another important aspect of Tibetan culture, its medicine. Like all medical systems, the way Tibetan doctors understand and treat disease reflects how they understand and relate to the world. Some of these influences are cultural, some come from religion, and others from the geographical conditions of the area. As the title suggests, the authors attempted to present material that is accessible and even useful to everyday people, as opposed to technical medical theories and techniques. It is the hope of the authors that this book will serve two purposes. One, to contribute to the understanding of Tibetan culture in those who are fascinated by it already. And secondly, to provide a framework for understanding health and some methods and theories that will help achieve good health.

At the same time, it must be remembered while reading this book that the medical system of Tibet grew out of and reflects a very unique culture and environment. Some of the treatments suggested in the text will sound strange to Western readers. Not all aspects of a traditional medical system are able to be transmitted to another culture. Differing tastes, social norms, and availability of certain resources can contribute to difficulty in transmission of a medicine.

With this in mind, it is better to approach this book from two angles, a cultural angle and a health angle. The entire book is a valuable and fascinating look at Tibetan medicine, gives insight into how it was shaped by the unique culture and geography of Tibet, and how medicine conversely helped to shape the culture of Tibet. The majority of the book is a valuable resource for those who wish to use the natural wisdom of Tibetan medicine to enhance their health. If some sections are encountered that seem strange or not useful to your health, simply look on them through the lenses of cultural education.

Carl Stimson

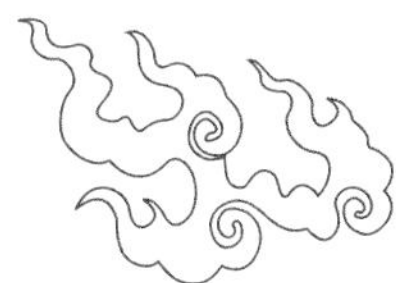

TABLE OF CONTENTS

Chapter 1 The Birth of Life

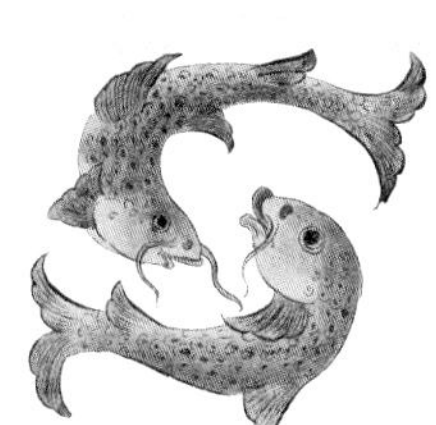

Chapter 2 General Knowledge of Life

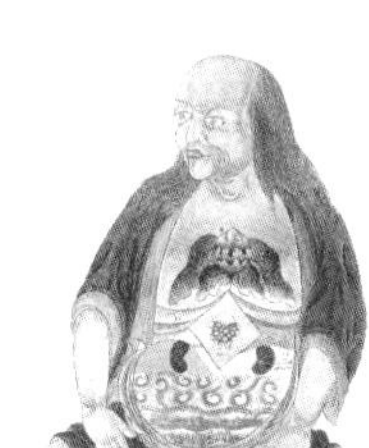

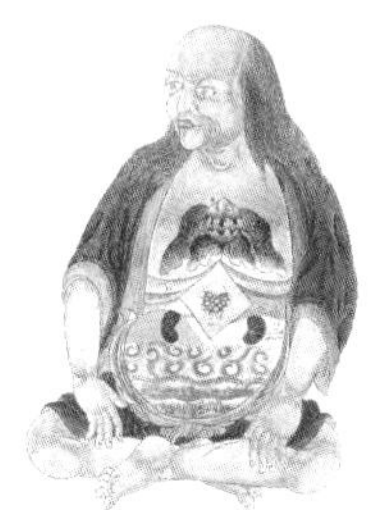

Chapter 3 Diseases

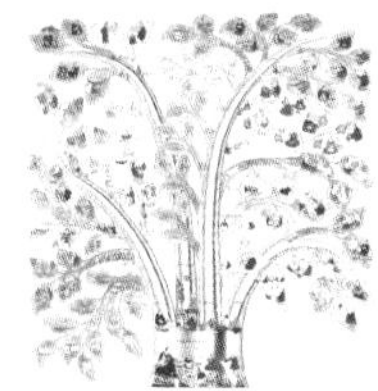

Chapter 4 Health Cultivation Habits

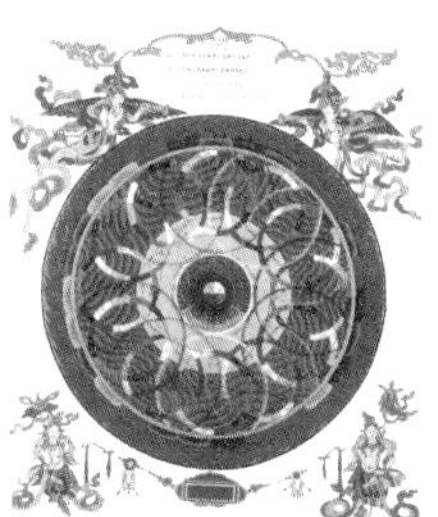

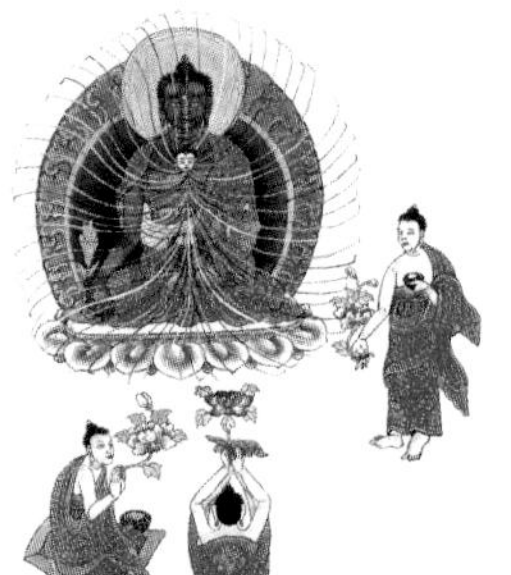

Chapter 5 Health Cultivation Through Diet

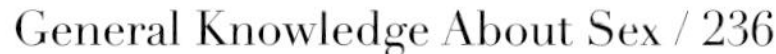

Chapter 6 Health Cultivation Through Sex

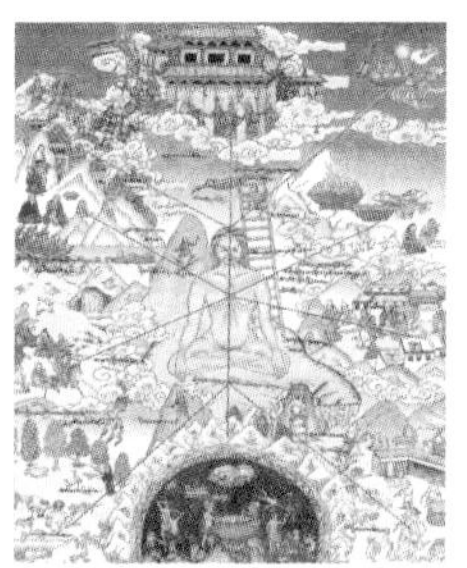

Chapter 7 Tibetan Medicinal Bathing

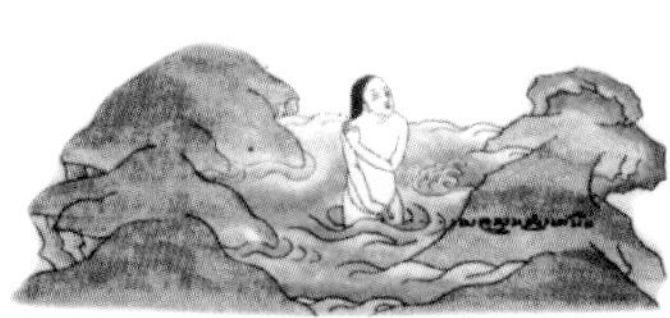

Chapter 8 Signs of Life

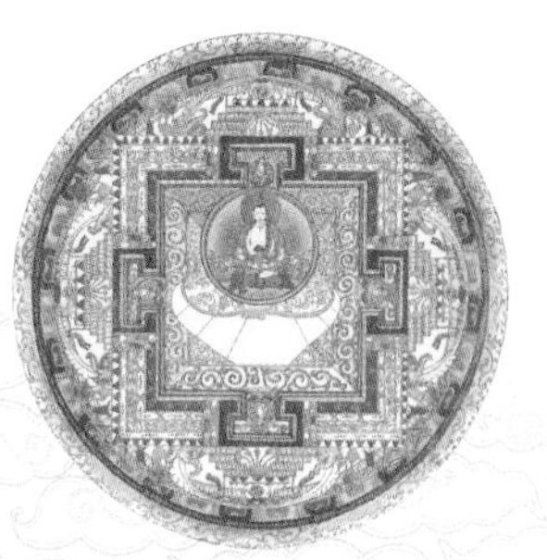

Chapter 9 Health Cultivation Advice

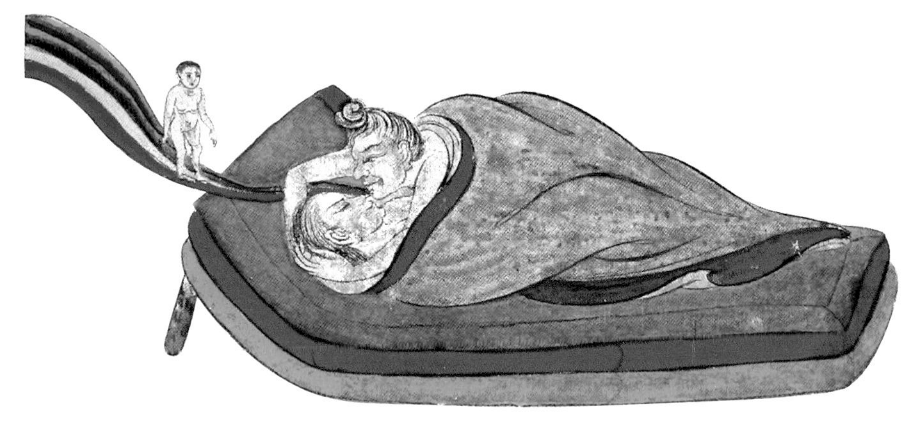

མངལ་ཆགས་དང་བཙས་པ།

CHAPTER 1 THE BIRTH OF LIFE

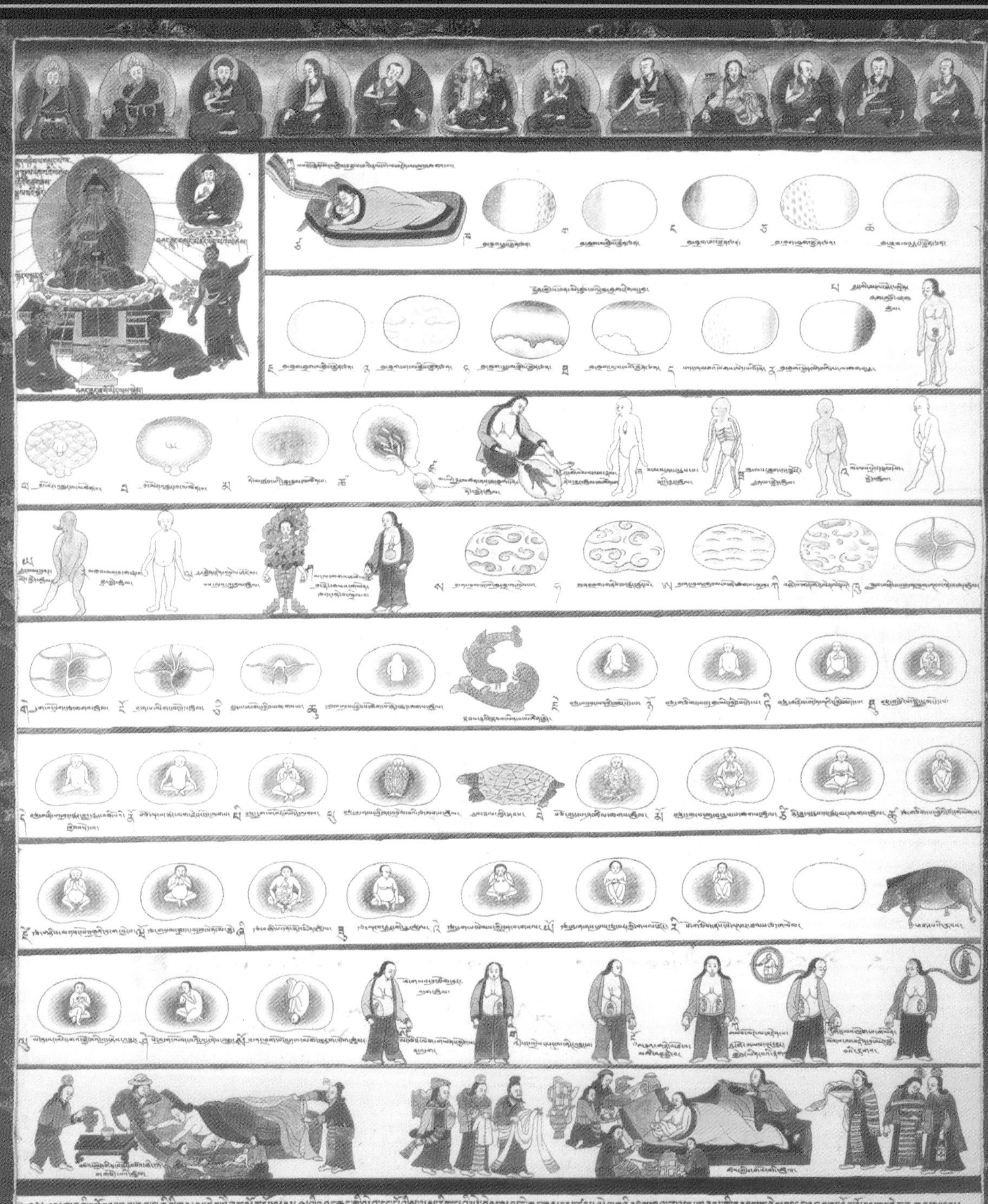

Thangkha Five in the *Sman thang* series. The *Four Medical Tantras*: the development of an embryo.

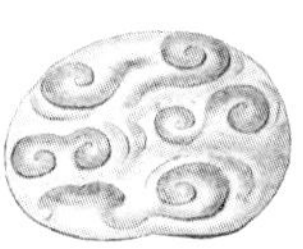

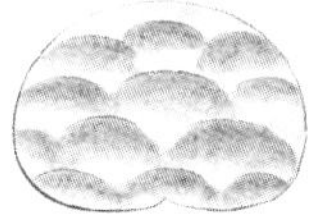

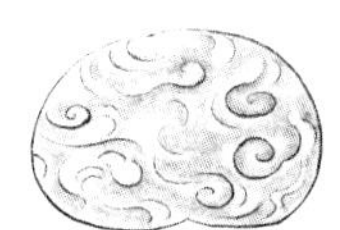

Where does life come from? From where does health commence? Tibetan medicine provides answers to these questions.

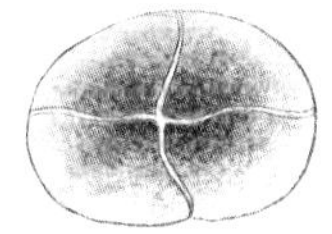

Based on extant ancient documents, it can be seen that the origins of a relatively mature embryology appear rather early in Tibetan medicine.

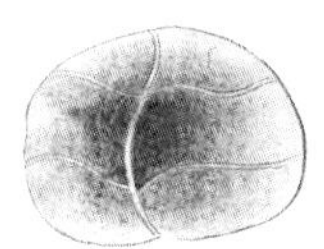

The Tibetan medical classic *Rgyud bzhi* (*The Four Medical Tantras*), compiled in the 8th century, describes the weekly development of the embryo. This achievement far surpasses other traditional medical systems, and is quite close to the conclusions made by modern embryology. Abundant records concerning conception, care for the pregnant woman, delivery, and postpartum care exist in the literature. In Tibetan medicine, life is well cared for and vigilantly protected from its very beginning.

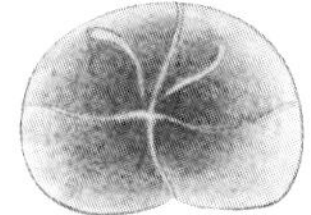

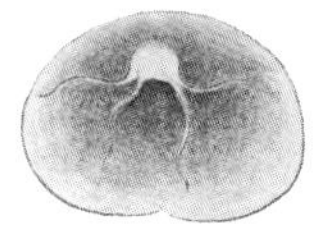

Here, we will explore the unique and meticulous healthcare of life, starting from fertilization.

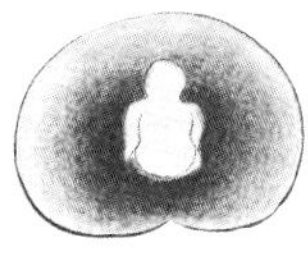

Formation of the Embryo

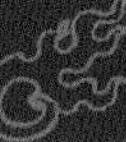

In the understanding of Tibetan medicine, it is essential to ensure a healthy embryo from the start, rather than treat problems in an embryo that has already been formed.

Tibetan medicine maintains that healthy semen-blood is the foundation of an embryo and an appropriate fertilization process is essential. Only with the existence of both can the journey of life proceed smoothly.

Healthy Semen-Blood

To obtain fire while drilling into wood a sharp drill and dry wood are indispensable. Naturally, a rough drill or wet wood will never yield fire. Similarly, proper fertilization requires healthy semen-blood.

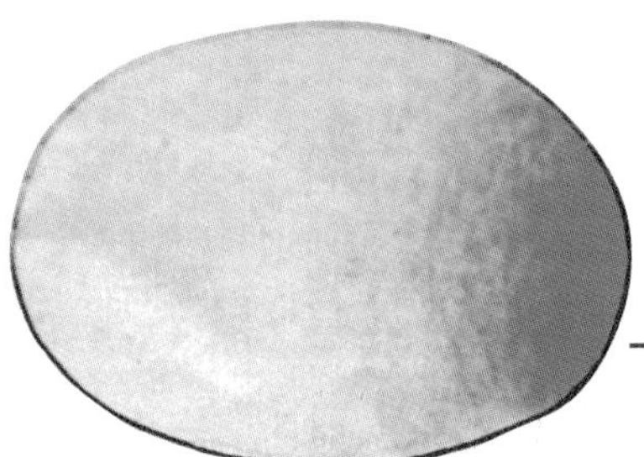

Paternal semen: white color, heavy quality, sweet taste, abundant quantity
Maternal blood: pink color

In Tibetan medicine it is said that when one takes grains and other food, the essence is absorbed and transformed in sequence into blood, muscles, fat, bones, and spirit. The residue of the spirit changes into two kinds of liquid, the red and the white. The white portion is the semen in males, and the red portion the maternal blood in females. What, exactly, is healthy semen-blood? According to *The Four Medical Tantras*, healthy semen is white in color, shinning as the morning dew, rather heavy in quality, plentiful, with a sweet and astringent taste. Healthy blood is red as rabbit's blood, pure and clear in quality, and can be washed away readily from cloth without leaving any trace.

Just like an excellent seed, healthy semen-blood will give rise to rich fruit, provided it is carefully fostered.

The Process of Fertilization

Healthy body

Procreation relies on semen-blood which, in turn, relies on the body. The body relies on food and medicine. If semen-blood is unhealthy or insufficient, the female will be unable to be fertilized even if intercourse is frequent. Hence, to produce a child, both partners should be in robust health. Therefore, training of the body and the taking of proper medicine is essential to having sufficient semen and abundant blood.

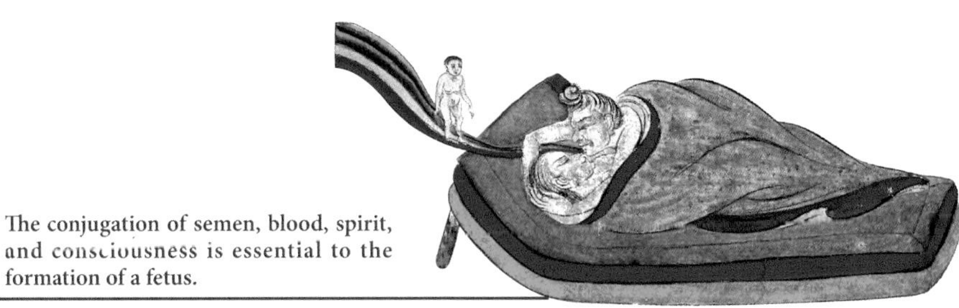

The conjugation of semen, blood, spirit, and consciousness is essential to the formation of a fetus.

Optimal time for intercourse

Tibetan medicine holds that menstrual blood flows into the womb through the two large vessels beside it on the 16th to the 30th days of each month, preparing to receive the sperm. If it fails to meet semen, under the action of the descending *rlung*, the mouth of the womb opens and the maternal blood flows out of the body with the uterine blood. This is menstruation. In girls younger than twelve years old, all material essence transforms to nurture the body so blood doesn't reach the womb. Similarly, in a woman over fifty years of age, due to the decline of the five sources, there is no chance for maternal blood to accumulate, so menstruation ceases to occur.

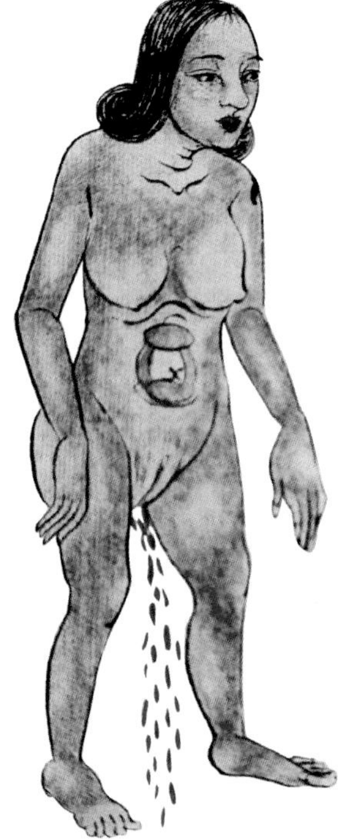

During the menstrual period, females feel lassitude, fatigue, have a pallid complexion, feel tremors in the waist, breast, neck, eyes, and coccyx, and have a strong sexual desire. In the twelve days after the opening of the womb-mouth fertilization is possible, except on the first three evenings and the eleventh day. If fertilization occurs on the first, third, fifth, seventh, or ninth days a male fetus will appear, whereas a female fetus will appear if the fertilization happens on the second, fourth, sixth, or eighth days. Beyond the above days, the mouth of the womb is closed like a lotus flower after sunset and no fertilization can happen.

Woman menstruate from 12 years old to 50 years of age.

Comfortable surroundings

Pleasant surroundings such as beside a picturesque pool, in a beautiful forest with moist and pleasant air, or a garden with blossoms and flowers will comfort one's mind and benefit semen production and sexual desire.

Formation of the Fetus

Signs of fetal formation

If fertilization takes place, the woman will feel lazy, heaviness in the body, tremulous extremities, have an accelerated heartbeat, and the small body hairs will stand on end indicating that the process of fertilization has been completed.

The last of the seven body essences (the essence from food, blood, muscles, bone marrow, bones, fat, and spirit) is now accumulated into the "pool" of *bsam-bse'u*, from where the spirit continuously flows into the "earth" of the fetus, or the womb, through two blood vessels. The fetus begins to grow when nurtured by the mother. The fetus absorbs the spirit from the mother once it appears in the womb and grows rapidly; thus beginning

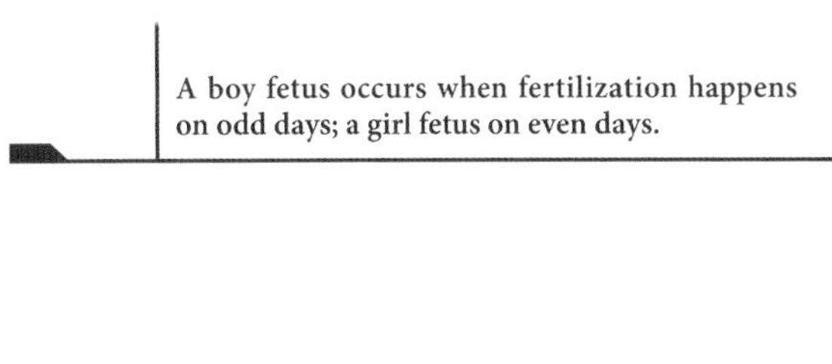

A boy fetus occurs when fertilization happens on odd days; a girl fetus on even days.

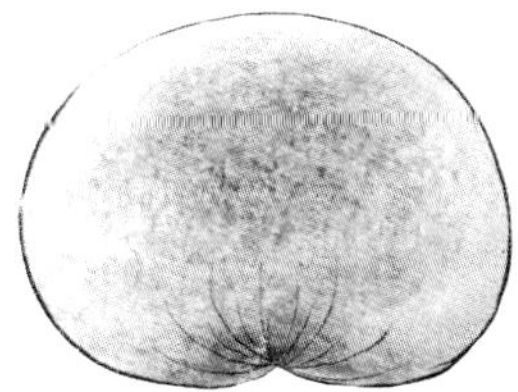

Predominant paternal semen results in a male fetus.

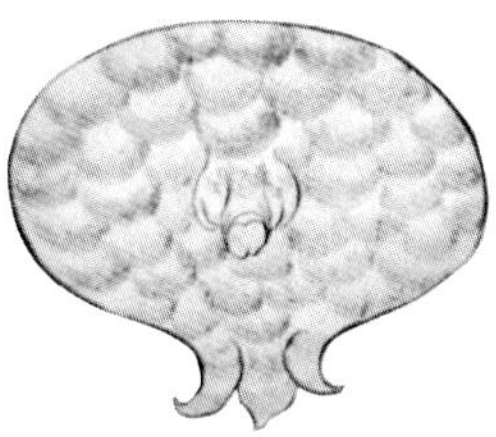

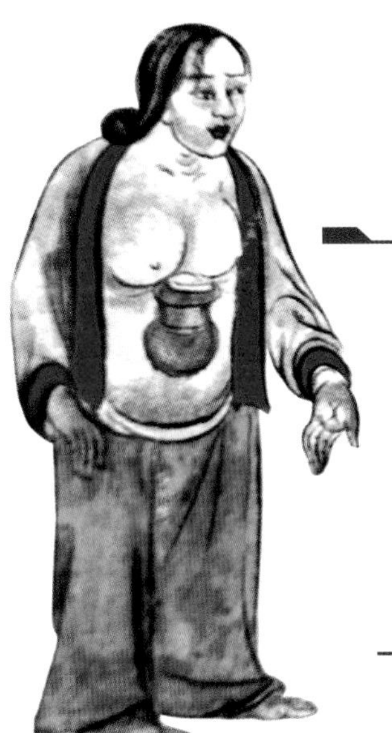

Predominant maternal blood results in a female fetus.

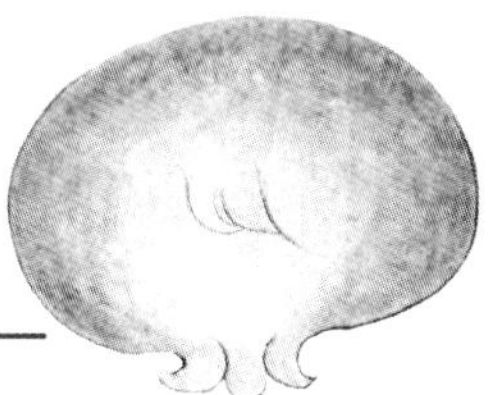

Like the irrigation of a field from a pool, the mother nurtures her fetus through the navel.

the 38-week journey within the mother.

During the process of fertilization, when more paternal semen is present, a male fetus is formed; a female fetus is formed when maternal blood is predominant. Equal amounts of both would result in a neutral fetus, including a stony girl (vaginal hypoplasia), a bisexual fetus, or a hermaphrodite.

If the conjugated and coagulated maternal-blood and paternal-semen multiplies, under the action of *rlung*, it will divide into two or three parts, and the embryo will become a twin or triplets. When paternal semen is predominant, a two-boy set of twins will be formed; and when maternal blood predominates, a two-girl set of twins will be formed. If both semen and blood are equally balanced, a set of twins with both a boy and a girl will be formed.

Impaired maternal blood or paternal semen will result in an animal embryo or simply a flesh mass. Even though this embryo may look like a human being, it will be born as a dwarf, lame, blind, or with other defects. The pathological basis for these is the contamination of the semen or blood with filth, or a lack of any of the five sources.

The five sources in the embryo

Following the conjugation of the semen and the blood, the paternal semen will generate the embryo's bones, marrow, and brain, while the maternal blood will generate the muscles, blood, and internal organs. Meanwhile, the embryo's own six consciousnesses will generate its own spirit and sense organs. Tibetan medicine applies the theory of the five sources to interpret the origins of the embryo's parts.

Earth source: generates the strong parts of the body, such as the muscles, bones, and the nose, from which the sense of smell is derived.

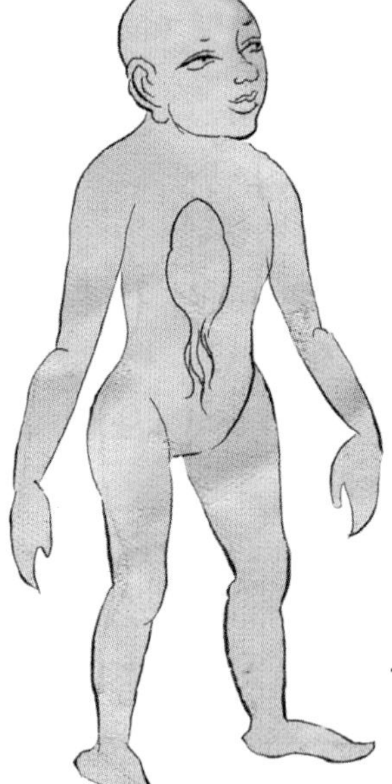

The embryo itself generates the five sense organs and the spiritual consciousness.

Water source: generates the blood, yellow fluid, and the tongue, from which the sense of taste is derived.

Fire source: generates warmth (temperature) so that the skin is lustrous, and the eyes, from which the sense of sight is derived.

Wind source: generates the function of breathing and the skin, from which sense of touch is derived.

Space source: generates the embryo's life, the orifices through which the seven essences pass, and the ear, from which the sense of hearing is derived.

All of the above factors, each playing its own role, are collectively responsible for the growth of the embryo.

The paternal semen generates the bones, brain, and marrow.

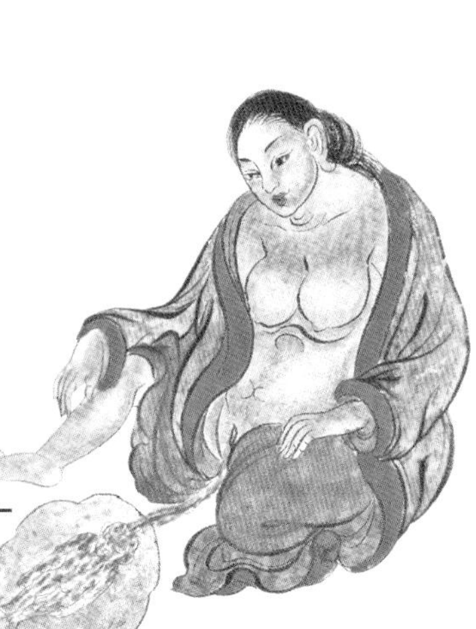

The maternal blood generates the blood, muscles, and internal organs.

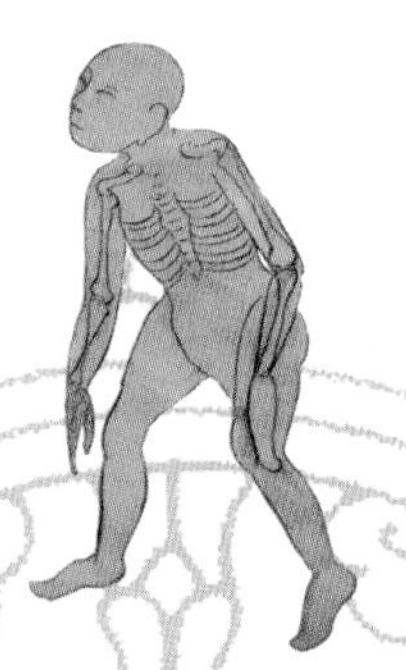

Earth source: generates muscles, bones, the nose and the sense of smell

Space source: generates the orifices and the sense of hearing

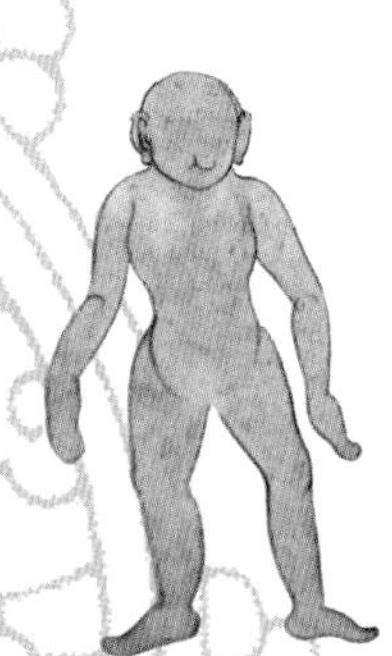

Water source: generates blood, the tongue and the sense of taste

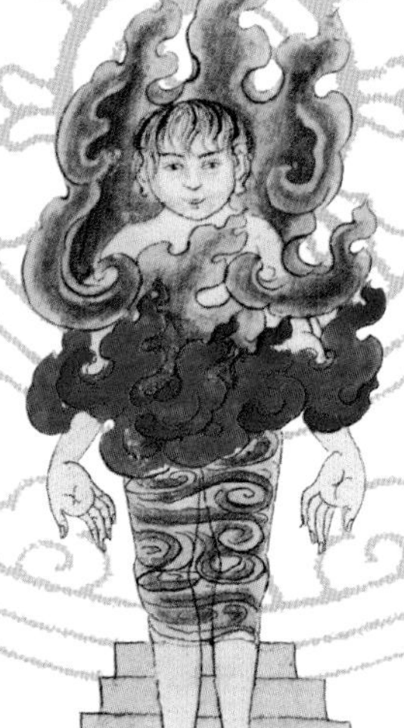

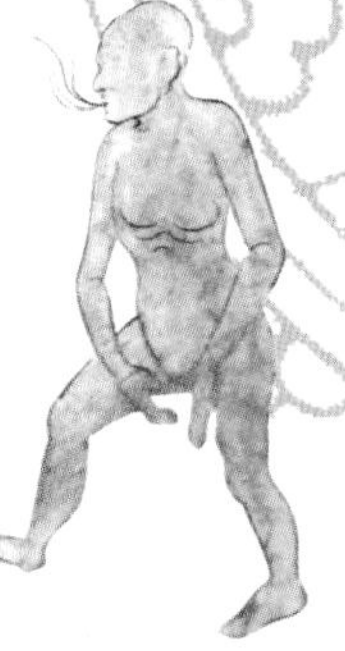

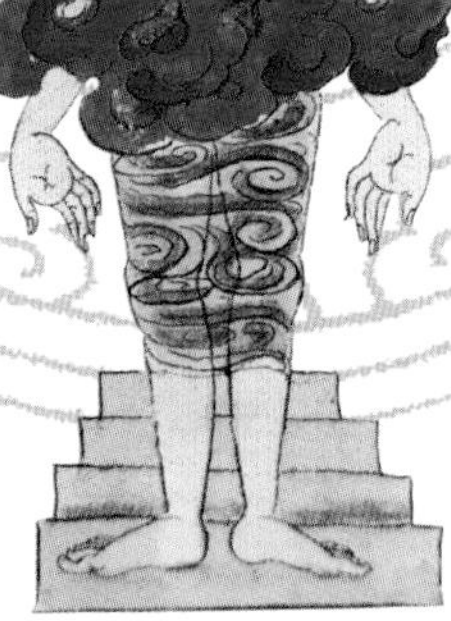

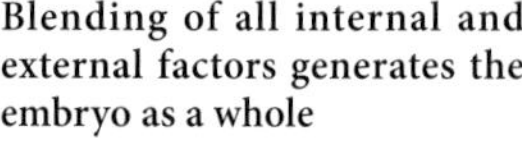

Wind source: generates the ability to breathe, the skin and sense of touch

Fire source: generates body temperature, the complexion and the sense of sight

Blending of all internal and external factors generates the embryo as a whole

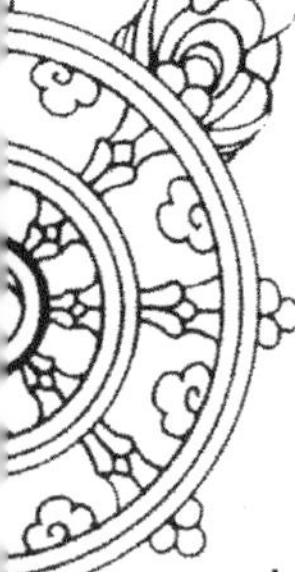

Illustration of the five sources in the embryo.

Early development of the embryo

This refers to the first month of embryonic development during which the pregnant woman feels her lower body is heavy, experiences a sudden loss of weight, frequent yawning, weakness, laziness, loss of appetite, nausea, a fondness of sour foods, relaxation of the uterine cervix, and enlargement of the breasts. The weekly changes of the embryo during this period include:

First week: the conjugated semen-blood is evenly mixed together like fresh milk that has been thoroughly stirred up.

1st week: **conjugation of semen and blood, similar to yeast mixed into milk.**

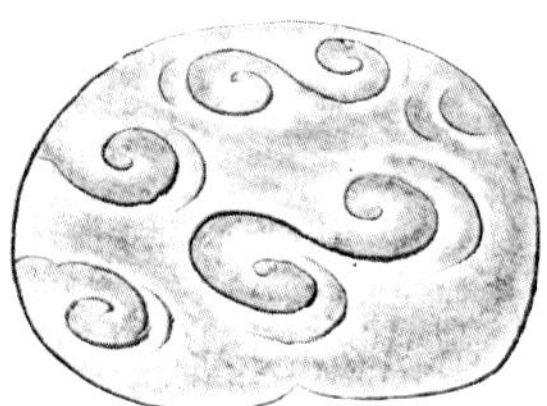

Second week: the conjugated semen-blood becomes thick and pasty, like a layer of butter floating on milk.

2nd week: **the coagulated semen-blood looks like a layer of butter floating on the surface of milk.**

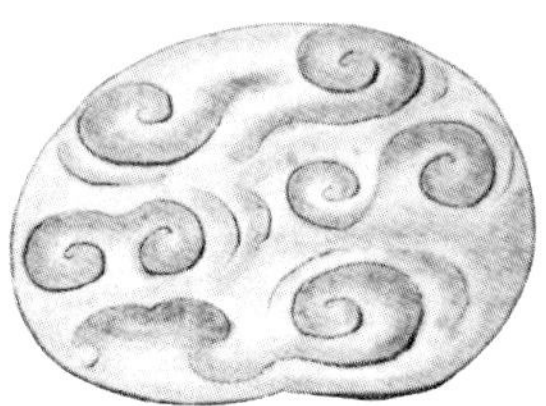

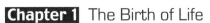

Third week: the mass becomes even thicker like coagulated cheese.

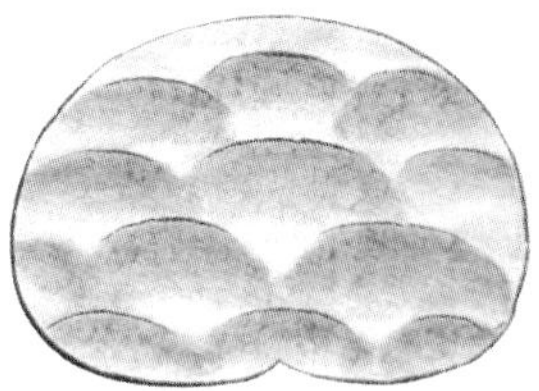

3rd ***week:*** further coagulation of the mass causes it to look like cheese.

Fourth week: the cheese-like mass becomes a fleshy mass. A harder mass will develop into a male fetus, a softer mass will develop into a female fetus, and a cylindrical mass will develop into a neutral fetus or hermaphrodite.

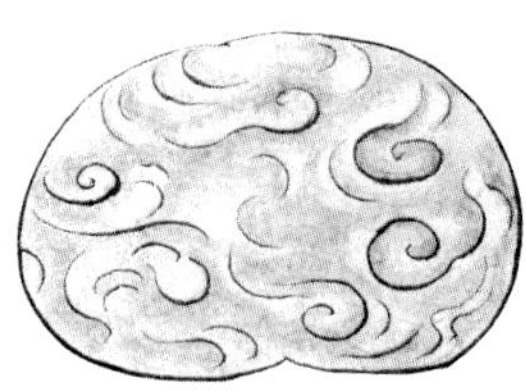

4th ***week:*** a hard mass means a male fetus; a soft mass means a female fetus; a cylindrical mass means a neutral fetus.

During this period, the pregnant woman should pay attention to her health, especially her daily habits, including avoiding frequent sexual activity, heavy physical labor, suppressing urgent desires of urination and defecation, or overstrain during such processes. She must avoid too much spicy food and stay away from foods of a sharp and heavy nature. Too much sleep in the daytime and little sleep at night, therapies that employ vomiting or purging, which increase the *rlung* element in her body and would threaten her fetus, should also be avoided.

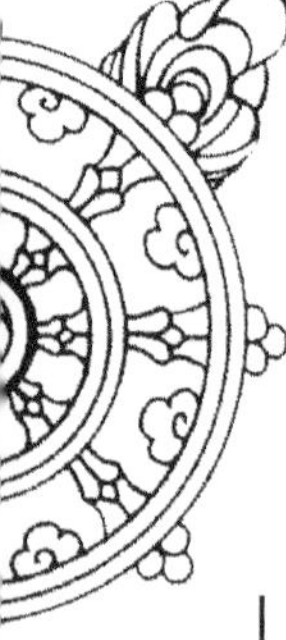

It is advised to satisfy a pregnant woman's desires, especially as to cravings for certain kinds of food. Even if such food might be harmful to the fetus, they can be eaten in limited amounts during regular meals so as to ensure the safety of the fetus and help the pregnant woman to be happy at the same time. By doing so, the healthy growth of the fetus can be ensured.

The Fish Stage of Development

From the fifth to the thirty-fifth week, the fetus undergoes the most important period of its development which is divided into three stages: the fish stage, the turtle stage, and the pig stage. Why these animal names?

Baidurya sngon po (*Blue Lapis Lazuli*) states that, "The embryo elongates in the first stage, which is called the Fish Stage. This leads to the four limbs with a head being formed and an appearance like a turtle, hence the Turtle Stage. Further development gives rise to different protrusions, forming the organs that can absorb food from the mother; hence this last stage is called the Pig Stage."

The fish stage includes five weeks, from the fifth to the ninth weeks, or the second month plus the remaining days of the first month.

The fifth week: the flesh mass becomes harder. This is called the hardening stage, during which the umbilical vessel wheel appears, with four strips radiating outward. This is the basic vessel plexus giving rise to all vessels and is situated in front of the fifteenth vertebra.

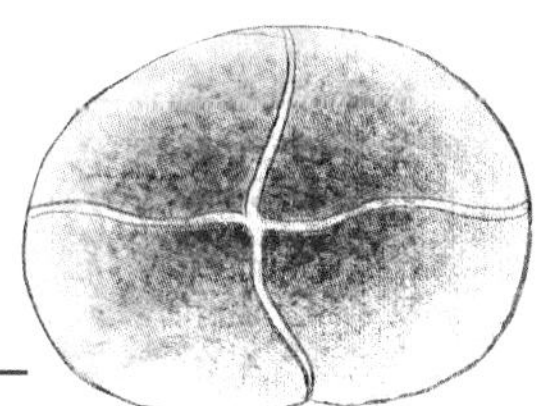

5th ***week:*** formation of the umbilical vessel wheel.

Tibetan medicine maintains that there are thirty eight weeks for the fetus to develop from the formation of the fetus to its delivery. During this period there are three stages, the Fish stage, the Turtle stage and the Pig stage. This idea of development of from fish, reptile, to mammal agrees with the modern concept of evolution.

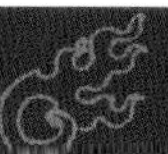

The sixth week: a vital vessel branches out from the center of the umbilical vessel wheel. This is the stem of all beating vessels (arteries) on which life and qi-blood rely on. The vessel measures sixteen times the length of the embryo itself, ascends upward and ends in front of the eighth vertebra.

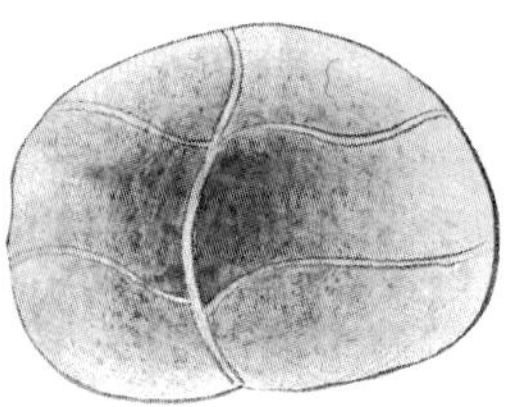

6th week: **formation of the vital gate near the navel.**

The seventh week: a vital vessel branches out from the heart vessel wheel. It runs upward thirty finger breadths and ends at the vertex to form the vertex vessel wheel. The eyes begin to take shape. Another vital vessel branches out from the umbilical vessel wheel and runs downward for a distance of fourteen finger breadths. It ends at the perineum to form the perineum vessel wheel.

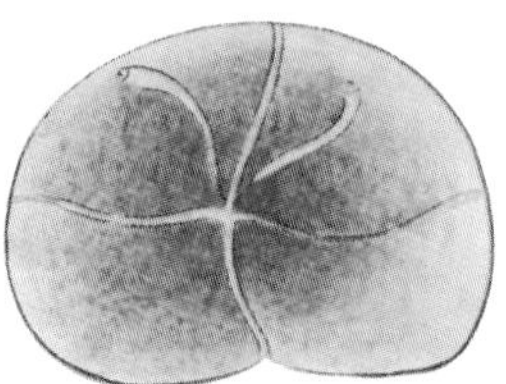

7th week: **formation of the eyes.**

The eighth week: the brain takes its shape, with the vertex vessel wheel and the eyes as its base.

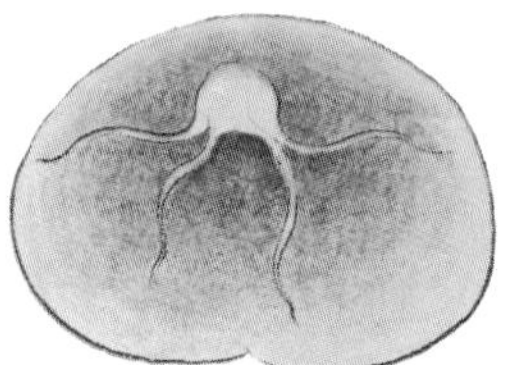

8th week: **the skull appears.**

The ninth week: the trunk of the fetus, or the upper and lower body cavities except the four extremities are formed.

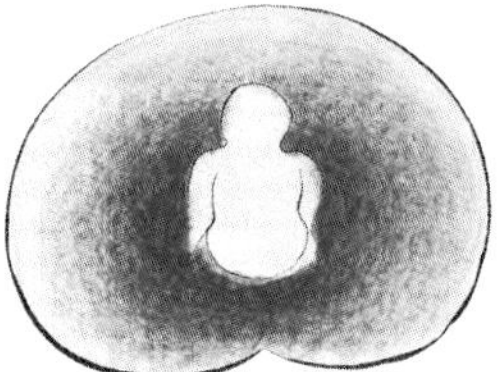

9th week: formation of the upper and lower body cavities.

In summary, during the five weeks in this stage the vital vessel is formed. Under the guidance of this vessel, the main body of the fetus grows continuously and the contour of life appears. Since the shape of the fetus is similar to a fish, this stage is called the Fish Stage.

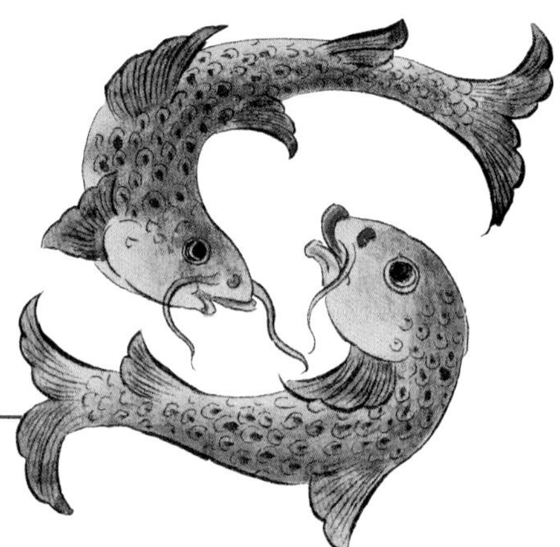

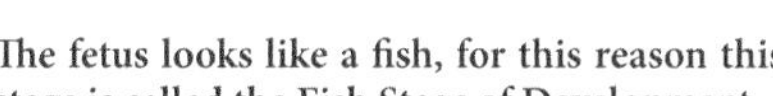

The fetus looks like a fish, for this reason this stage is called the Fish Stage of Development.

Hints for protecting the fetus:

- Moderate sexual activities and stay away from spicy food or foods of a sharp or heavy nature.
- Avoid overstrain when defecating and urinating, and washing with cold water.
- No blood-letting treatments.
- All taboos must be obeyed for eight months. If not, miscarriage or a dead fetus will be the result.

The Turtle Stage of Development

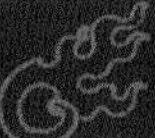

There are altogether four weeks in this stage, all except three days of which occur in the third month of development, the remaining days are part of the second month of development.

The tenth week: the fish-like fetus grows two upper limbs and the beginnings of the thighs.

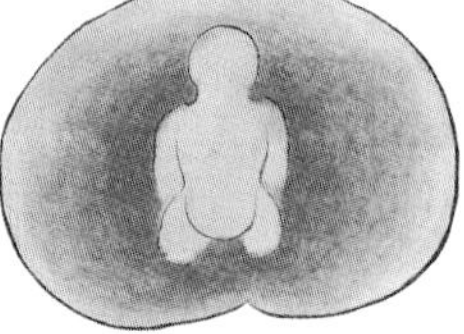

10th week: initial form of the thigh appears.

The eleventh week: the nine orifices, including the eyes, nostrils, ears, genitals, and mouth are formed.

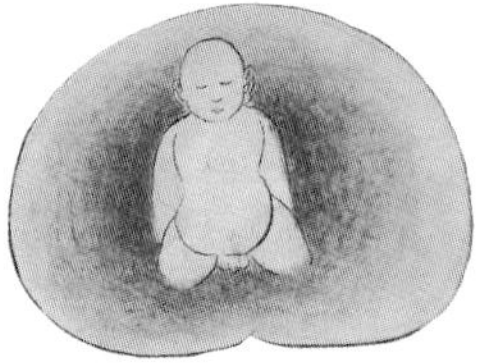

11th week: formation of the nine orifices.

The twelfth week: the five solid internal organs (heart, liver, spleen, lung, kidney) begin to form.

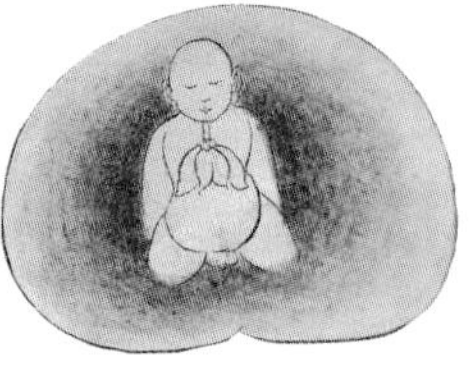

12th week: formation of the five solid internal organs.

Characteristics of a pregnant woman: heavy abdomen, loss of appetite, frequent yawning, lassitude and laziness, enlarged breasts, fond of sour foods. Attention must be paid to the satisfaction of her desires and to the administration of tonic foods.

The thirteenth week: the six hollow internal organs (stomach, large intestine, small intestine, gallbladder, urinary bladder, essence mansion) begin to form.

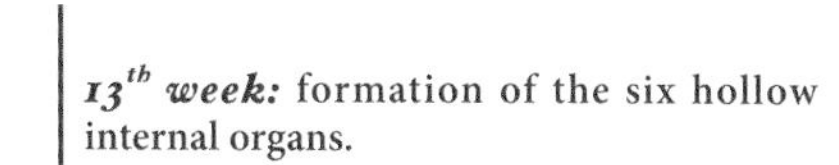

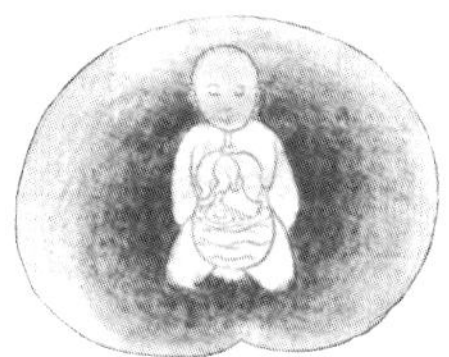

13th week: **formation of the six hollow internal organs.**

The fourth month: altogether four weeks plus two days.

The fourteenth week: the two arms and the two thighs begin to form.

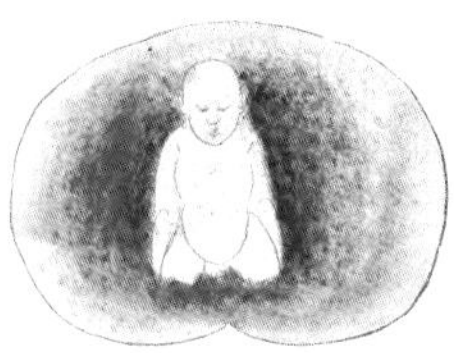

14th week: **formation of both arms and thighs.**

The fifteenth week: both forearms and legs begin to form.

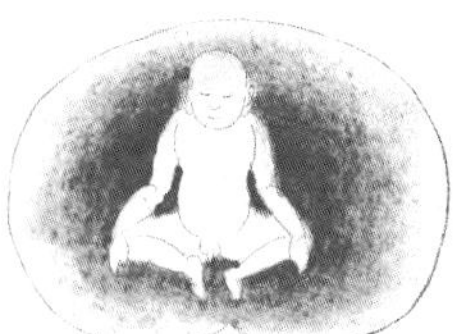

15th week: **growth of both forearms and legs.**

The sixteenth week: the fingers and the toes are formed.

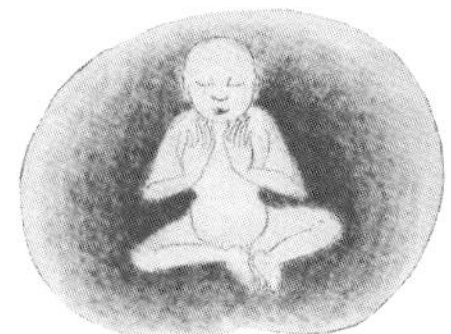

16th week: **formation of the fingers and the toes.**

Records on the development of the embryo appear in the literature of Chinese Medicine rather early. The *Tai Chan Shu (Book of Pregnancy and Delivery)* of the Han dynasty unearthed in the Mawangdui caves and the *Zhu Yue Yang Tai Fang (Nurturing the Fetus Month by Month)* of the Southern-Northern dynasties described the development of the fetus. However, month by month, it is not as precise and detailed as that of Tibetan medicine.

The seventeenth week: the sixteen visible vessels on the body surface and the numerous invisible vessels inside the body are formed.

Since the fetus is shaped like a turtle, this stage is called the Turtle Stage of Development.

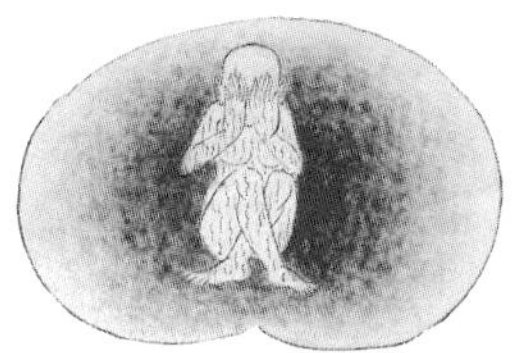

17th week: **formation of the vessels inside and on the body surface.**

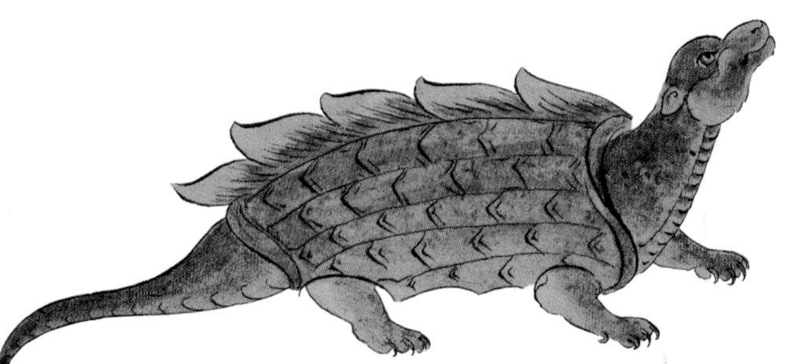

Since the fetus is shaped like a turtle, this stage is called the Turtle Stage of Development.

In Western embryology, the theory of "pre-formation" prevailed for a long time, believing that there was a "minute man" identical in form to a human being inside the woman and its development is nothing more than the continuous increase in size. It was not until 1628 that the Englishman William Harvey established a new theory, claiming that the fetus is formed by an evolutionary process from an ovum to a worm-like creature and eventually to a human form. The scientific description of human embryology was finally achieved in the 18th century by a Russian scientist.

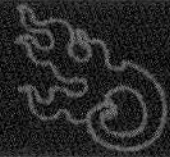

The Pig Stage of Development

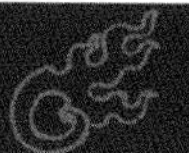

There are four weeks plus several days in this stage.

The eighteenth week: the fat and muscle tissues are basically formed.

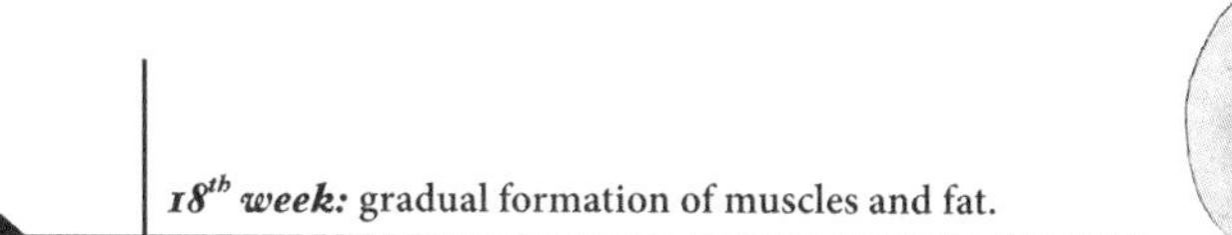

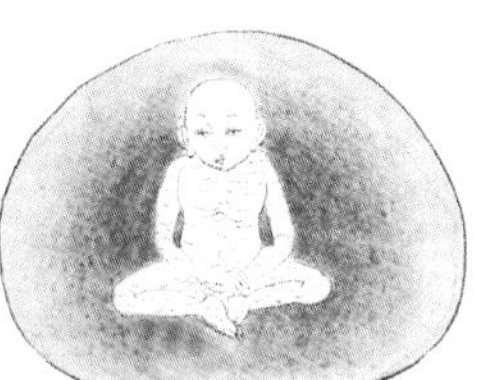

18th week: gradual formation of muscles and fat.

The nineteenth week: the ligaments and tendons begin to form.

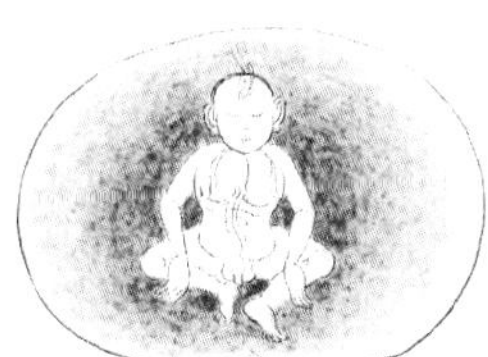

19th week: formation of ligaments and tendons.

The twentieth week: all bones and bone marrow are formed.

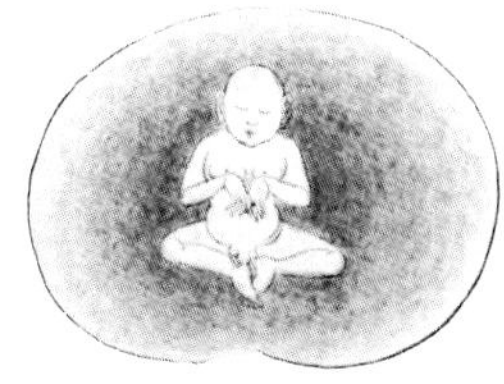

20th week: formation of the bones and bone marrow.

The twenty-first week: the skin membrane over the whole body begins to form, just like the layer of cream floating on the surface of milk.

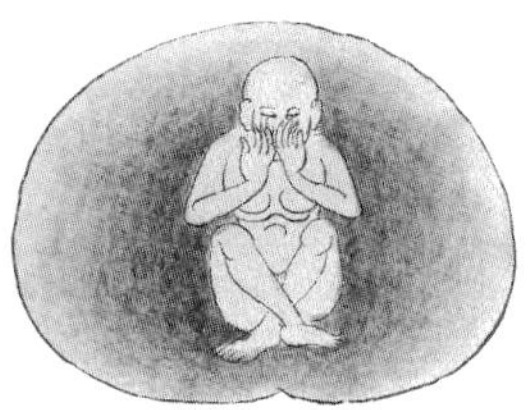

21st week: appearance of the external skin.

The following refers to the sixth month plus two days from the previous month and three days from the next month, making five weeks altogether.

The twenty-second week: all nine orifices, including the five sense organs, are open.

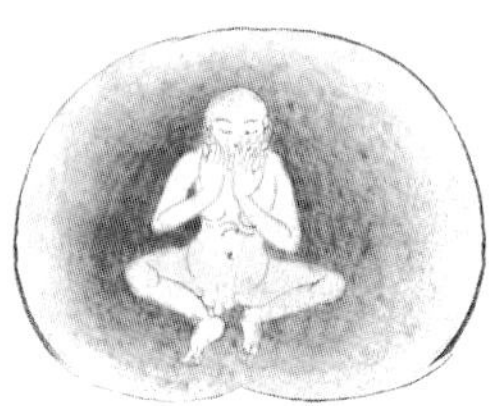

22nd week: opening of the orifices.

The twenty-third week: the fetal hairs, fine hairs, and nails begin to form.

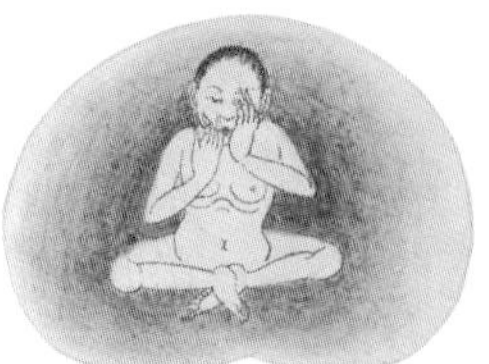

23rd week: hairs, fine hairs, and nails.

The twenty-fourth week: all the organs previously formed become mature. Sensation appears, and the fetus is aware of comfort and misery.

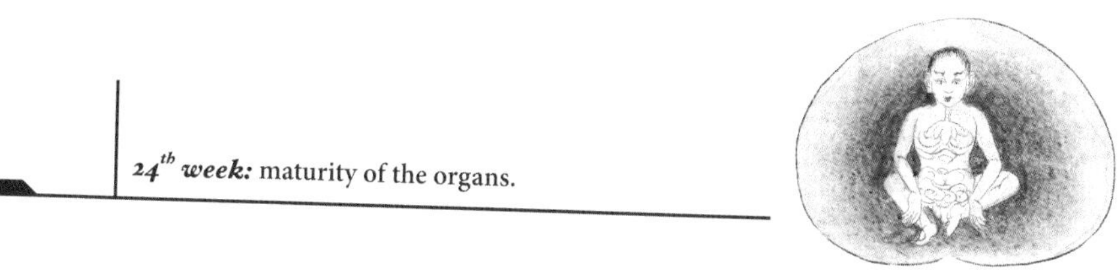

24th week: maturity of the organs.

The twenty-fifth week: qi begins to flow through the orifices. In other words, this is the beginning of respiration.

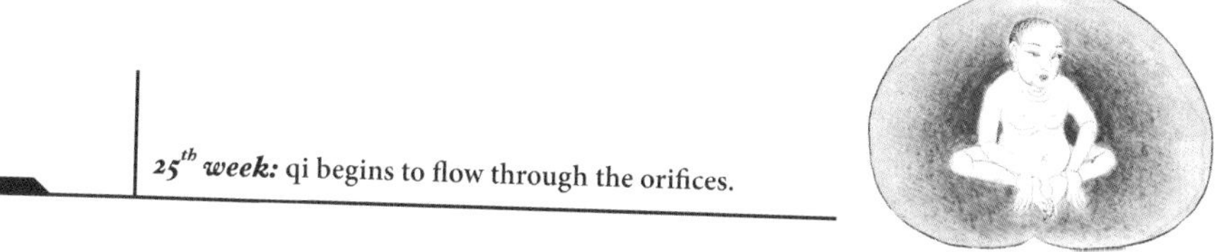

25th week: qi begins to flow through the orifices.

The twenty-sixth week: the consciousness of the fetus becomes increasingly clear.

There are four weeks in the seventh month. All tissues and organs become even more mature and some fine tissues begin to appear.

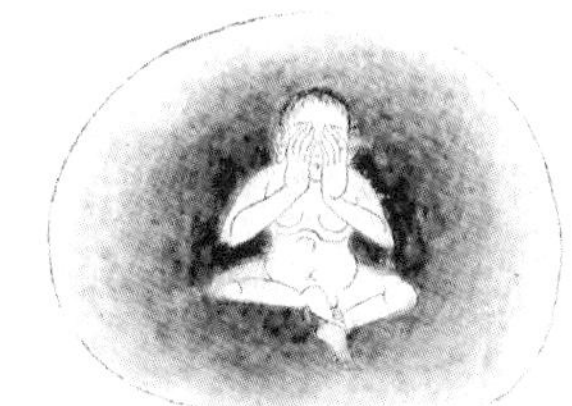

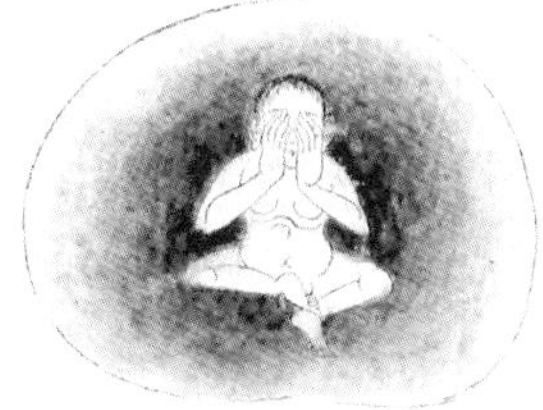

26th week: consciousness begins.

There are five weeks in the eighth month plus five days from the previous month. The fetus grows further from the thirty-first to the thirty-fifth weeks.

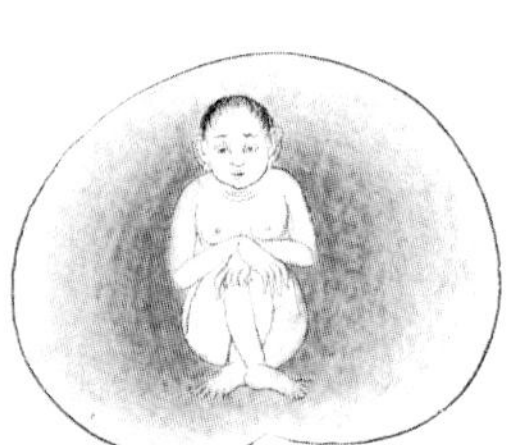

27th-30th *weeks:* the organs mature.

During this stage, the organs and tissues mature. The fetus looks like a pig, hence it is called the Pig Stage of Development.

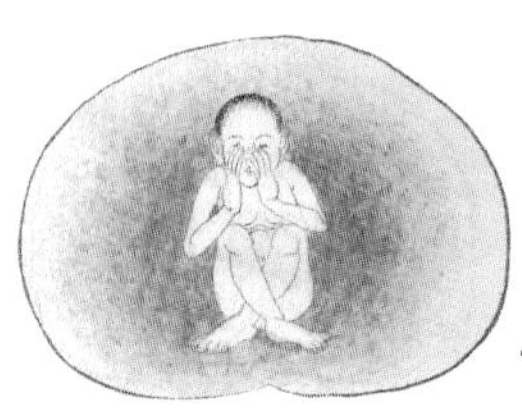

31st-35th *weeks:* the fetus grows.

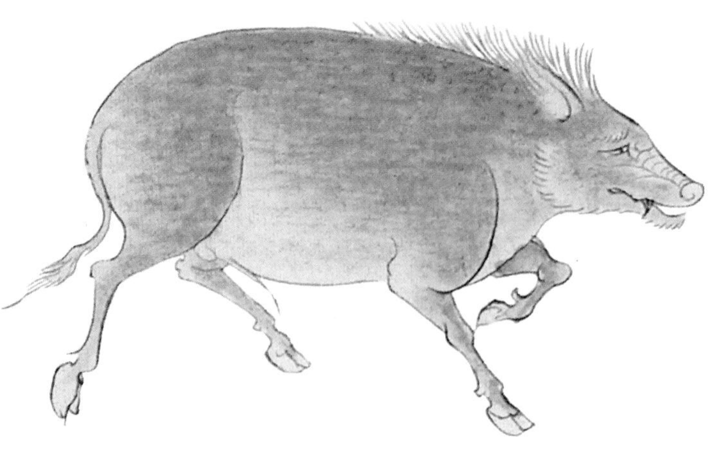

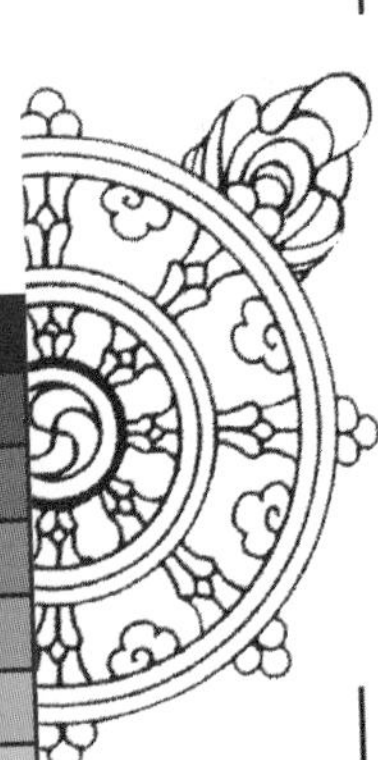

The fetus looks like a pig, hence it is called the Pig Stage of Development.

Modern science holds that human life begins and develops gradually from the conjugation of a single cell ovum and sperm. The process of development of a fetus repeats the evolutionary process from a lower class animal to a higher mammal. As said by Engels, the evolutionary history of embryo inside the mother is nothing but a miniature imitation of the body evolving from a small worm over millions of years. The descriptions of stages as fish, turtle, and pig in the embryo exactly coincide with evolutionary stages of fish, reptiles, and mammals. Because of this, it can be said that Tibetan embryology stands at the forefront in the history of all traditional medical systems.

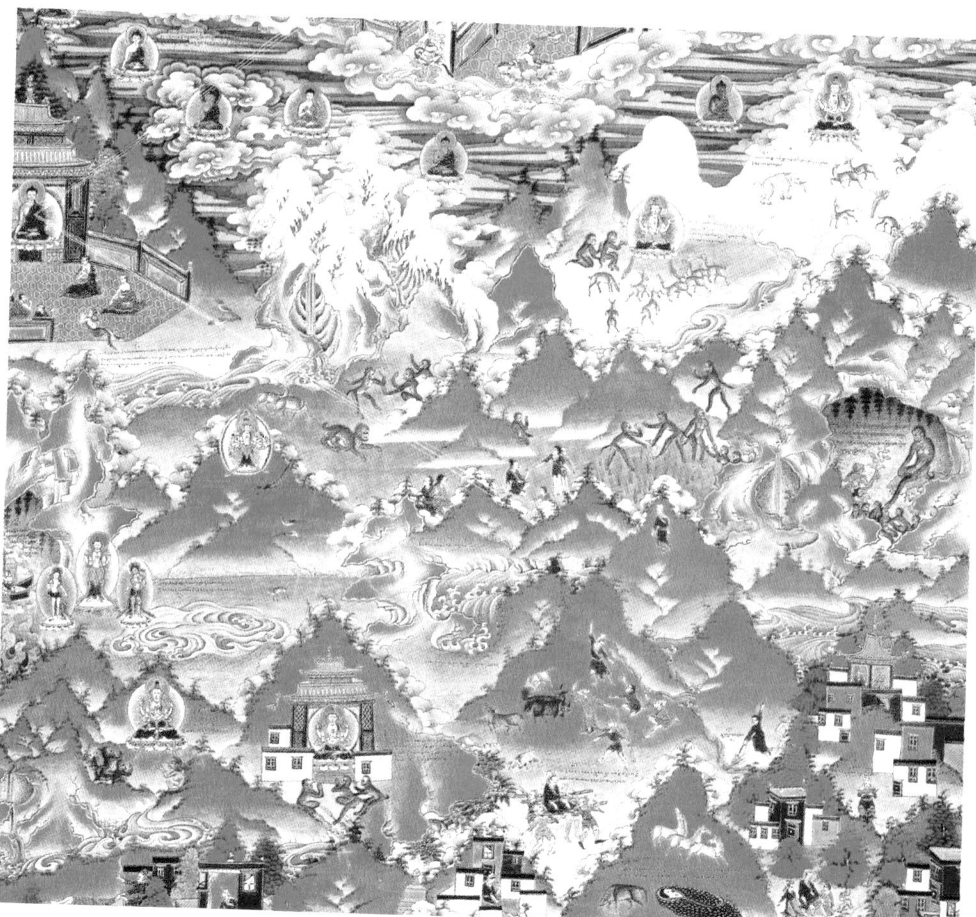

Legends tell that the Tibetan people came from the monkey, manifesting a primitive idea of evolution. (The image is part of the *thangkha* on the origin of the Tibetan people)

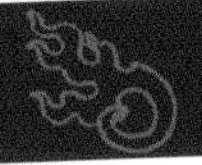

Preparations for Labor

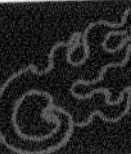

Preparation for delivery begins from the thirty-sixth week. Normally, this stage covers about three weeks. During this period, one must pay close attention to the changes happening in the pregnant woman. She should undergo all necessary pre-delivery exams and regulate her meals and daily habits so as to welcome the advent of a new life.

Pre-delivery Period

In the 9th month, there are altogether three weeks plus four days, because the first three days of the month belong to the previous stage. The development during this month includes the following in succession.

The thirty-sixth week: beginning from the first day of this month, the fetus begins to feel uncomfortable in the womb, developing a feeling like it is trapped in jail. It feels much aversion to its situation.

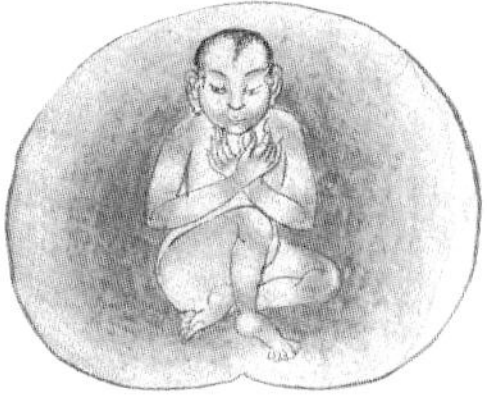

36th week: **the fetus feels abhorrent of its situation.**

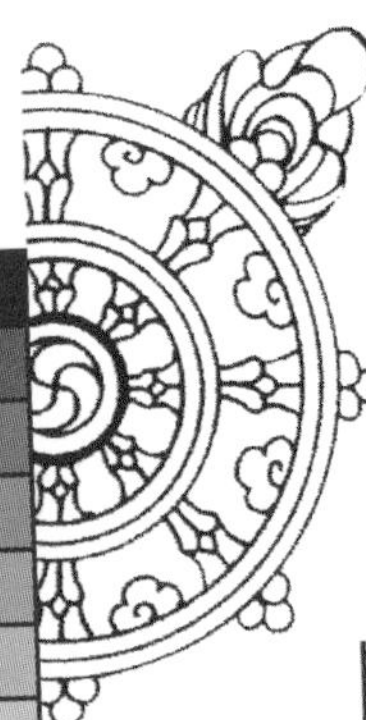

The thirty-seventh week: the aversion of the fetus reaches a high point and it begins to desire to change its environment – by leaving the womb.

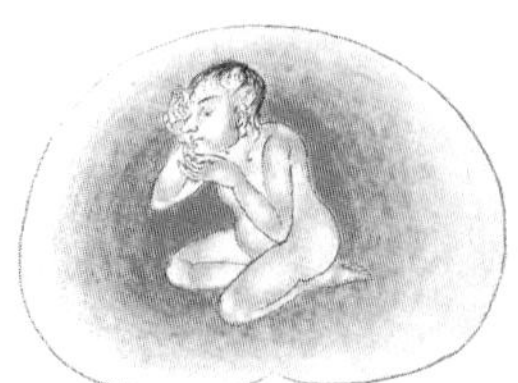

37th week: **dislike of the mother (womb).**

Sign of the birth: laziness, relaxed pelvis, heavy lower body, stinging pain in the lower abdomen and navel, frequent urination, sudden pain in the coccyx region.

The thirty-eighth week: the fetal head turns upside down and faces outward, preparing for delivery.

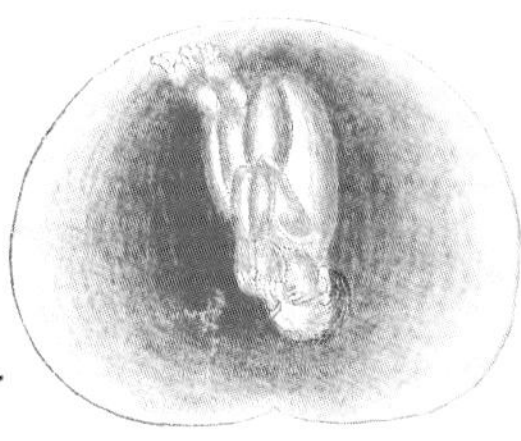

38th week: **the fetus faces outward, preparing to be delivered.**

Thirty eight weeks is the ideal length of pregnancy. The longer the pregnancy is, the closer relationship between the fetus and the mother. During the 31st-35th weeks, a lustrous complexion alternates between the fetus and the mother. As said by the *Nectar Stream*, "There is mutual generation among all essential materials in the body. Sometimes the essence of the mother is absorbed by the fetus and the fetal complexion becomes lustrous while the mother's complexion becomes dim. Sometimes the essence of the fetus is absorbed by the mother and the mother's complexion becomes lustrous while the fetus's complexion becomes dim. A fetus born when the mother's complexion is lustrous is liable to die due to the absence of essence in the fetus. However, the life of the mother is safe."

Even though the time might not be right for delivery, some external factors may lead to early labor. When this happens at the time when the mother's complexion is lustrous and her face glows, a delivery may give rise to a dead fetus and the mother will be safe. If the mother's complexion is dim when she begins labor the baby will be safe but the mother may be in danger. During this last stage, due to the presence of the fetus, the mother may have edema.

In summary, the best time for delivery is between the ninth month minus ten days at the earliest and the tenth month at the latest. Specifically, after the ninth month plus ten days is the best time for delivery.

Signs of Delivery

Prior to delivery, there are signs that indicate the sex of the fetus, male, female, or neutral.

Signs of a male baby: a male fetus is situated over the mother's right hip, and the right side of the mother's abdomen is more prominent. She feels comfortable and relaxed and dreams of a boy. She has no sexual desire. Milk first leaks out of the right breast.

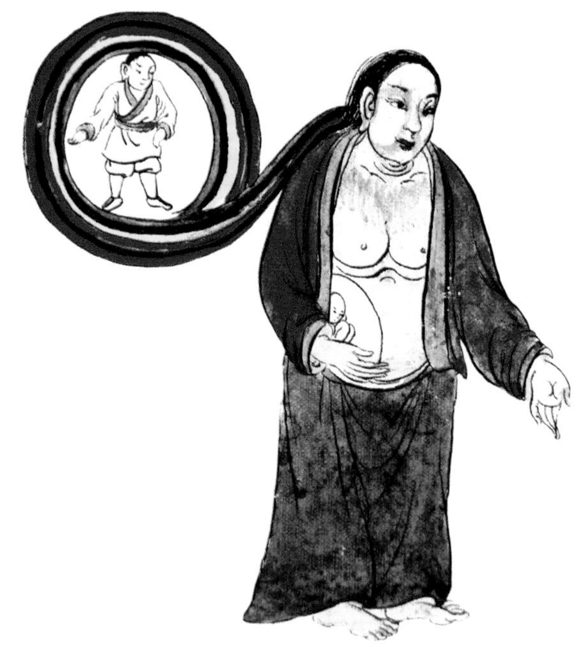

Protrusion of the right side of the abdomen and milk appearing at the right breast signify a male fetus.

Signs of female baby: the mother likes to chat with males, to dance and sing, wear jewelry, and dress nice. The left side of the abdomen is more prominent and she feels her body is heavy, dreams of girls, and milk leaks out of the left breast. All these signs are the reverse of those that indicate a male baby.

Protrusion of left abdomen and milk leaking out of the left breast signifies a female baby.

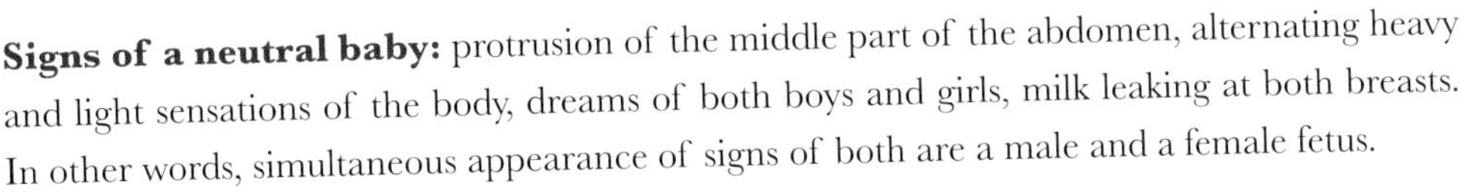

Signs of a neutral baby: protrusion of the middle part of the abdomen, alternating heavy and light sensations of the body, dreams of both boys and girls, milk leaking at both breasts. In other words, simultaneous appearance of signs of both are a male and a female fetus.

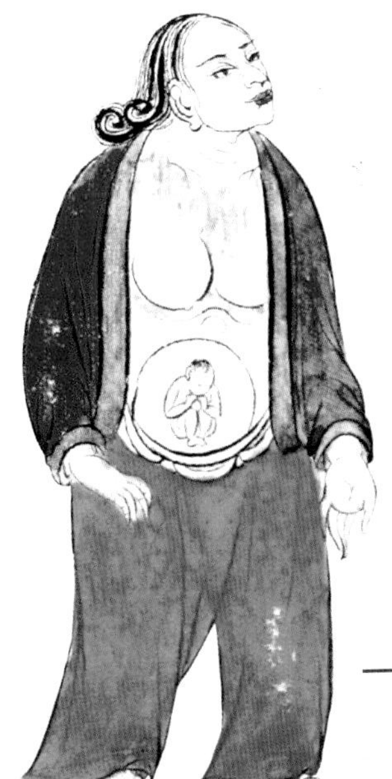

When the fetus is situated in the middle of the abdomen, a neutral baby will be born.

Signs of twins: the abdomen of the mother reveals protrusions on both sides and a depression in the middle. A set of male twins reveals all the signs of a male baby as described above. Likewise a set of female twins shows all the signs of a female baby as described above. When there are mixed signs of male and female, there is a set of twins that includes both a male and a female.

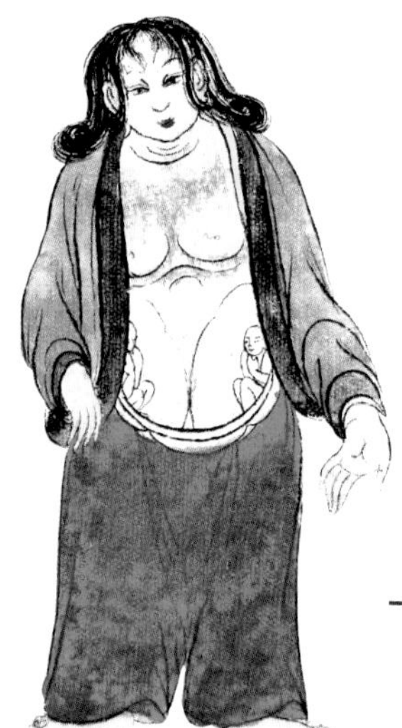

the abdomen reveals protrusions on both sides of the abdomen with a depression in the middle.

Once the above signs appear, all measures to prepare for delivery must be completed, aided by an experienced midwife. The mother should be taught how to lie and how to best use her strength.

Pre-delivery Examination

Tibetan medicine maintains that there are three causes of delayed delivery. When the mother loses too much blood the fetus will not receive enough blood in the womb to grow normally and require more time to grow. An overweight fetus will cause difficult delivery even there is enough there has been enough time for growth. Finally, when the delivery orifice is blocked, the fetus can't be born even though it is already nine months old.

Because of the possibility of complications, Tibetan doctors give importance to pre-delivery exams. Generally, from the third month after fertilization, monthly exams are called for. Beginning from the eighth month, twice monthly exams are necessary. For a woman pregnant for the first time, a very comprehensive physical exam must be performed, including inquiry into any present illness, examination of the pulse, breasts, and advice on diet and physical activity. Immediate measures should be taken if there is any illness, and only low doses of medication can be administered if necessary. Women who have previously given birth, especially those who experienced difficult delivery, should receive a careful examination because their abdominal muscles may be very loose, the elasticity of the delivery orifice may not be satisfactory, and are liable to excessive bleeding after delivery.

There are four kinds of fetal positions that can be found in the pre-delivery examination:

- Normal fetal position is with the head in a downward position. This position is good for delivery.
- In some cases the head is facing upwards. Normally it will turn itself upside down prior to delivery.
- Reversed position is when a fetus has its head in an upwards position and does not turn downwards prior to delivery. The legs will appear first during delivery. This is a difficult situation. Inappropriate handling may lead to the death of the fetus.
- Transverse position: this is a very abnormal fetal position. The fetus lies transversely in the womb. This position may threaten the lives of both the mother and the fetus.

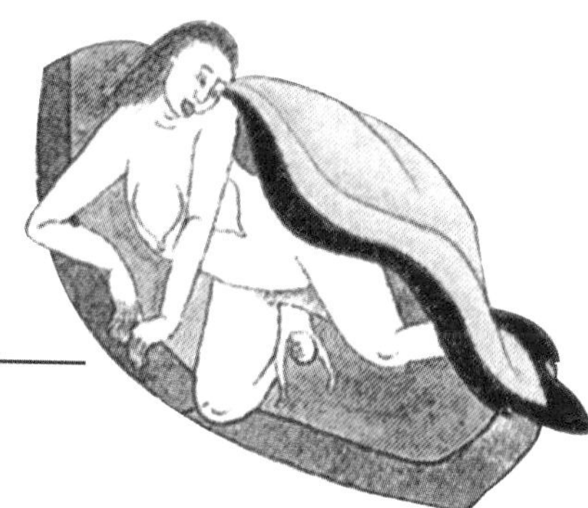

A fetus delivered with the head first in a supine position. This is a smooth delivery.

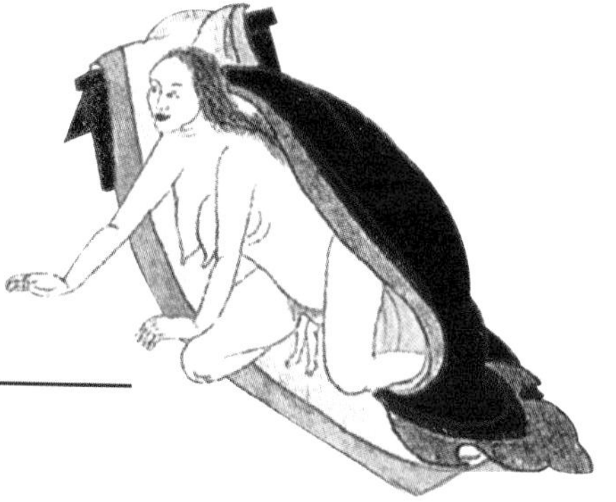

A reversed presentation with the feet first indicates a difficult delivery.

Methods for examination include:

- Palpation of the fundus of the womb to check for the head or legs.
- Palpation of the upper margin of the pubic symphysis to check for the fetal head. A positive result signifies a transverse fetal position.
- Palpation of both sides of the abdomen to check the fetus' vertebral column or upper extremities. A head at one side with the feet at the other side signifies a transverse position.
- When the head descends into the pelvic cavity, the examiner can touch the head with their sterilized hands.
- The doctor can detect whether it will be a difficult labor by extending the fingers into the womb.
- A twin fetus can be detected by the mother's abdominal shape, characterized by a depressed middle part and protruded sides.

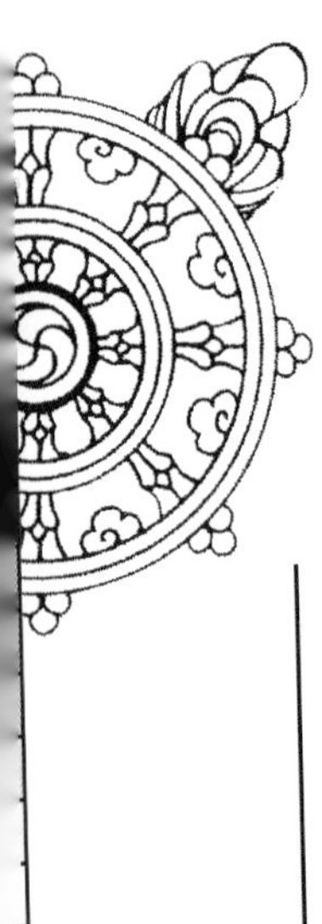

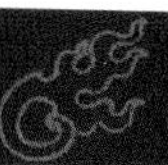

The Advent of a Life

The process of the departure of the fetus and placenta from the mother is called delivery (labor). At the beginning of labor, the upper body of the mother feels relaxed, but feels heavy in the lower body. She will also experience loss of appetite, a pulling sensation in the medial aspect of the thigh when walking, and a dislocated feeling in the lumbar vertebrae. The labor orifice is open and there will be frequent urination and profuse labor secretions. All the above signs signify that a new life is coming to this world very soon.

Labor

Let the mother lie comfortably in a quiet room, relax her whole body and comfort her. Cover her body with clothes and massage her *feng* point. Find an experienced midwife to help with the delivery and prepare all necessary materials.

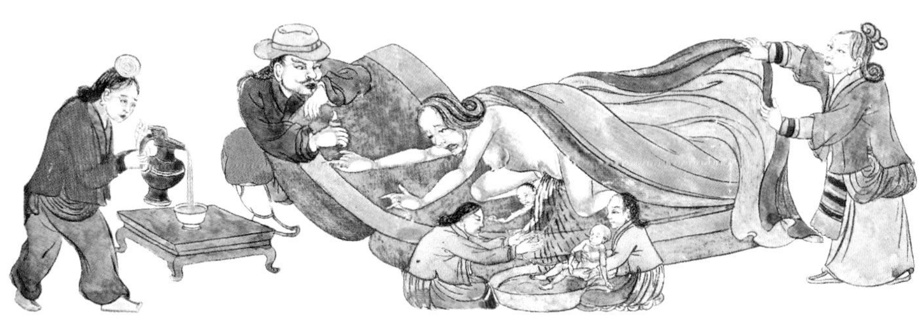

Let the mother relax both body and mind. Keep her warm with clothes and blankets and prepare all necessary instruments.

At the beginning, when the contractions begin, use mild and neutral formulas, such as *Powder that Can Disperse with Eleven Ingredients, Powder that Can Disperse with Six Ingredients* or simply long pepper steeped in hot water.

The effect of these formulas is similar to the butter-needling method mentioned in *The Four Medical Tantras*. For first time mothers, *Opening the Womb Orifice Decoction* can be given to prevent laceration of the delivery gate. When rapid delivery is required, the above formulas can be given repeatedly.

When the abdomen becomes hard, pain from contractions worsens, and the delivery gate opens, delivery is coming soon. At this time the midwife should kneel on the delivery bed and press the mother's abdomen to assist delivery. Overstrain at this point will injure the fetus and should be avoided. The posture of the mother should be adjusted if bleeding is serious.

If the amniotic sack doesn't rupture at the beginning of delivery, it is essential to cut open the sac to let out the amniotic fluid so as to facilitate the delivery of the fetus. When this is done the fetus will be delivered readily.

There will be some pain when the placenta is delivered. Let the mother hold her breath to press out the placenta, assisted by pressing the abdomen from above downward by the hands. In the meantime, let the mother lie supine and take great care of her. Burn *Nine Ingredient Incense Recipe* to fumigate the room and dissolve borneol in warm water to wash the perineum. Prevent wind from attacking the perineum, and apply some medicine for preventing *rlung* diseases.

If the placenta is still retained in the womb, the doctor may find it manually if it is stuck to the womb. Generally, adhesion occurs at the upper part of the womb, only a few adhere to the lower part. The latter condition is more dangerous.

Normally, the placenta is delivered right after the birth of the fetus. However, a too early descent of the placenta is also dangerous.

Birth

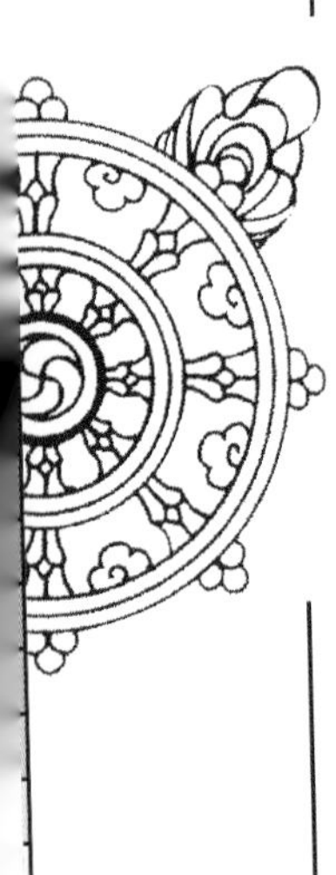

After the baby is delivered, squeeze the umbilical blood into the newborn. Use wool to make two knots about four inches from the baby's navel. Cut the umbilical cord in between the knots. When no more blood appears, hold the newborn and wash it with aromatic warm water and rub the inside of the mouth with a wet clean cloth, then put an incantation written with safflower on the baby's tongue, and feed it a little musk water with butter and bee honey.

Then let the newborn suck his/her mother's breast. Cow's milk can be used if the mother's milk is insufficient. Rub the newborn's navel with a paste made of butter and costusroot .

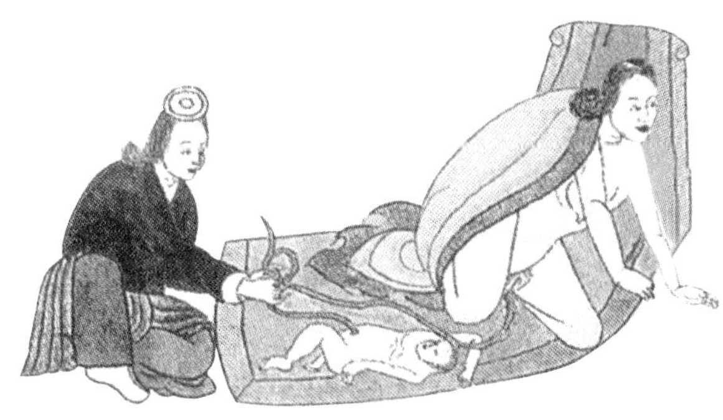

After the baby is delivered, squeeze the umbilical blood into the newborn's body. Make two knots over the umbilical cord with wool and cut it between the knots.

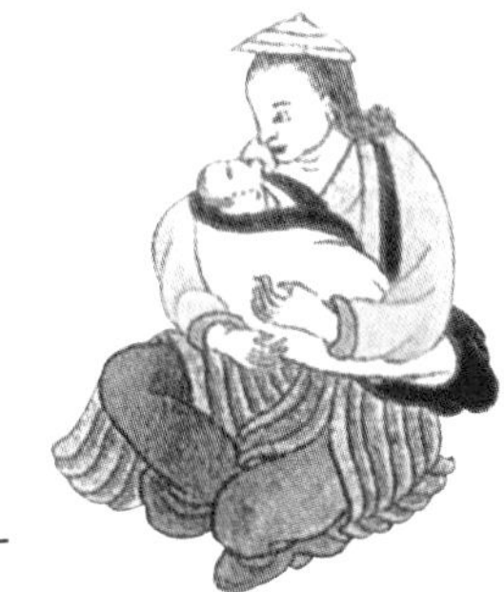

After no blood can be squeezed from the cord, place the newborn in the mother's arms.

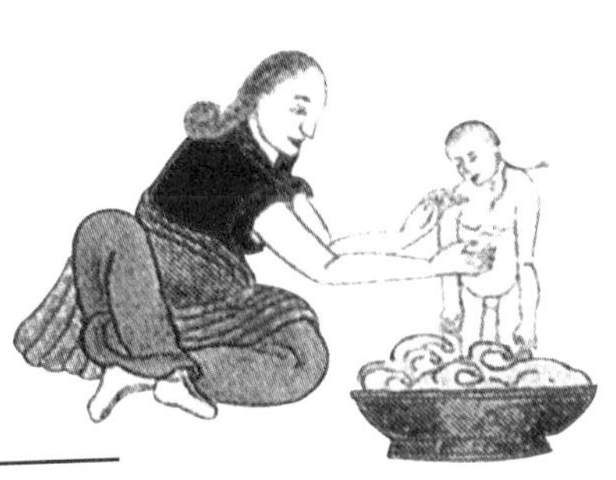

Wash the newborn with aromatic medicinal water.

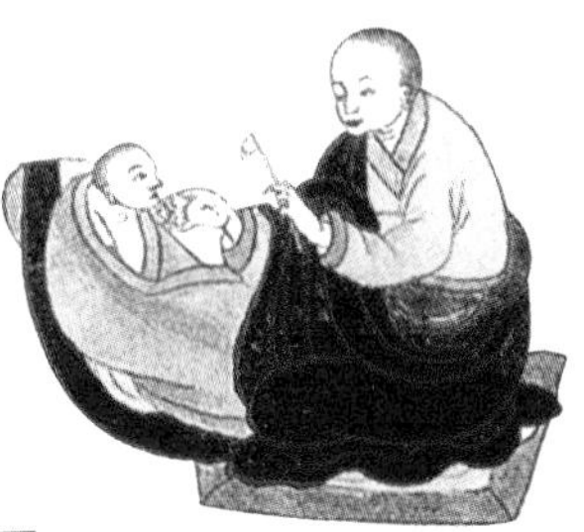

Put an incantation written with safflower on the newborn's tongue.

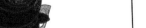

According to Tibetan medicine, when the fetal head comes out first, with the body in a supine position, the umbilical cord around the upper body, and the fetus has a loud crying voice, an elongated skull, small fontanels, a high nose ridge, a high hair line, large ears, strong sucking power, rapid response to outside stimuli, and keen reactions, the signs are auspicious, reflecting the baby will be easy to raise.

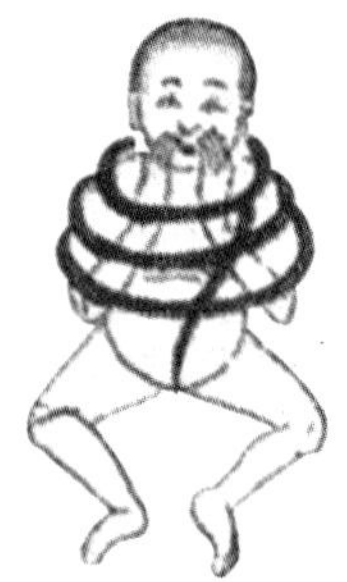

The umbilical cord around the upper body, a loud crying voice, a sharp skull, small fontanels, high hair line.

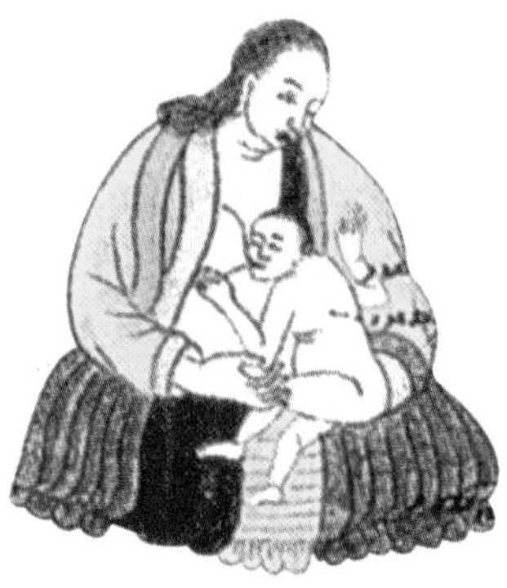

Strong sucking power and keen reaction to stimuli are auspicious signs.

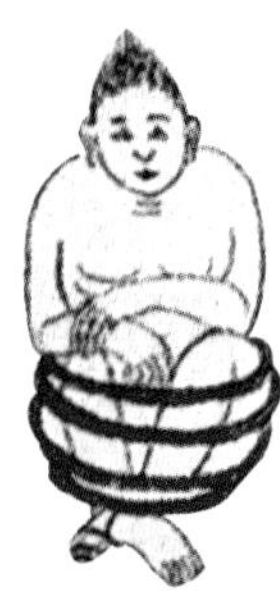

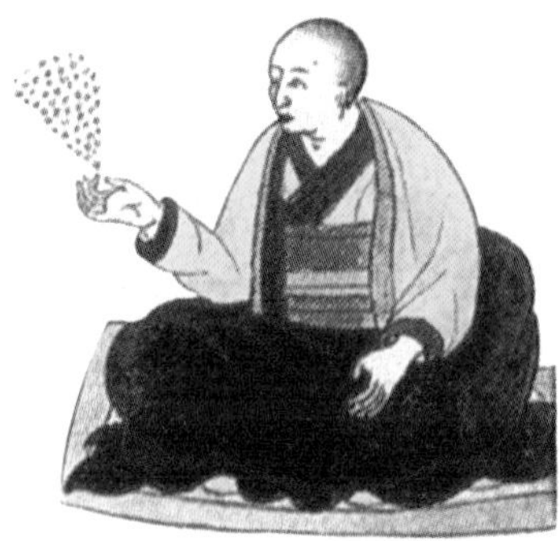

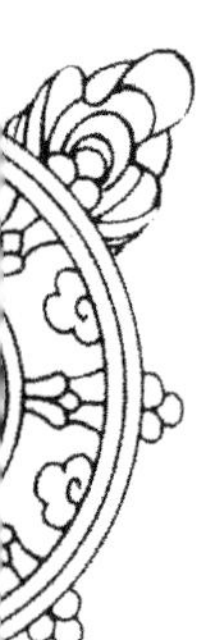

Newborns with the cord around their lower body, a weak crying voice, large fontanels, and a low hair line must be prayed for and receive best wishes right away.

Care for the Newborn

Since a newborn is not yet mature, and its adaptation to the environment is not perfect, care and protection are very important. Inappropriate care may cause low intelligence, a weak physique, and diseases like lameness, blindness, deafness, and muteness. Proper care for the newborn includes:

Breast feeding: in the first couple of days, the mother often does not secrete milk. Give the baby three meals of butter, honey, and xanthium boiled in water. Though the first milk secreted is very nutritious, it shouldn't be given in large amounts, and the amount fed to the baby should increase gradually. Medicine and food that promote lactation can be given if necessary. If the mother fails to make breast milk, breast feeding from a wet-nurse, cow's milk or sheep's milk can be used as substitutes. Butter plus bee honey diluted with warm boiled water can be also be used to substitute for mother's breast milk. The amount of boiled water and breast milk can be increased after the child is one month old.

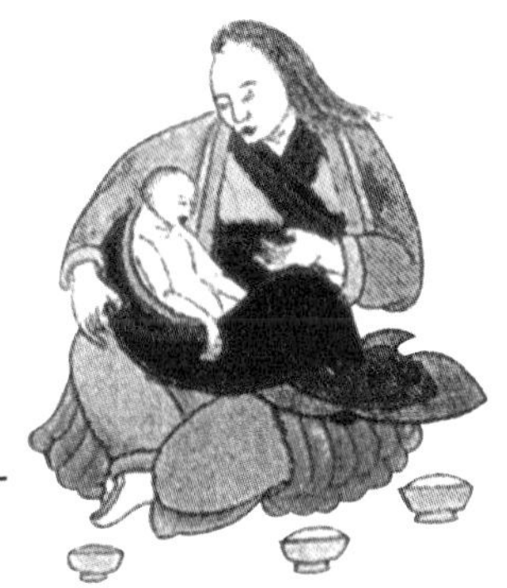

In case the mother fails to begin lactation several days after delivery, feed the baby a small amount of fresh butter, bee honey, and xanthium boiled in water, taken three times a day.

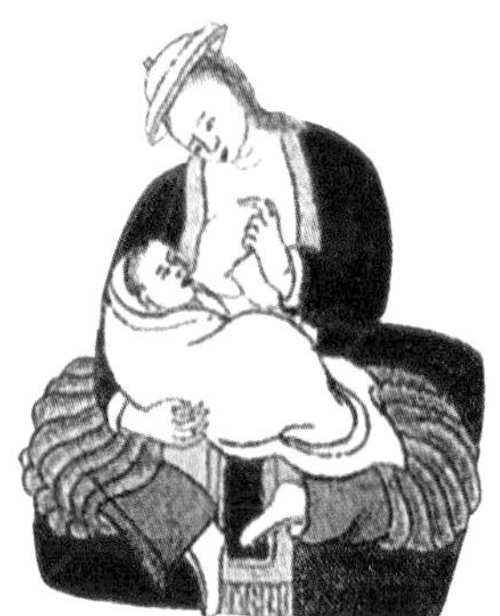

For mothers who do not lactate, a wet nurse can be employed.

Sleep: premature newborns should be kept in a warm bed with the head facing a clean place, covered with soft clothes, smooth quilts, and a cap.

Naming: the parents and relatives should choose the baby's name based on the baby's birth time. The name should be auspicious. If the mother's former child died early, the baby's name can be changed frequently, and call him/her Tsering, Puntsho, and Tsashi. If the baby is male, his name should be said frequently after he is one month old.

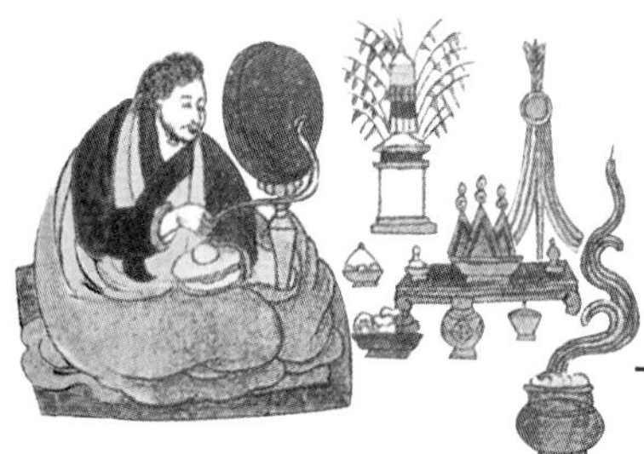

Celebrations for the child reaching one month old should include giving a name, wearing nice clothes, and praying for auspiciousness.

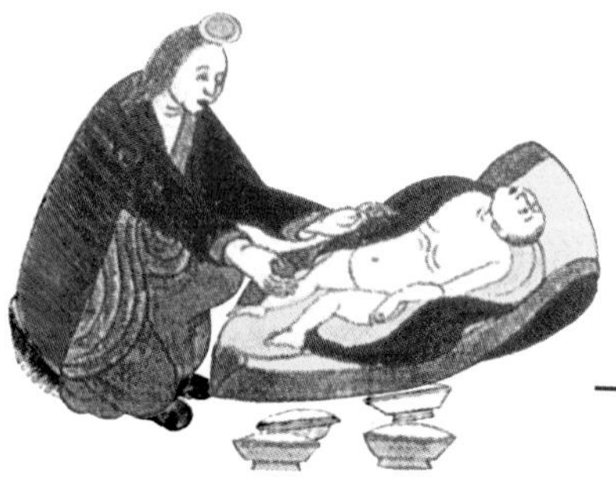

The cut surface of the navel should be rubbed with a paste made of butter possibly combined with costusroot.

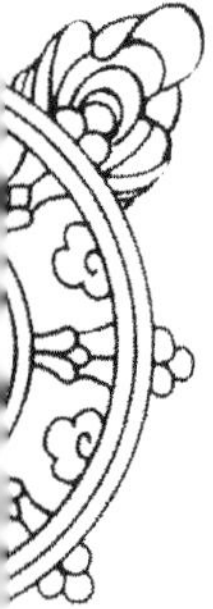

Medicinal care: the cut surface of the umbilical cord should be rubbed frequently with a paste made of butter and costusroot. To achieve a long life for the baby, beginning on the second day after birth, use a powder made of detoxified gold and tiger claws. To render the baby clever, use a powder made of bovine bezoar, acorus, and costusroot. To render the baby energetic, use a powder made of peacock's feather, musk, and gymnademia. All the above should be made into powder, mixed with sugar and hemp seeds and taken every day in the morning. Musk mixed with fresh wine and myrrh soaked in water; or asafetida, charcoal of peacock feather, sulfur, and costusroot may also be given. By doing so, the baby can be given a good spirit, made clever, wise, brave, mighty, and active, and achieve longevity. This therapy also heals or prevents diseases.

Diet: feed the baby with soups containing sugar, honey, meat, and vegetables to eliminate skin diseases. Furthermore, a powder made with chebulae, asafetida, acorus, costusroot, juniper, and purple rock salt powdered and boiled in goat's milk and butter should be administered once a week. This can cause the baby to be clever, have a clear and rapid voice, and a good memory.

Immediately after the birth of the baby, one must pray for its happiness, "My darling, may you have a long life and be wealthy, remain free from disaster and diseases, do good deeds, prosper in wealth, happiness, and auspiciousness."

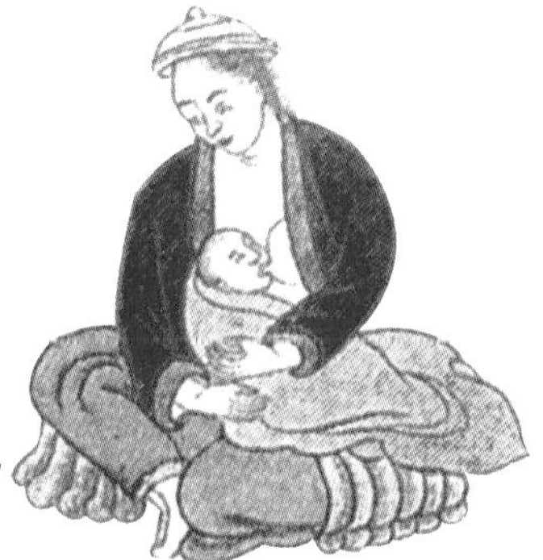

Pay attention to the method of breast feeding and holding the baby. Avoid hunchbacked and curved neck positions.

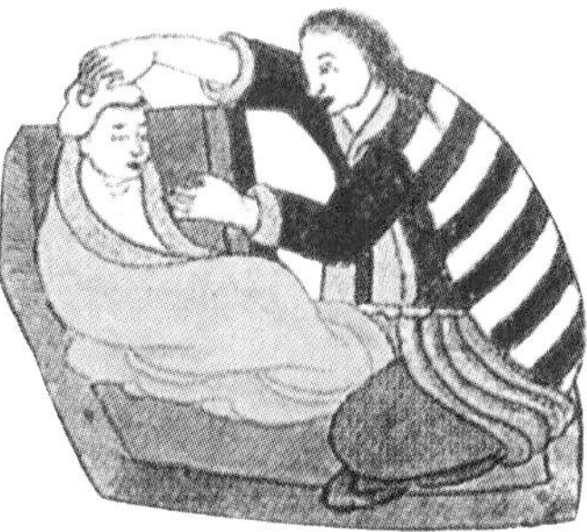

Ensure the baby develops correct posture. Rub and massage daily.

Daily life: prevent the baby from having a flattened head, wry neck, or a deformed head due to unsuitable sleeping positions. The mother should massage the baby's skull to prevent deformity. Avoid strong light that may injure the eyes, cause crossed eyes, or blurred vision. The vision may be injured when the sole of the foot and the fontanel are under direct sunlight. Frequent colds may cause deafness. Inappropriate positions of holding the baby may cause hunchback or a curved neck. Premature standing may cause prolapse of the liver. Avoid burns, animal bites, infectious diseases, and fright. Frequently massage the baby and expose it to an appropriate amount of sun. The above methods of caring for the newborn baby will render the baby healthy and bring positive effects and happiness for its whole life.

This completes the whole processes of pregnancy and reproduction, how a new life comes to this world, and the protection and care for the life just begun.

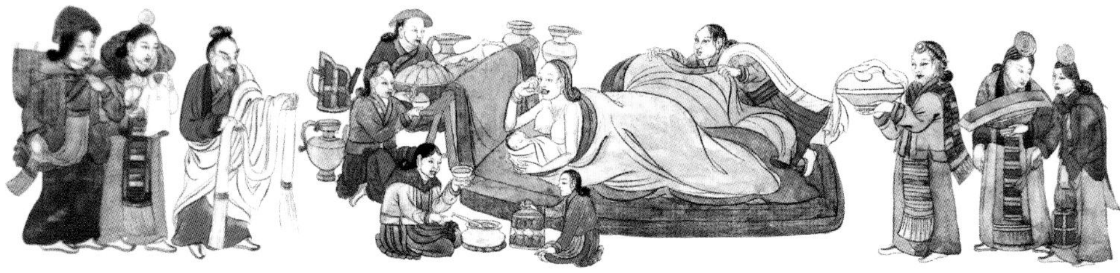

The mother finishes the whole process of pregnancy and reproduction. Careful protection must be given to both the mother and the baby.

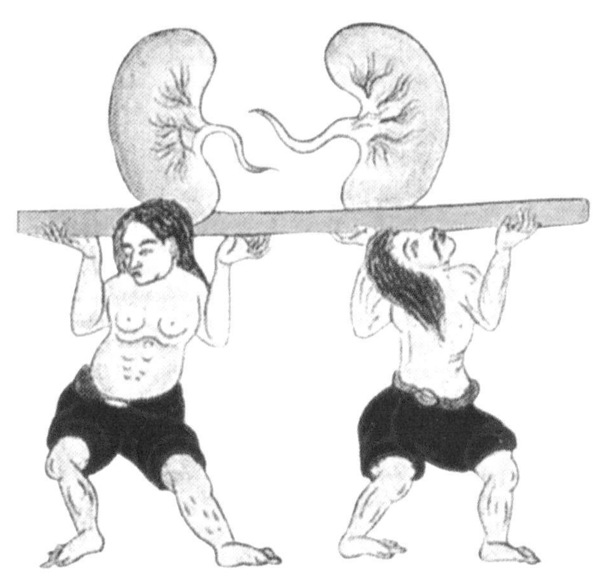

ཚེའི་རྒྱུན་ཤེས།

CHAPTER 2 GENERAL KNOWLEDGE OF LIFE

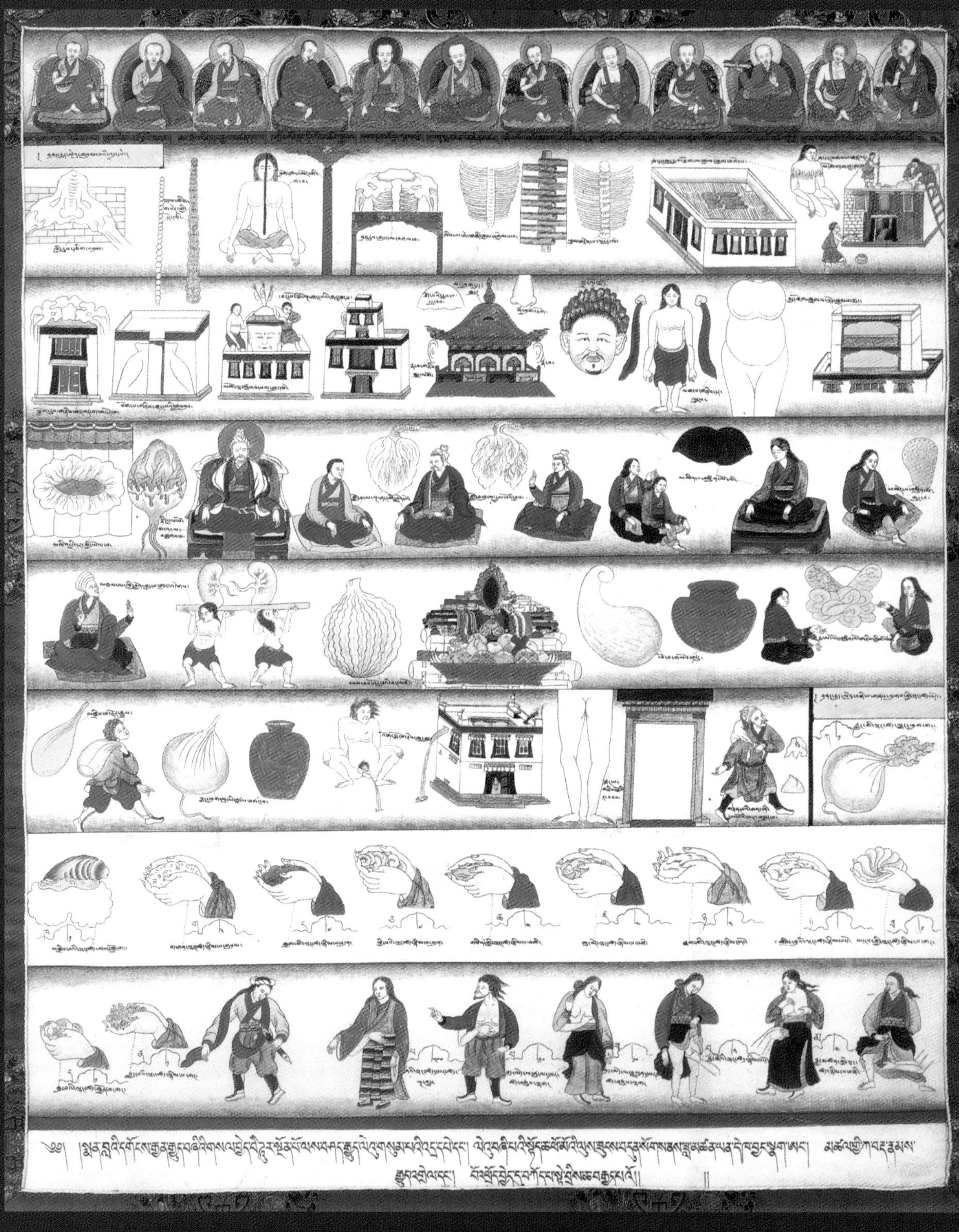

Thangkha eight in the *Sman thang series* of *The Four Medical Tantras*, the metaphors of the organs and measurement of materials.

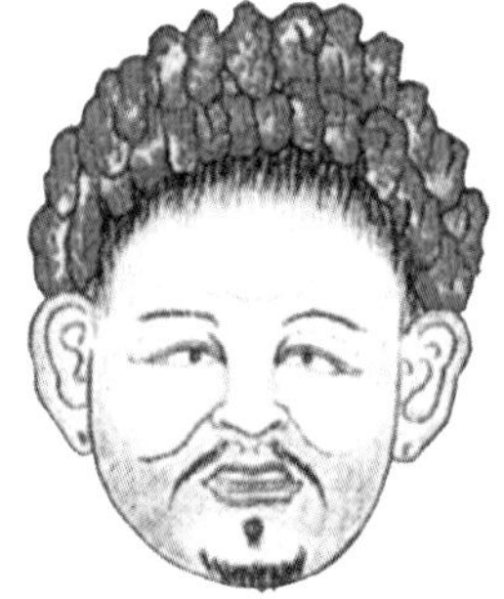

What is life?

Throughout history, different opinions have been put forward by various academic schools and scholars. Born on the roof of the world, the philosophy of life that forms the basis of Tibetan medicine is based on natural conditions of the plateau, the native population, and religious teachings. Through these lenses, the questions of life are analyzed and deciphered.

Based on these conclusions, it is possible to comprehend the process of life and understand the methods of health cultivation put forth by Tibetan medicine.

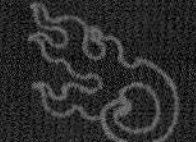

Body Metaphors

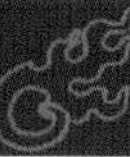

On the basis of anatomical knowledge, Tibetan medicine offers a rich, vivid, and extensive field of metaphors dealing with all of the organs of the body. The metaphors are related to daily life and deal not only with the shape and structure of the organs, but also with their functions. It should be noted that most of the metaphors are unique to Tibetan culture, which give them a unique flavor.

Body Metaphors

The head is like the loft of a building. The five sense organs are likened to skylights and windows, the skull to a roof, the fontanels to a chimney, the two ears to decorative Rocs* at the sides of the roof, the nostrils to a golden roof, and the hair to overlapping tiles.

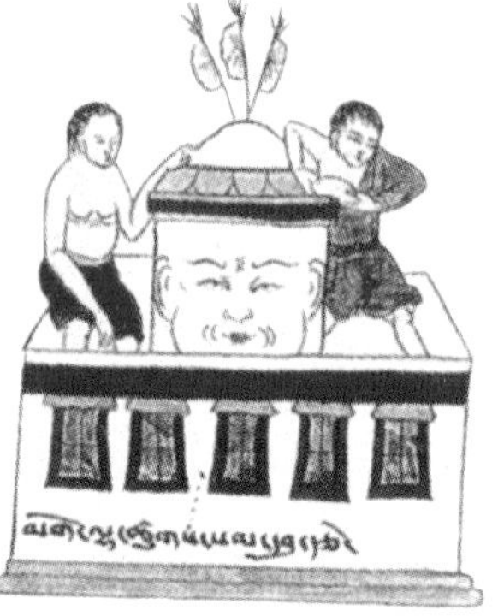

The head as a dignified loft.

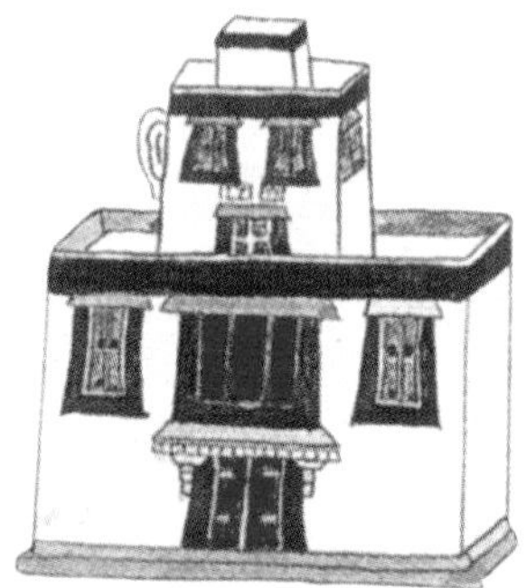

The five sense organs as doors and windows.

The spine is likened to gold coins piled one on the other, the vital vessel to an agate pillar that supports the whole palace, the square breastbone to the beam, the twenty four ribs to neatly arranged rafters, the cartilage connecting the breastbone and spine to wood pads supporting the rafters, the scapula to the lateral pillars of the house, the clavicle to

*A Roc is a legendary giant bird with a wingspan of thirty paces that is capable of carrying off an elephant in its claws.

The flower of health gives rise to the fruits of faith and wealth.

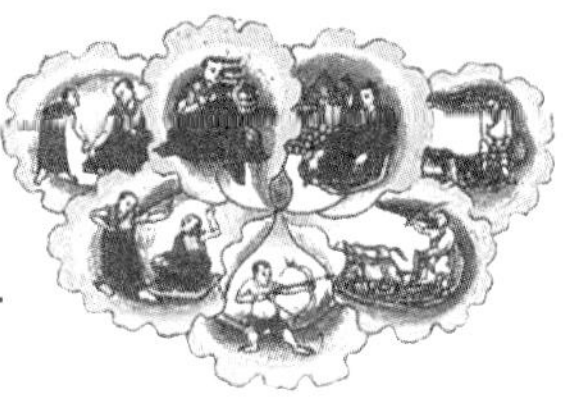

The flower of longevity gives rise to the fruit of extraordinary happiness.

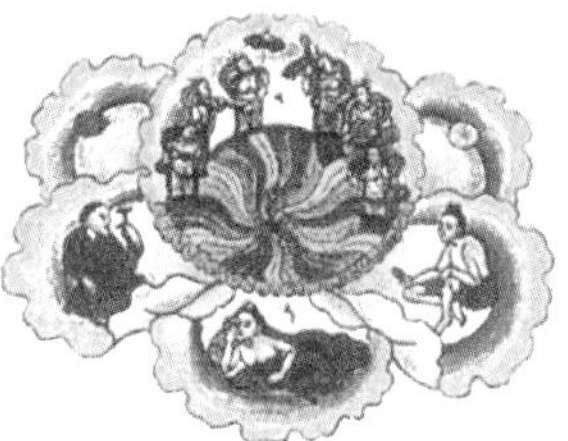

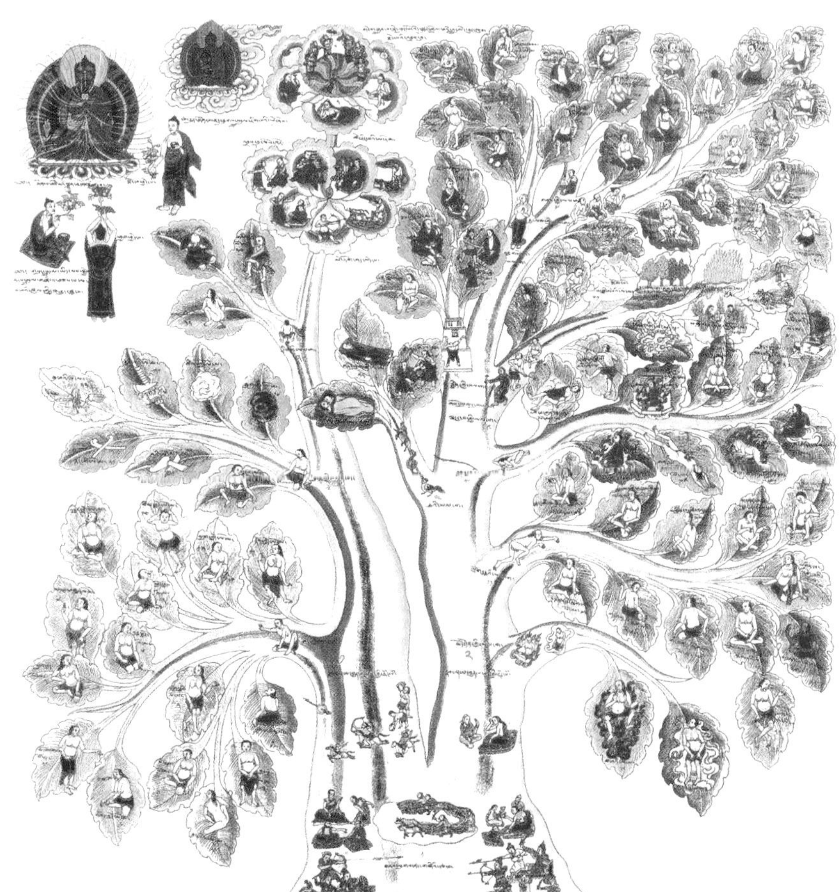

Tibetan medicine uses a tree to describe life. With its two trunks, twelve branches, eighty-eight leaves, two flowers, and two fruits the basic relationship between health and disease can be explained. The above two illustrations are the flower of health and the flower of longevity. (*Thangkha* two in the *Sman thang* of *The Four Medical Tantras*).

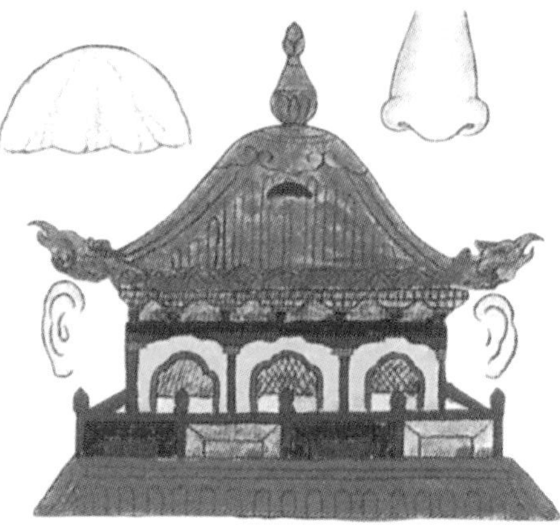

The skull bone is the roof of a house; the two ears are decorative Roc heads, the fontanel is the chimney, the nose is the roof's decoration.

flying eaves on the windows, the arms to flying streamers hanging outside the house, the vessels and tendons to branched rafters, the skin and muscles to cement and paint, the hip bones to the walls of the house, and the two legs to solid door pillars.

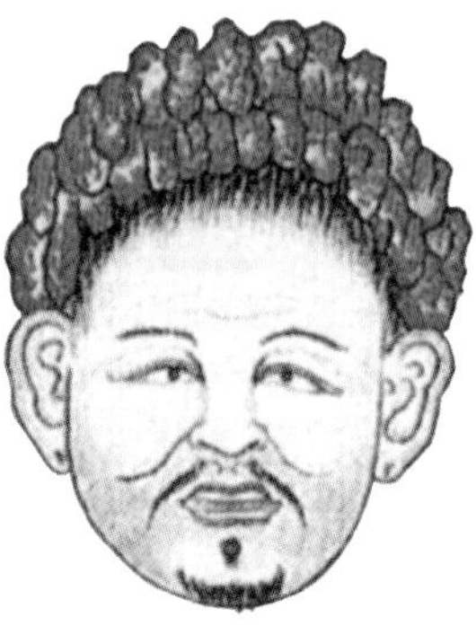

The hairs are the overlapping tiles.

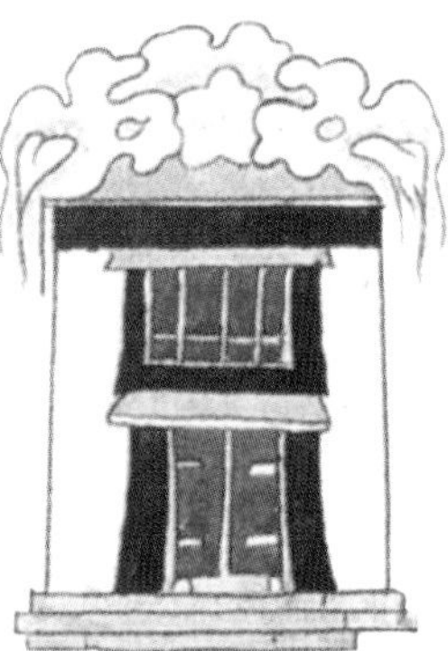

The clavicles are the flying eaves.

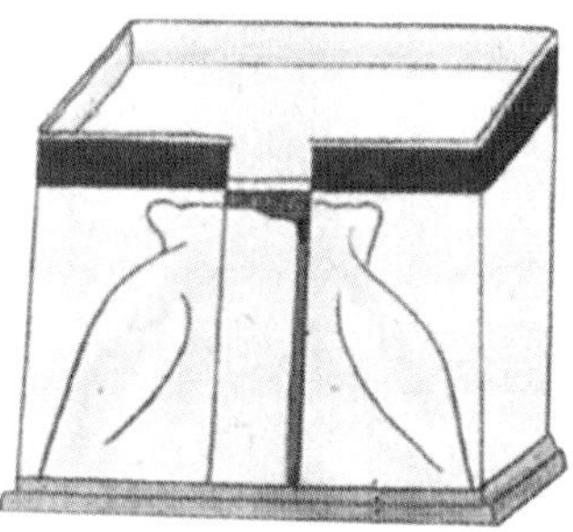

The scapulas are the lateral pillars.

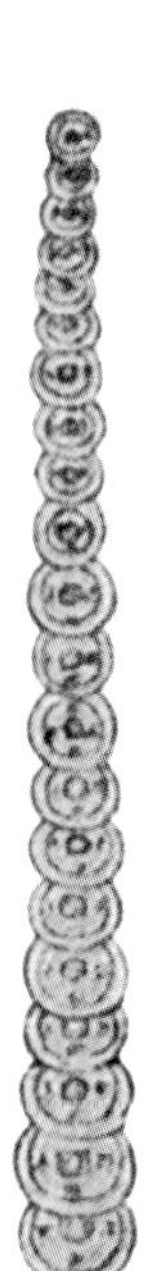

The spine is a pile of gold coins.

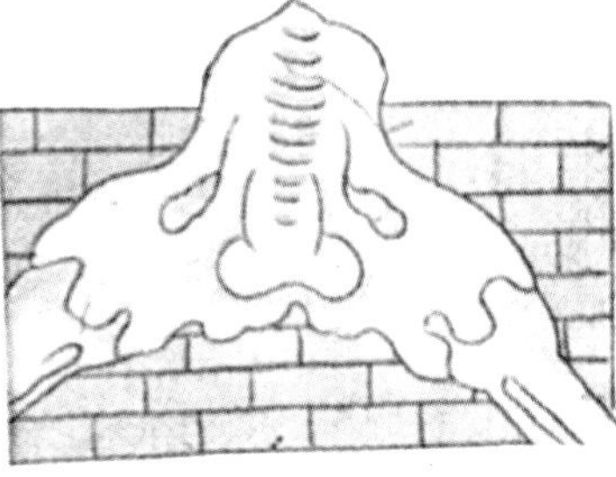

The hip bones are the walls.

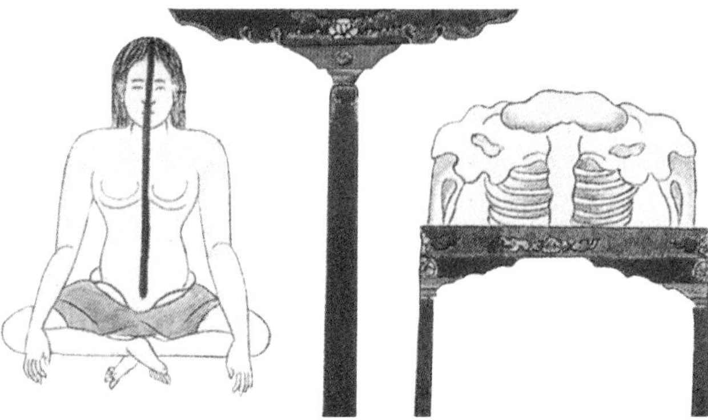

The vital vessel is the agate pillar.

The chest is the beam.

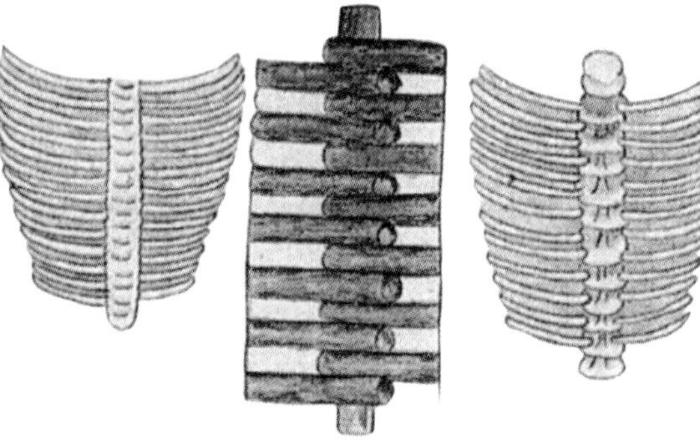

The ribs are the rafters orderly arranged.

The cartilage connecting the breastbone and spinal column are wooded pads between the rafters.

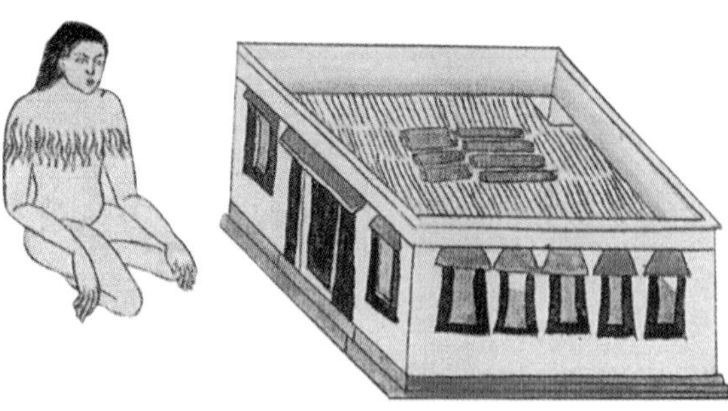

The tendons and vessels are the branches on the roof.

The muscles and skin are the mud and cement that cover the walls.

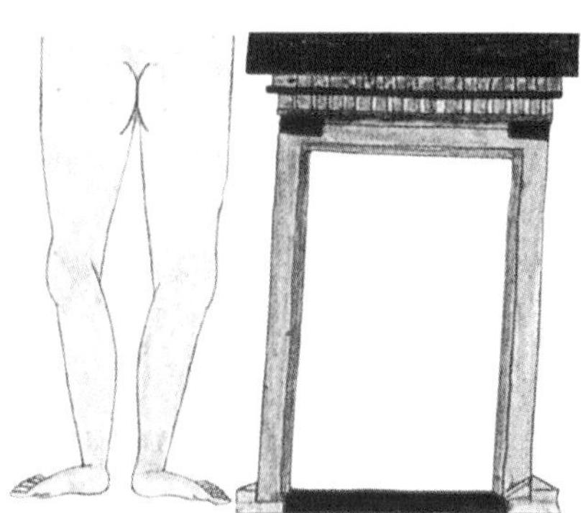

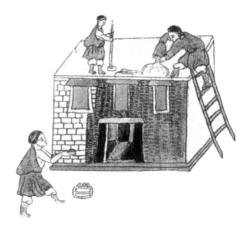

The two legs are the door pillars.

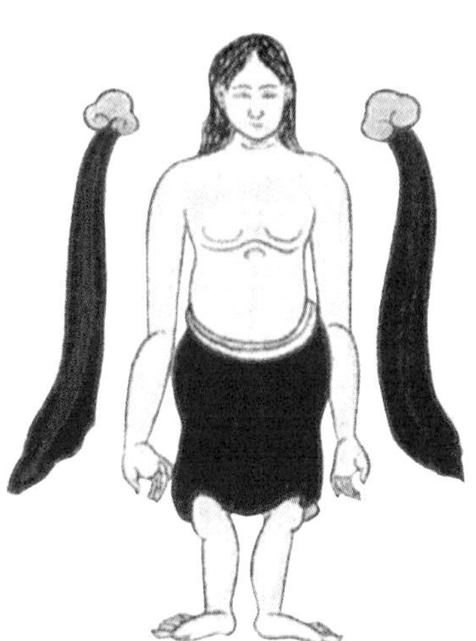

The arms are hanging streamers.

Metaphors for the internal organs

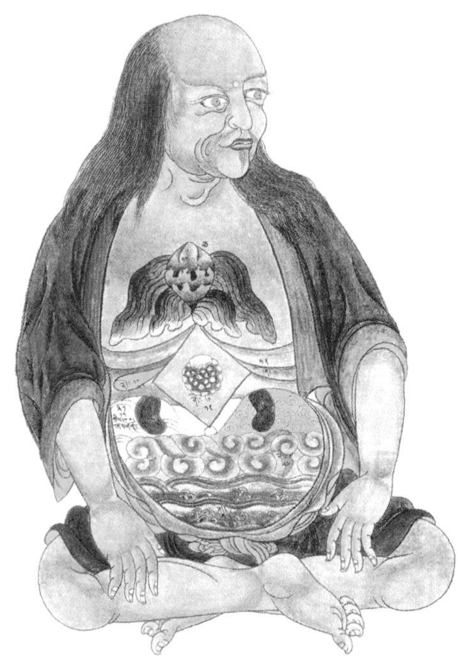

The metaphors used for the internal organs are even more vivid and figurative.

The chest and abdomen are likened to a double layered corridor, the diaphragm to a piece of silk, the heart to a king on his throne where life is attached, the five-lobed child lungs to princes that protect the king, the five-lobed mother lungs to ministers that support the king or to a mother holding her child, the liver to a queen, the spleen to the concubines. All of these are in protected positions so they will not be injured. The two kidneys are likened to ministers of the queen supporting the house like pillars, the essence mansion (*bsam bse'u*) to a treasure-house, the stomach to a cauldron for cooking, and the gallbladder that sits beside the liver and between the liver and stomach to a bag of seasoning or to a blacksmith's bellows. The functions of the large and small intestines are likened to the passages for conducting dregs or to attendants to the queen, the bladder to a water vessel, and the two yin orifices (urethra and anus) to the outlets of a sewer. All the vital points are like envoys dispatched by the king to certain tasks at certain posts and should be carefully protected from injury. If the envoy at their post is injured the heart will sooner or later be involved and the result will be grave.

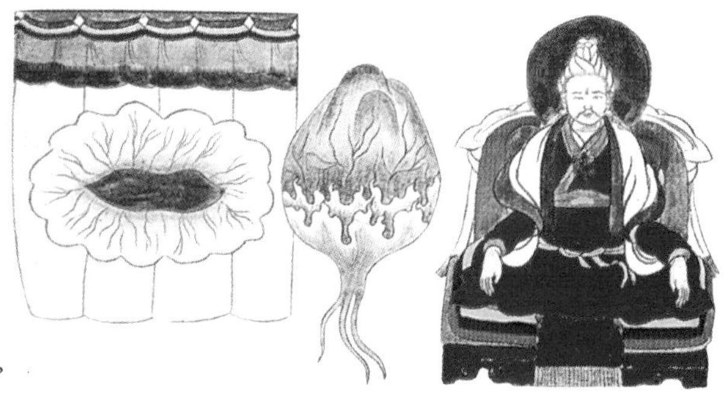
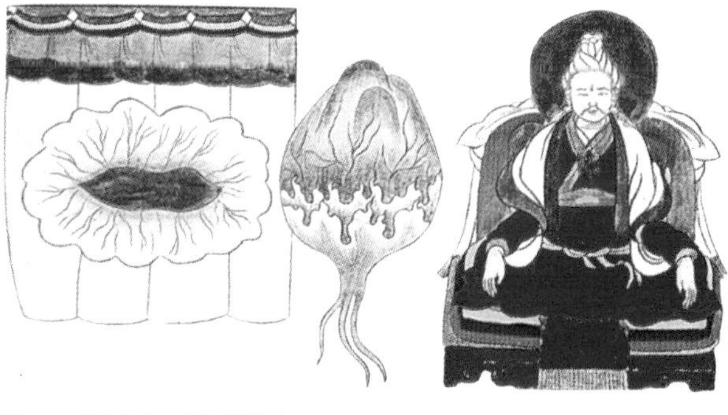

The diaphragm is a curtain,
the heart is a king.

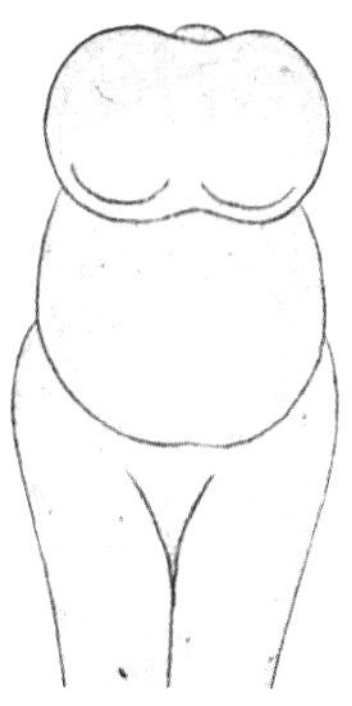
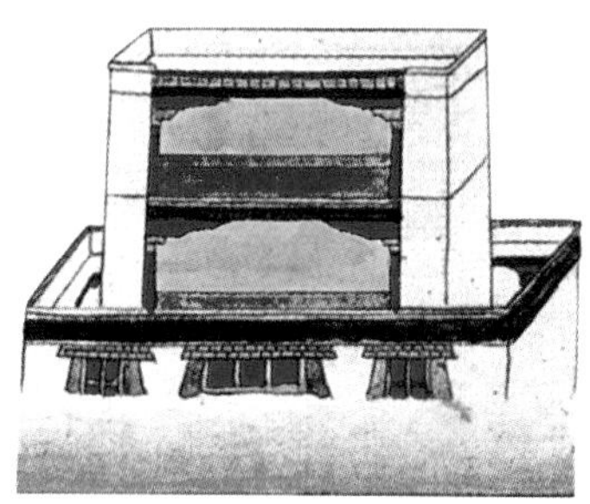

The chest and abdomen are a double layered corridor.

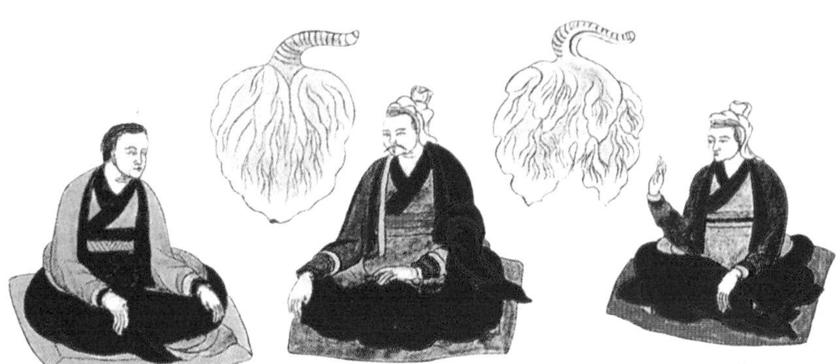

The five-lobed mother lungs are the ministers. The five-lobed child lungs are princes.

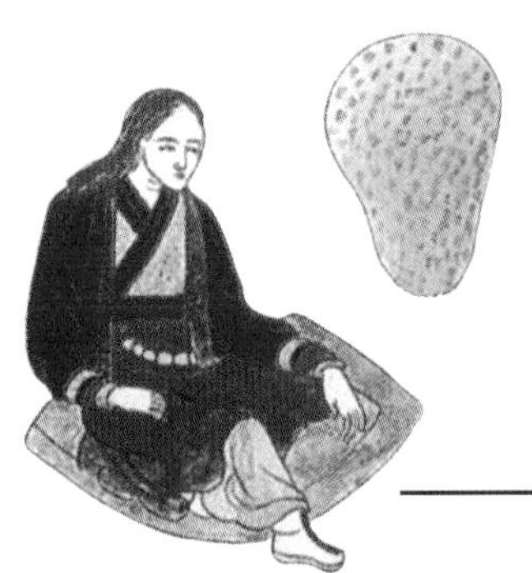

The spleen is a concubine.

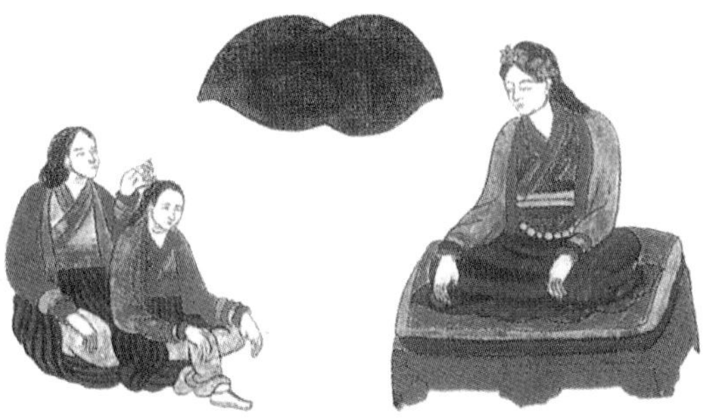

The liver is the queen.

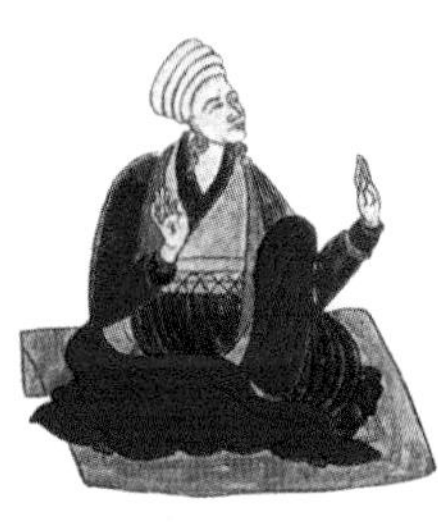

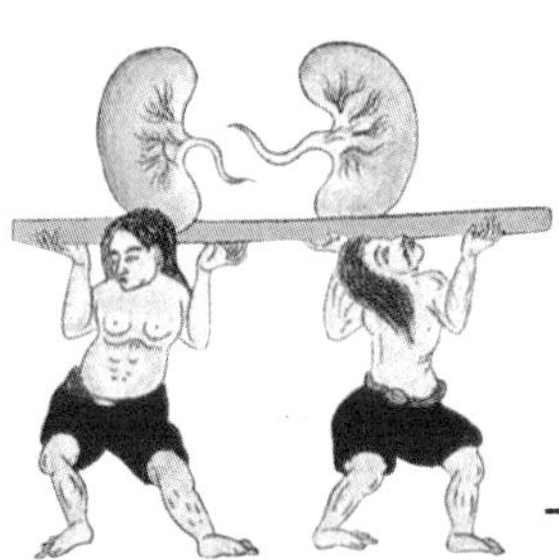

The kidneys are men with incredible strength.

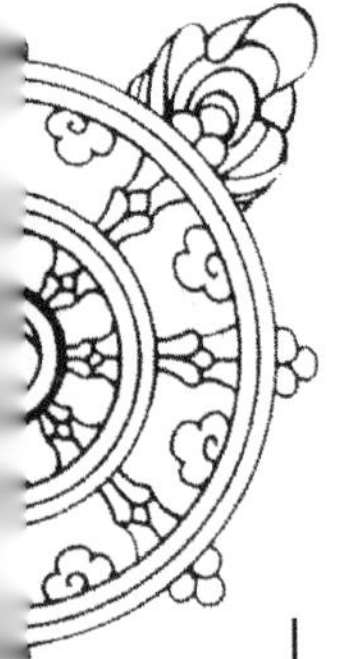

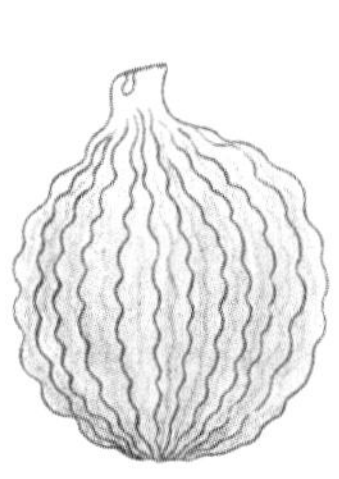

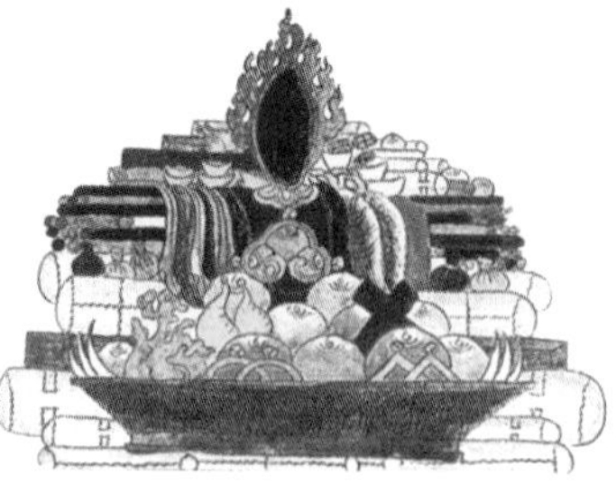

The testicles and ovaries are treasure-houses.

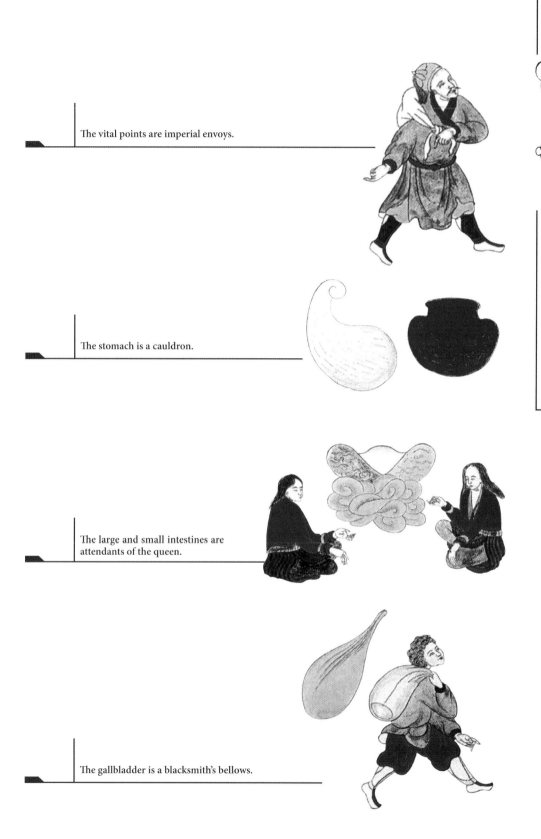
The vital points are imperial envoys.
The stomach is a cauldron.
The large and small intestines are attendants of the queen.
The gallbladder is a blacksmith's bellows.

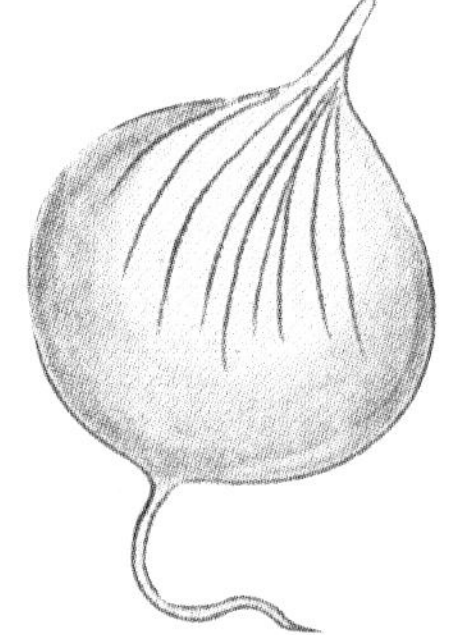

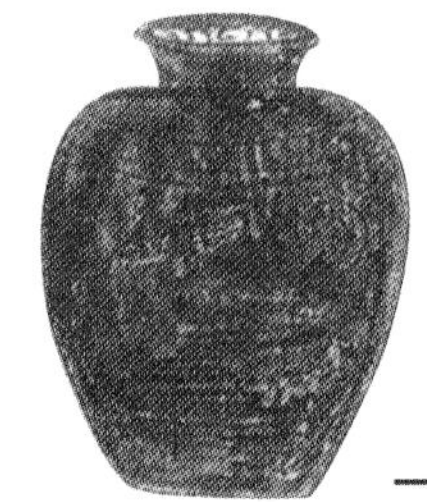

The bladder is a water container.

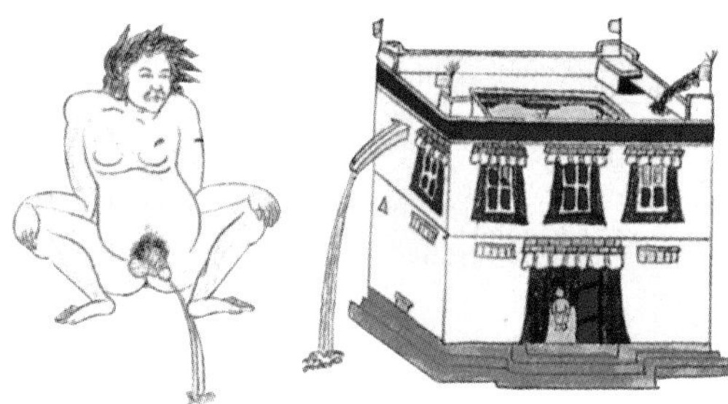

The two yin orifices are the sewer outlets.

Ancient Tibetan medicine uses common items and people as metaphors to describe the functions and structures of the parts of the body and its organs. It is vivid and figurative, though rather rough.

The Three Factors

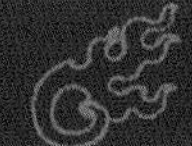

In all mature traditional medical systems a systematic and unique theoretical basis must be established as its core to explain the process of life. The theoretical core is always composed of a small number of basic elements, which possess material connotations and also special functions. The relationship among them and the complexities they lead to are used to explain the process of life. In Tibetan medicine the three factors form the basis of the system. They not only explain all life processes but also guide treatment and diagnosis.

The three factors are *rlung*, *mkhris pa* and *badkan*. Many scholars have attempted to define these terms in their own language. In English they were often written as follows: *rlung* as wind or air, *mkhris pa* as fire, gallbladder, or bile, and *badkan* as earth, water, phlegm, or mucus. Since the paraphrased terms fail to capture the meaning of the original, most scholars now simply use the transliteration of the original Tibetan terms.

Rlung

This is the power of movement in life. It corresponds to active-wind in the five sources. Having a cold nature it travels everywhere in the body's tissues. It is found mainly below the navel but also in the head, chest, heart, stomach and genitals. Its functions include respiration, blood circulation, all movements (physical movements as well as speaking and consciousness). *Rlung* is responsible for maintaining the powers of vision, hearing, smell, taste, touch, and consciousness, the secretion of sweat and excretion of urine and feces, the digestion and absorption of the essence from food, the nourishment of the whole body, maintaining the movements of the body, prolonging life, fostering semen-blood, and maintaining sexual desire and reproduction. In total, there are five kinds of *rlung*:

The three factors refer to *rlung, mkhris pa and badkan.* Tibetan medicine holds that these are the material and energetic basis of life.

Health cultivation *rlung*

Attached to the muscles, bones, and the brain, converging at the vertex, and circulating in the throat and in the chest, this type of *rlung* maintains normal physiological activities, keeps the vital vessel regulated, maintains swallowing, breathing, the secretion of saliva, sneezing, and belching, keeps the brain clear, strengthens the memory, and makes a person wise and clear-minded.

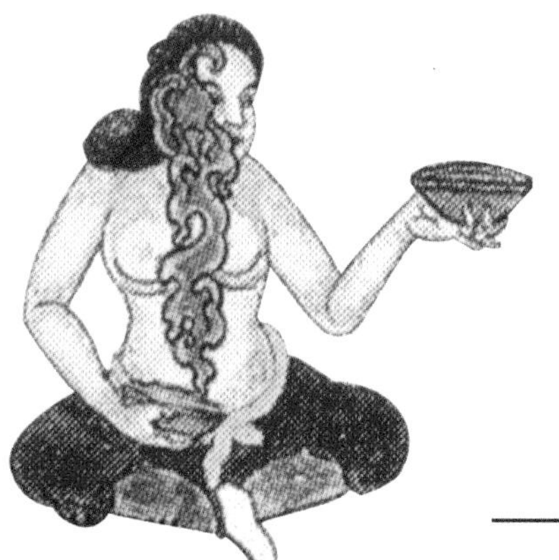

In charge of swallowing, breathing, a strong memory and keen sensation.

Ascending *rlung*

Attached to the chest, it circulates through the nose, tongue, the vocal cord, esophagus, and trachea. The ascending *rlung's* functions include the ascension of qi and blood, speaking, the voice, the ability of to think, memory, and vigorous bodily activities. It also makes one appear energetic, lustrous, gives endurance, and reflects the overall spirit of the body.

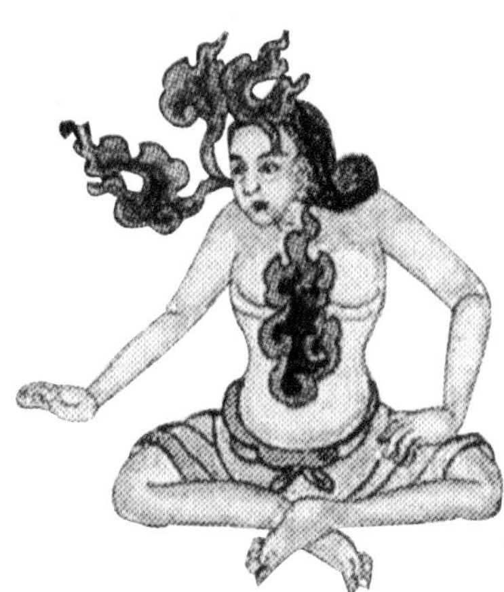

In charge of speaking, moistening of the skin, and energizing the spirit.

Pervasive *rlung*

Attached to the heart, and circulating in the blood vessels and channels. Its functions include the regulation of all *rlung*, and transportation of food essence throughout the body, blood circulation, moving the extremities, mouth, and eyes, walking and governing thinking and language. Movements of the body basically rely on this *rlung*.

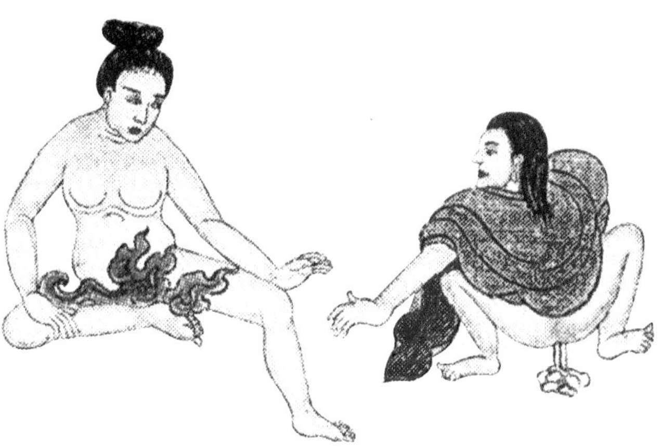

Responsible for urination, defecation, ejaculation, menstruation and birth.

Fire accompanying *rlung*

Attached to the lower part of the stomach, it circulates through all the internal organs, including the large and small intestine, and transports nutrients in the vessels. It is one of the three stomach fires, and is in charge of digestion, increasing the strength of intestinal movement, separating the essence from the dregs and transporting them to the proper locations for metabolism, resulting in the production of the seven essences, three excretions and the generation and maturation of the blood.

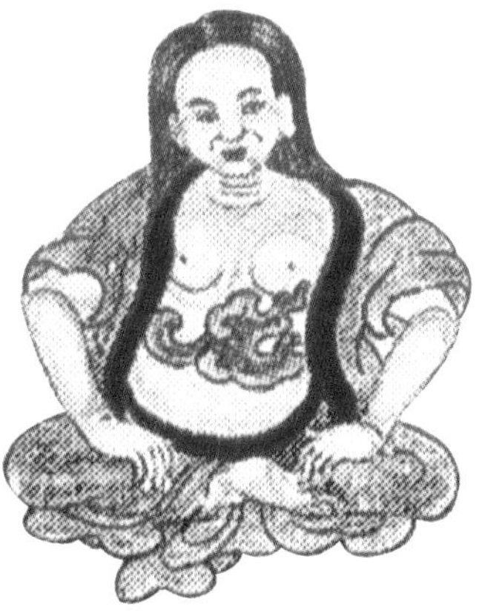

In charge of digestion, absorption and blood circulation.

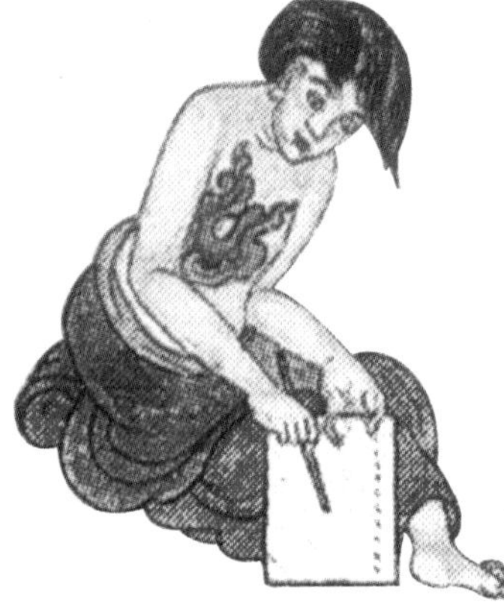

Responsible for movements, speech, and the opening and closing of the orifices.

Descending *rlung*

Attached to the anus, it circulates through the lower body, including the large intestine, bladder, genitals and the medical aspect of the thigh. Its functions include excretions such as ejaculation, menstruation, urination, defecation, sweating, birth, descent of the placenta, and expulsion of post-delivery diseases. In short, all functions of lower body are belonged to this *rlung*.

Mkhris pa

This is the heat energy of life. *Mkhris pa* belongs to warm fire in the five sources, distributes throughout the body, and mainly attaches to the liver and gallbladder, or the middle part of the trunk from the heart to the navel. It produces heat, maintains body temperature, promotes digestion, regulates the appetite, absorbs essence and medicinal substances, promotes the maturity and transformation of the seven essences, makes the face and skin lustrous, and makes one ambitious, wise, and considerate. There are five kinds of *mkhris pa*:

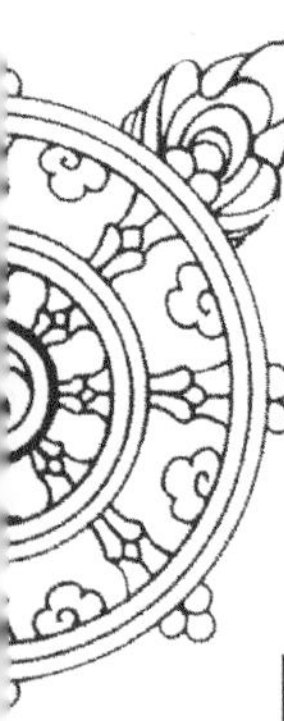

Digestive *mkhris pa*

Attached to the digestive tract, it is the most important of the three stomach fires. Its functions include the production of heat energy, digestion of food, and decomposition of food into essence and dregs. With its production of heat it assists other types of *mkhris pa* to ensure normal functions are strengthened. It also warms and dries the fluids in the body.

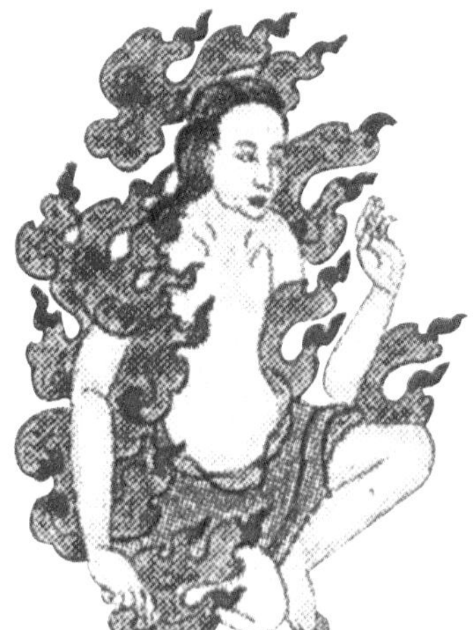

It breaks down food to produce energy.

Color changing *mkhris pa*

Attached to the liver, and circulating in the seven essences, its functions include the transformation of the pigments in essence into the colors of the body, such as the red of blood, the yellow-green of bile, the yellow of urine and the brown of feces.

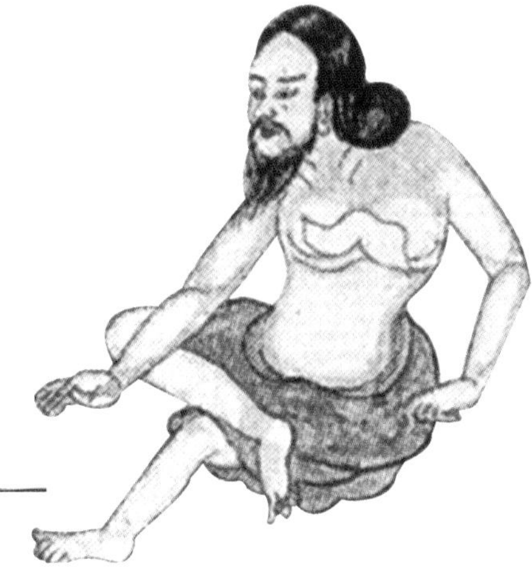

Transforms the essence from food to maintain the color of all bodily materials.

Action *mkhris pa*

Attached to the heart, it controls the mind, consciousness, emotions, and is responsible for one's wisdom, boldness, strategic ability, desire, and makes one courageous.

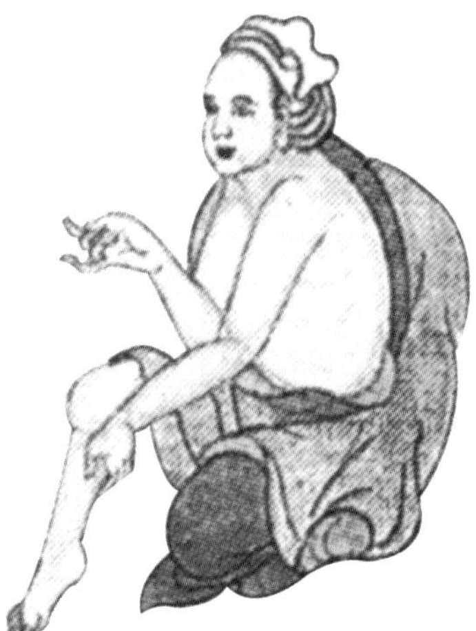

Responsible for ambition, emotions and strategy.

Visual *mkhris pa*

Attached to the eyes and the vessels, controlling visual perception, it is responsible for distinguishing shape, size, dimension and color.

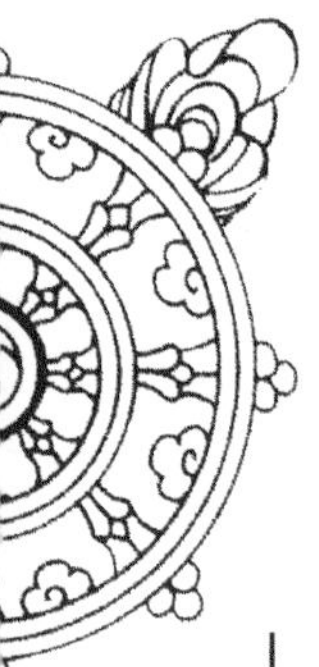

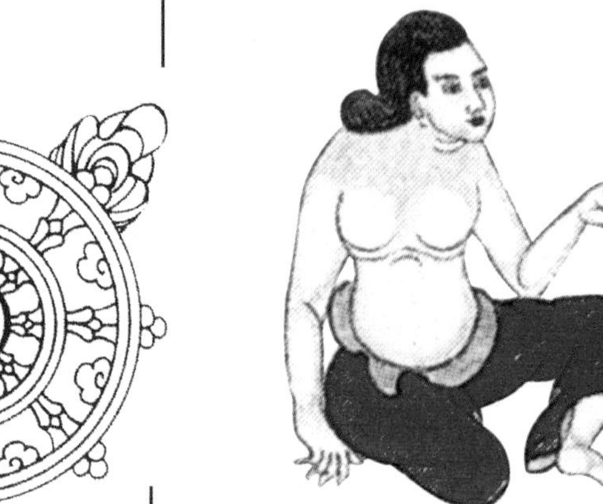

Responsible for the vision and the differentiation of colors.

Color differentiating *mkhris pa*

Attached to the skin, its functions include maintaining the moisture, texture, and luster of the skin.

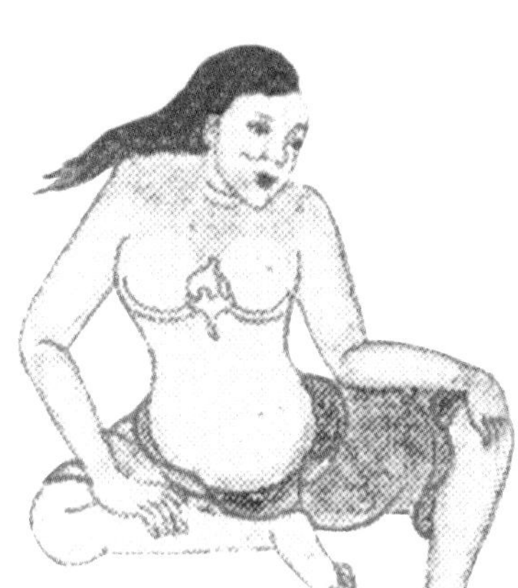

Responsible for moistening the skin.

Harmony among the three factors keeps the body healthy. Exuberance or declination of any of them will result in disease.

Badkan

Badkan is responsible for the functions of fluids, belonging to solid-earth and wet-water in the five sources. Its nature is cold (or cool) and moistening. It attaches to the brain and lung, and is responsible for the growth of the body, prolongation of life, and the regulation and production of body fluids. It breaks down food, increases stomach secretions, and helps with the digestion and absorption of food. It is responsible for taste, the distribution of nutrients in the body, the maintenance of water, moistening, lubricating and solidifying the joints, regulating the size of the body, making the skin moist, elastic and soft. It is especially responsible for emotions, makes one tender, stable, courageous in front of danger and produces sleep. *Badkan* is also divided into five different types:

Dependable *badkan*

Attached to the chest, more specifically the cartilage at the junctions of the breastbone. It is responsible for the coordination among other *badkans*. When the body fluids are abnormal, either excessive or deficient, it works to restore a normal balance. It regulates the moisture of the body.

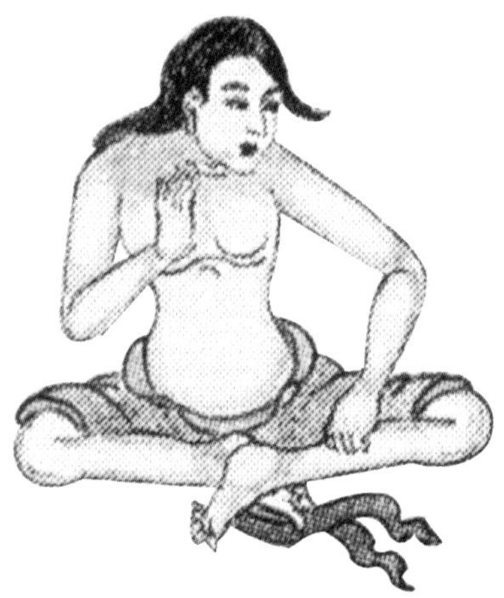

Responsible for regulation of body fluid.

Transformation *badkan*

Attached to the upper part of the stomach where food is not yet digested. Its functions include grinding and cooking food, so that the food ingested is readily decomposed and easily digested. This is the last of the three stomach fires.

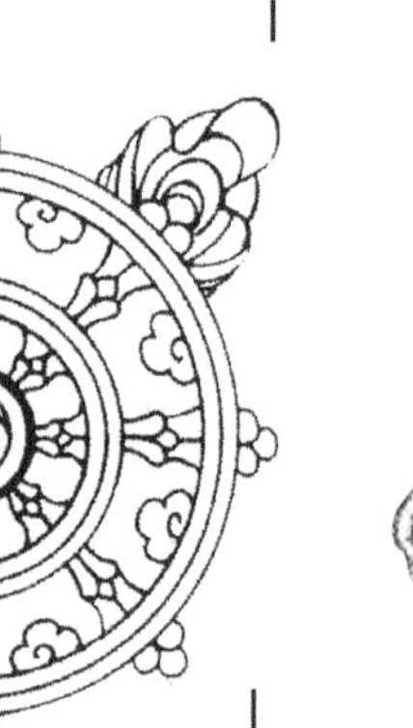

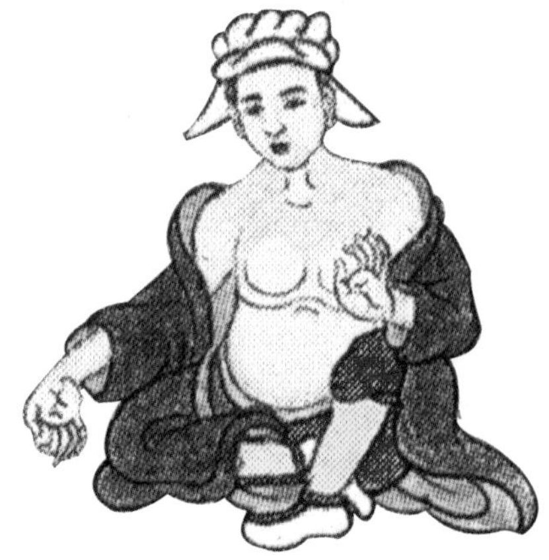

Responsible for cooking and grinding the food.

Taste *badkan*

Mainly attached to the tongue, it differentiates tastes.

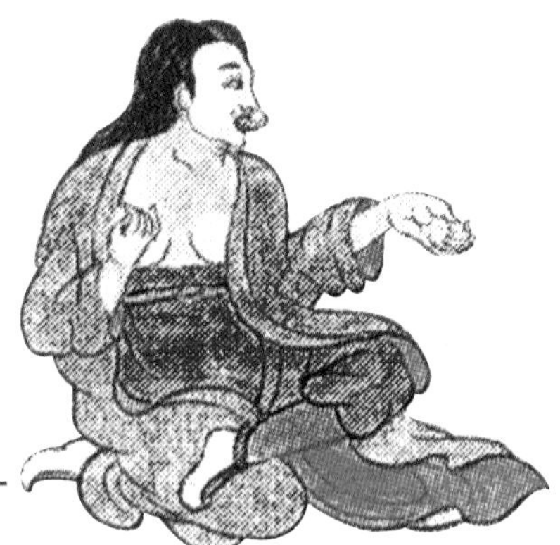

Responsible for tasting and differentiating the six tastes.

Satisfaction *badkan*

Attached to the head, it is responsible for the sense organs like the eyes and ears. By receiving the sensations from color, sound and taste, it yields the emotion of satisfaction.

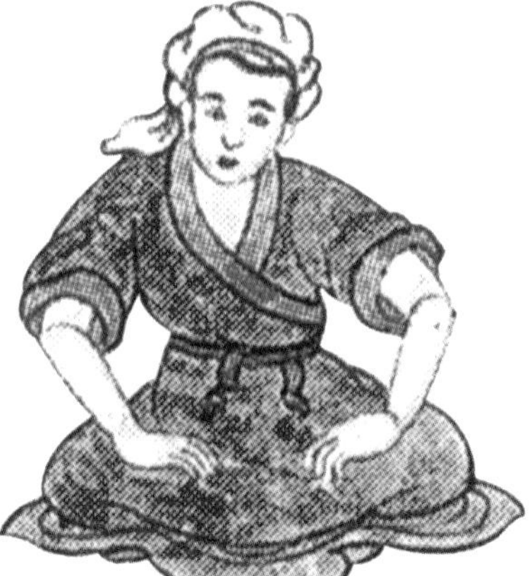

Responsible for the sensation of the ears and eyes, and the emotion of satisfaction.

Unified *badkan*

Attached to the joints, it is responsible for the union, lubrication, and movements of the joints.

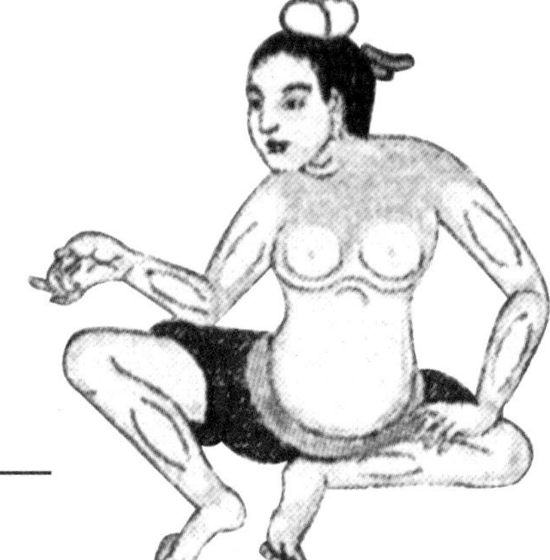

It is responsible for the lubrication, extension and flexion of joints.

Tibetan medicine holds that when *rlung*, *mkhris pa* and *badkan* are harmonious, life is stable and normal. Once the balance is broken, disease will occur. Therefore, the three factors not only demonstrate normal life activities, but also reflect disease processes.

Diagnosis involves the identification of the external signs produced by disharmony of the three factors. Treatment measures are then adopted to restore the original harmony and balance.

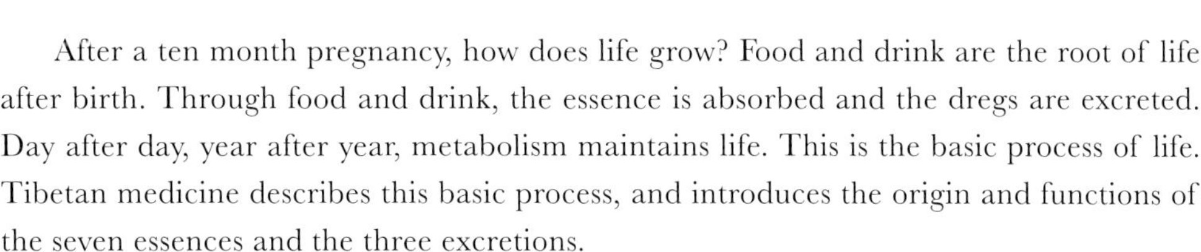

Life Process

After a ten month pregnancy, how does life grow? Food and drink are the root of life after birth. Through food and drink, the essence is absorbed and the dregs are excreted. Day after day, year after year, metabolism maintains life. This is the basic process of life. Tibetan medicine describes this basic process, and introduces the origin and functions of the seven essences and the three excretions.

The basic process

After being thoroughly chewed, food passes through the throat and into the stomach. It is then immersed in and softened by the gastric juice, the fire accompanying *rlung* blows at the digestive *mkhris pa* and causes the gastric juice to boil, grinding and smashing the food. In this way food turns into a foamy material and is digested by the high temperature digestive *mkhris pa*, and sweet food is transformed into sour. At last, the fire accompanying *rlung* separates this foamy material into essence and dregs, and the sour is changed into bitter. This process illuminates the importance of stomach fire in the digestive process. Normal stomach fire ensures a good appetite, smooth excretion, and a strong body with a lustrous appearance, whereas weak stomach fire causes a bad appetite and indigestion.

The dregs that are left after food is broken down enter the small intestine, and are further decomposed into a dilute part and a concentrated part. The former enters the kidneys to become urine, while the latter enters the large intestine to become feces.

The essence that is the result of digestion in the stomach under the action of heat energy and the pervasive *rlung* enters the liver through the nine major vessels and is further decomposed into finer essence and dregs. These dregs become bile and are sent to the gallbladder. The bile is further decomposed into spirit and dregs and the spirit is the yellow fluid lubricating the joints, while the latter enters the bladder to become urine. The essence that stays in the liver becomes blood and circulates through the vessels throughout the body. This blood transforms into muscle, which is again broken down into essence and dregs. The former becomes fat, and the latter becomes bodily substances like ear wax, nasal excretions, saliva and other such materials. Fat is decomposed into essence and dregs, the latter enters the joints to acts as lubrication and also becomes sweat, and the former becomes the bone which is further divided into essence and dregs. These

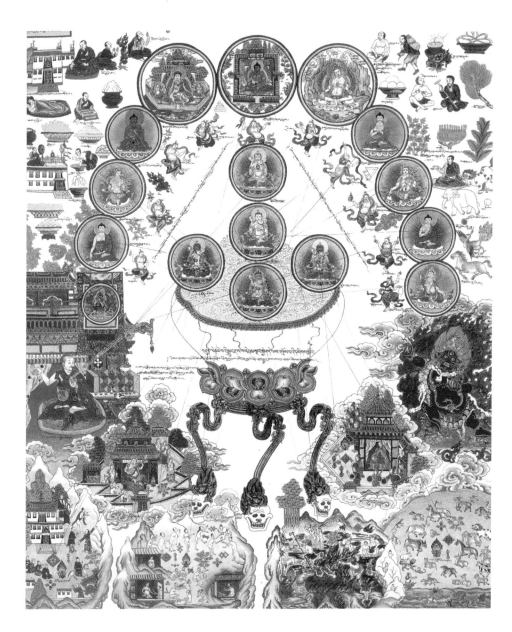

Health cultivation extends life, practicing Buddhism works to purify *samsara* (the round of rebirths). Practicing Buddhism is a form of health cultivation and its process is a part of samsara. The Buddhist interpretation of life gives Tibetan medicine a unique viewpoint on health cultivation. At the upper right and upper left the various health cultivation practices are illustrated, and in the center lies the western paradise. The lower part shows the six forms of *samsara*. (*Thangkha* fifty-four on health cultivation in the *Sman thang* series of *The Four Medical Tantras*)

dregs become teeth, finger and toe nails, and body hair, while the refined part becomes marrow that promotes growth. This marrow is again divided into essence and dregs. The dregs become the fat around the anus and hair follicles, and the essence passes through the channels to enter the essence-mansion to become the semen. This is further broken down into essence and dregs, the essence becoming the lustrous spirit, which is the basis of health and longevity, and the dregs become white semen (semen of the male) and red semen (the female menstruate and ovum).

The seven essences

This includes essence from food and drink, blood, muscle, fat, bone, marrow and semen-blood. Essence from food and drink is the root of the other six, and is especially connected to blood, which nurtures the body and maintains life, and is also one of the carriers of *mkhris pa*. The muscles cover the body and are the source material that forms the organs and limbs. Fat provides luster and moisture and maintains the body temperature. The bones form the framework, and support and strengthen the body. The marrow produces the spirit-essence (male semen and female blood) and is important in reproduction and making the life full of energy and the body robust.

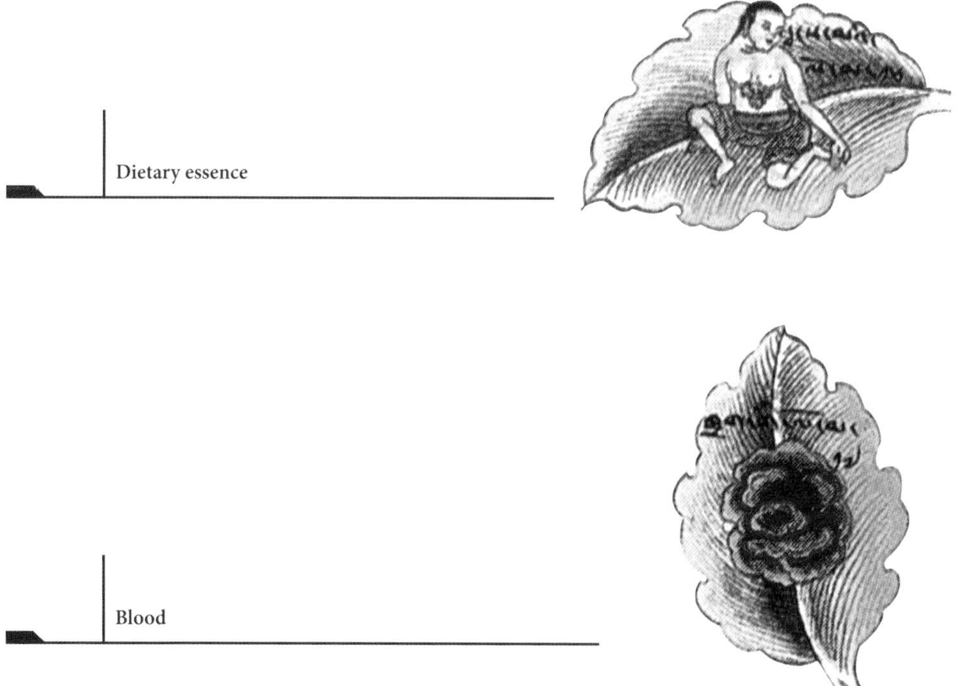

Dietary essence

Blood

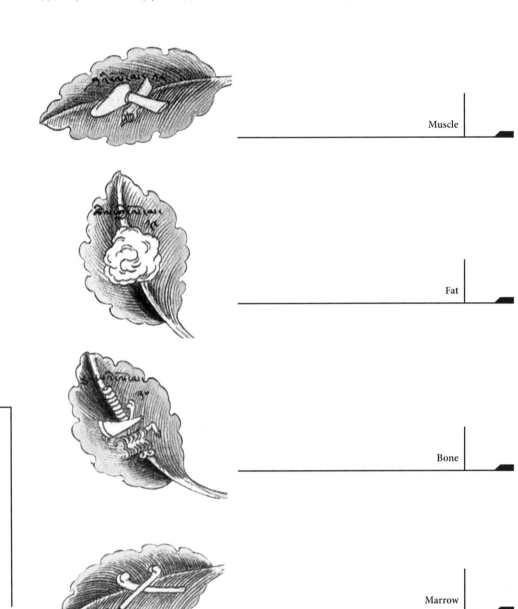

Muscle

Fat

Bone

Marrow

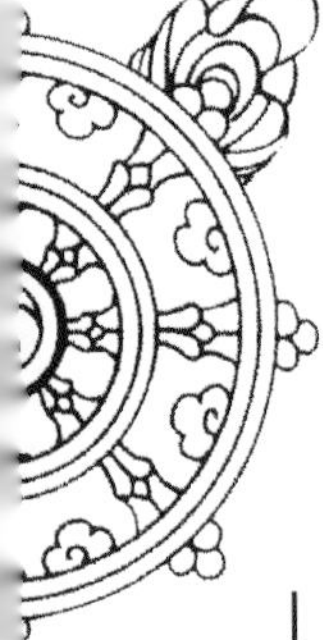

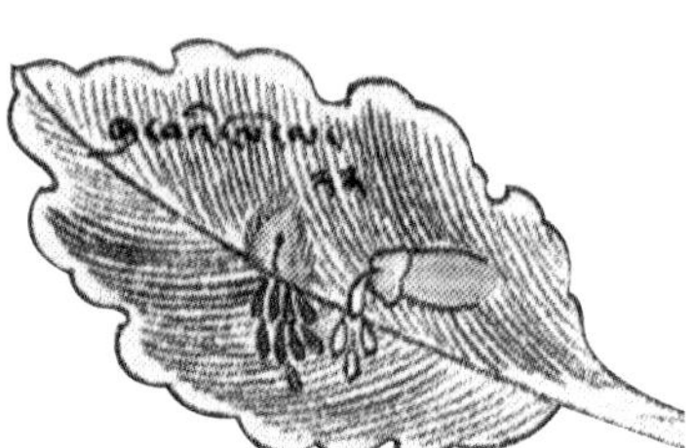

Semen

Three excretions

This refers to the feces, urine, and sweat, and also includes the teeth, finger and toe nails, ear wax, mucus, tears, and hair. Feces are the dregs of food that are left after its nutrients have been absorbed. Urine facilitates the excretion of the dregs from the internal organs. Sweat moistens the skin and also protects the body surface, and is also the way for internal waste to be excreted.

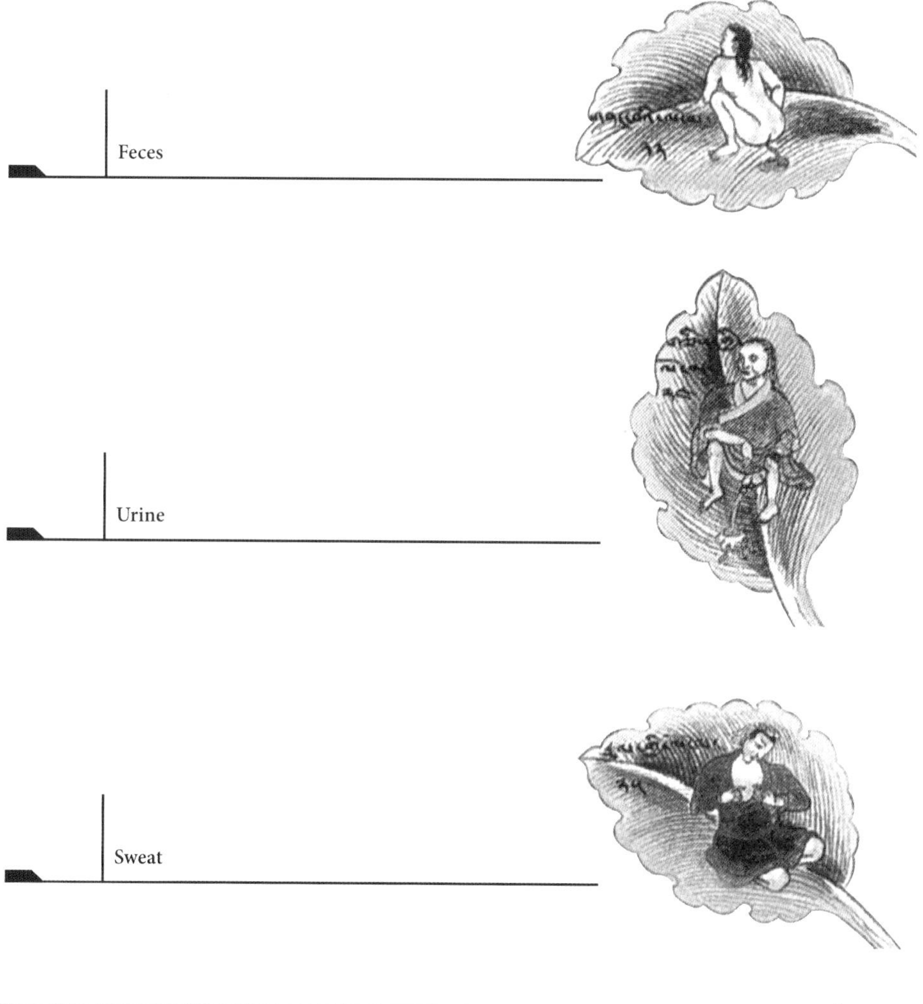

According to Tibetan medicine, after food is digested its essence becomes blood on the first day, becomes muscle on the second day, becomes fat on the third day, becomes bone on the fourth day, becomes marrow on the fifth day, and becomes essence on the sixth day.

Constitutional Types

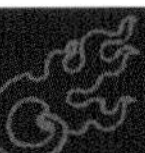

The three factors come from maternal blood and paternal semen. The embryo possesses all three factors even in the womb. Since the quantity and quality of semen-blood is different for everyone and the quantity and quality of *rlung*, *mkhris pa* and *badkan* taken from the outside world by the mother and the baby is also different, the physical constitution will vary with each individual.

Simple types

Based on the quantity of three factors, people are divided into simple and mixed types. There are three subtypes in the simple type, which are summarized in *The Four Medical Tantras* as follows:

Rlung type: *rlung* is predominant, a hunchbacked posture, greenish gray complexion, averse to cold, the joints make a sound when walking, lack of wealth, short life span, shallow sleep, short body height, slender, likes to sing, talk and laugh, good at the bow and arrow, likes sweet, sour, bitter and spicy food, with the temperament of a vulture, crow and fox.

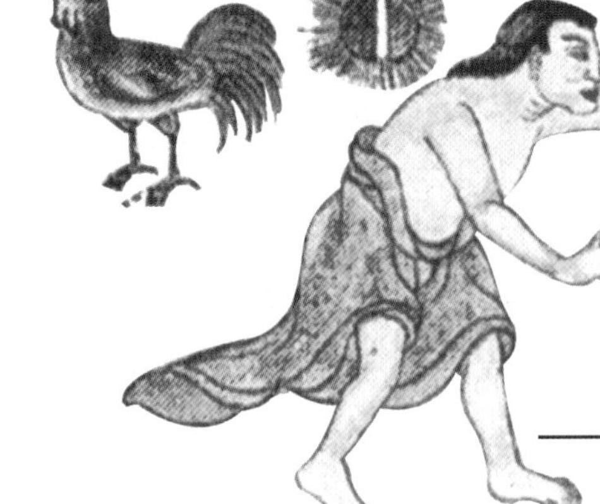

Short and slender, hunchbacked, grayish green complexion, likes to talk.

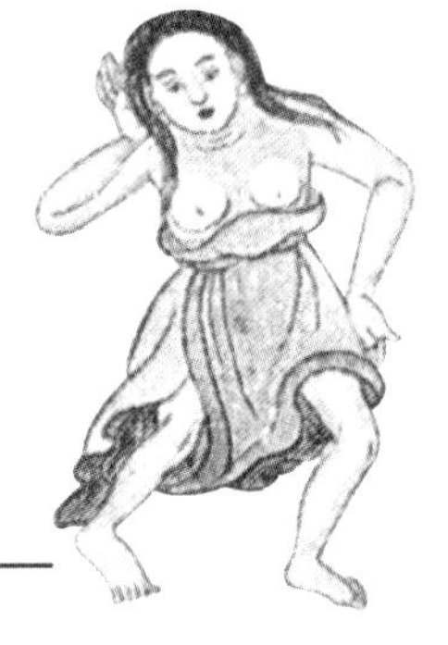
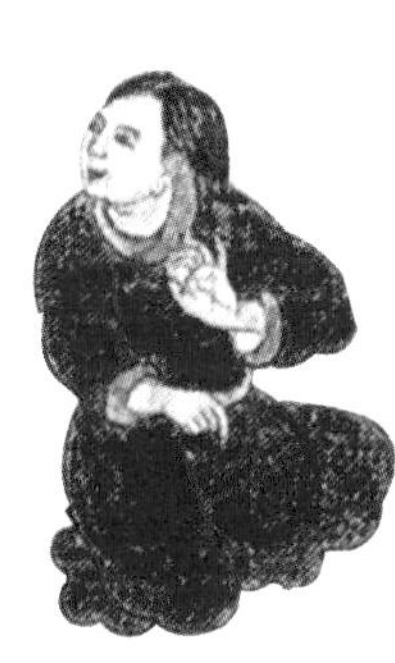
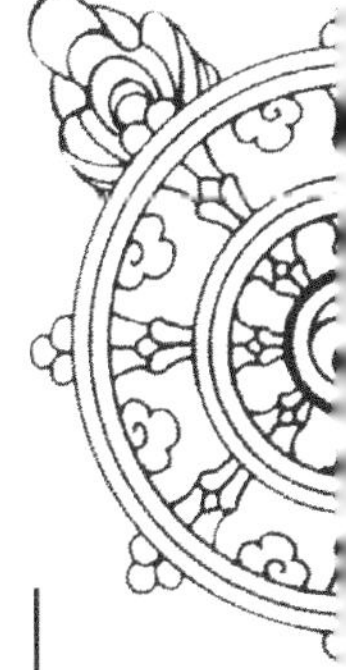

Enjoys singing, dancing, and humor.

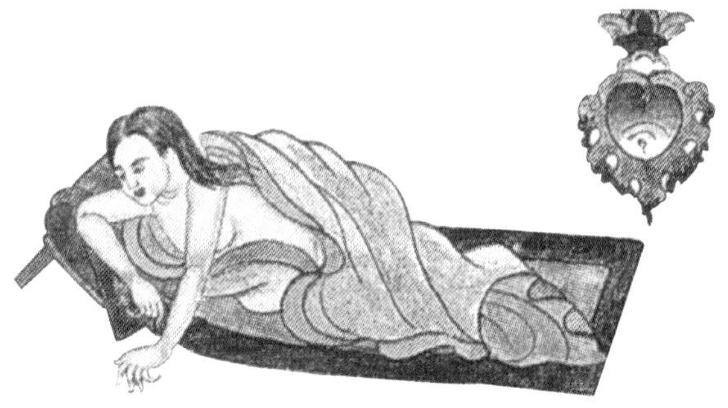

Averse to cold, thirst and hunger, susceptible to insomnia, lack of good fortune, short life span.

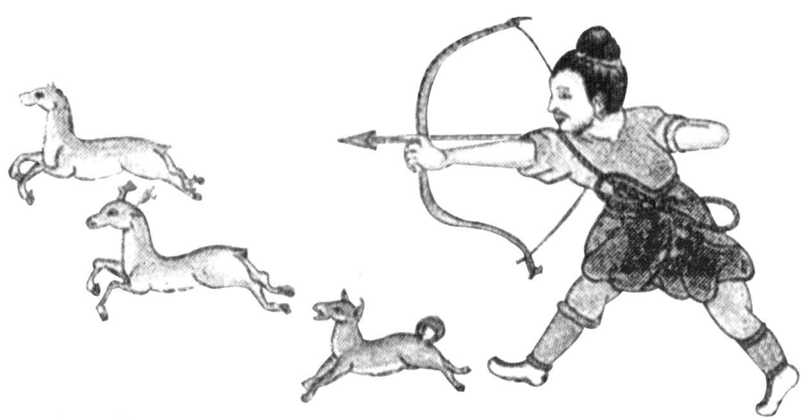

Likes to play and hunt.

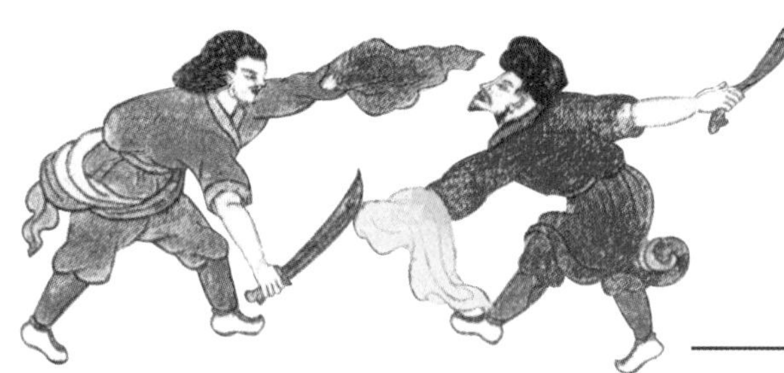

Tends to fight with others.

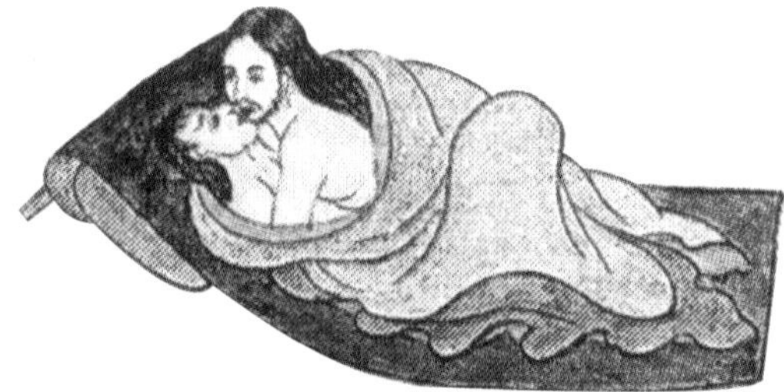

Strong sexual desire.

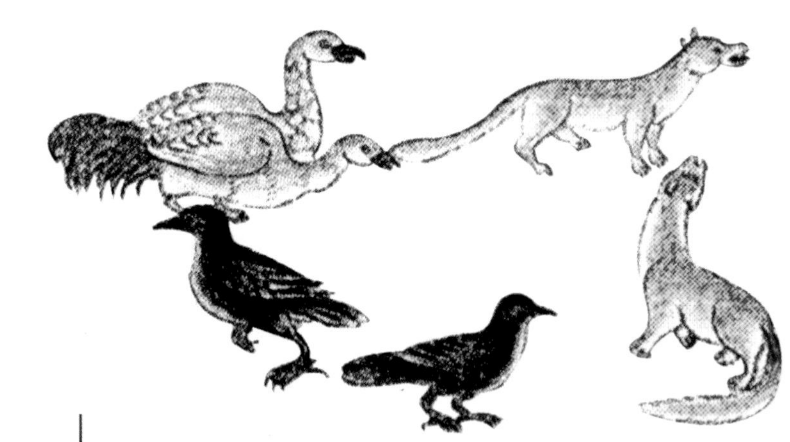

Like the crow with the ugly voice, they tend to hurt others.

Like a fox, they can not be trusted.

Mkhris pa type: *mkhris pa* is predominate, always thirsty and hungry, yellow hair and skin, very clever and arrogant, always sweating, long life, with moderate wealth, fond of sweet, bitter, astringent tastes and cool food, the temperament of a tiger, monkey and yaksha (malevolent spirit).

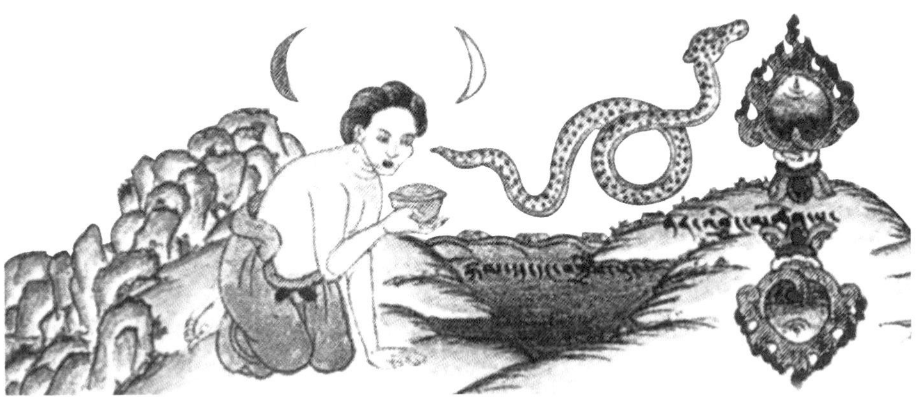

Exuberant inner fire, always hungry and sweating, light red and yellow hair and skin, moderate stature and wealth.

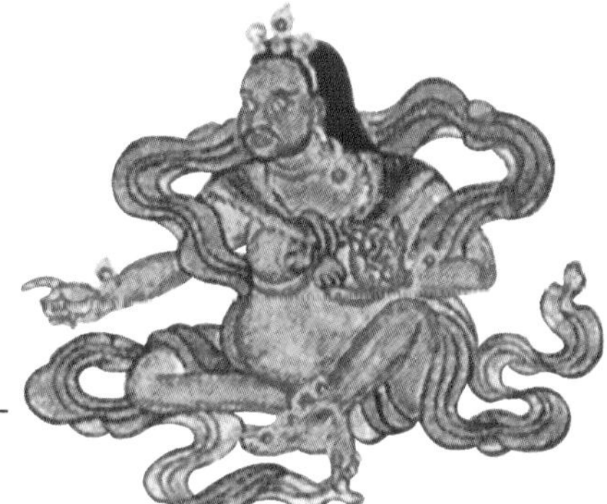

As arrogant as a yaksha, uncontrollable.

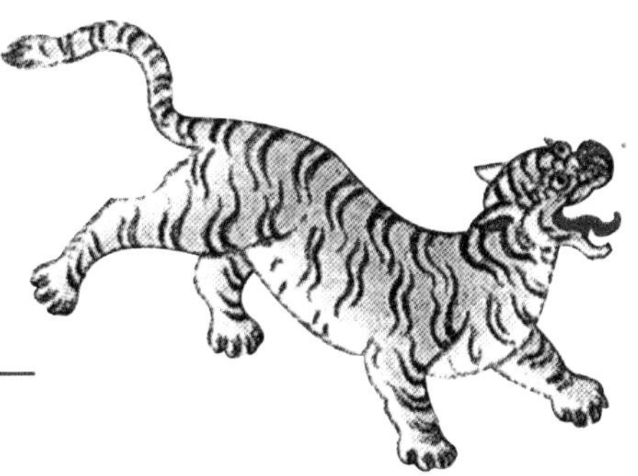

As powerful as a tiger and easily enraged.

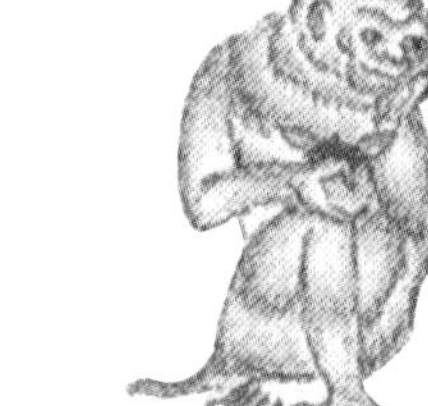

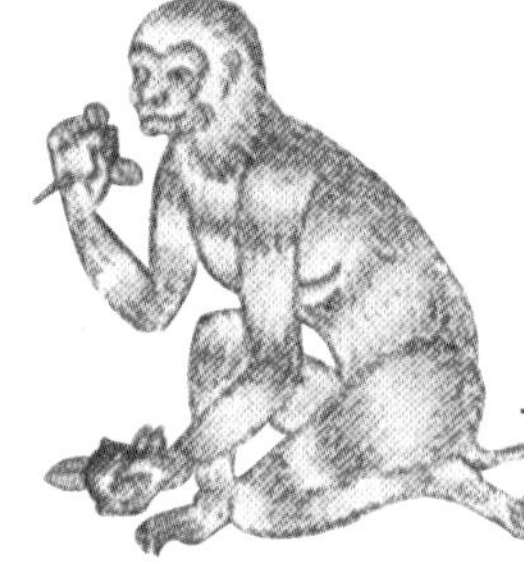

As clever as a monkey with rapid reactions.

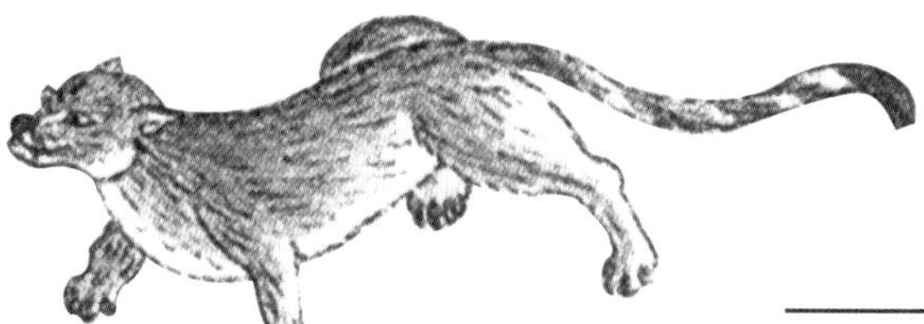

As keen as a cat.

Badkan type: *badkan* is predominant, with a low body temperature, indistinct hip joints, muscles well developed, white skin, straight posture, tolerant to hunger and thirst, resistant to vexation, misery, and drought, rather fat stature, long life, wealthy, strong internally but gentle exterior, always kind hearted, fond of spicy, sour, astringent, and crude food, with the temperament of a lion.

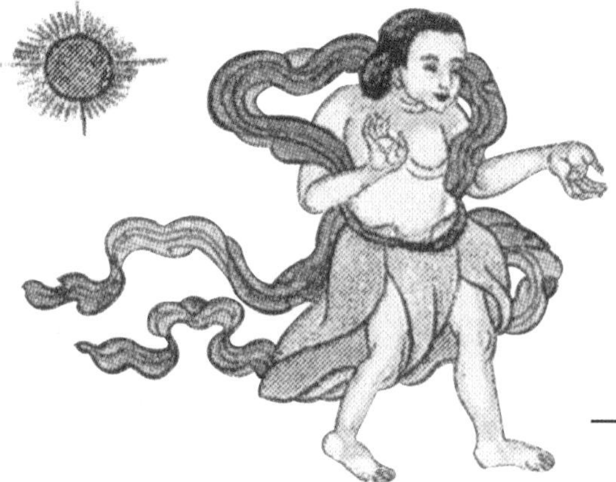

Tall and strong, well developed muscles, white skin, peaceful and gentle.

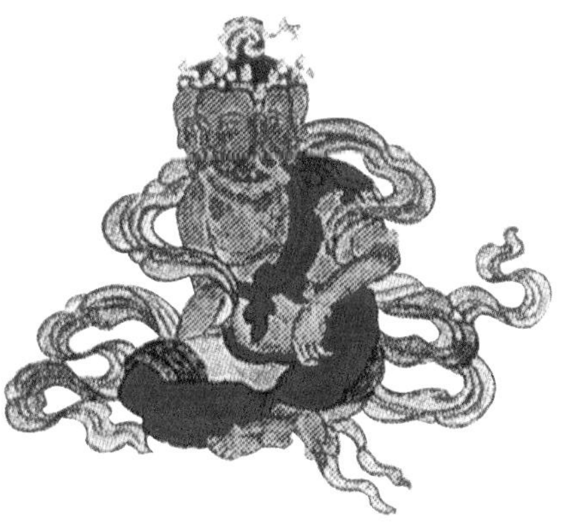

A man of distinguished achievements.

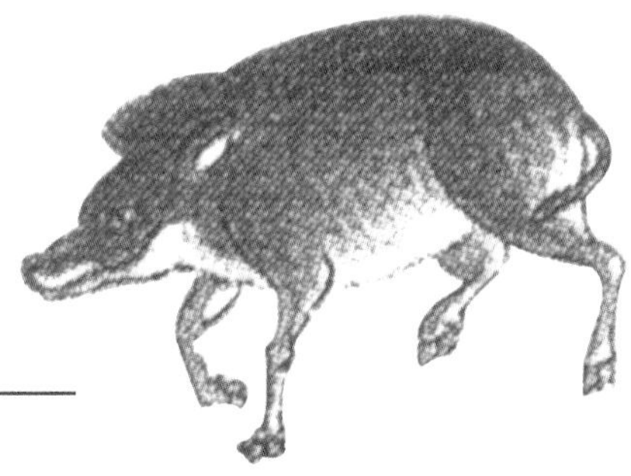

Unlikely to move about.

Tibetan medicine classifies man in to three basic types, *rlung*, *mkhris pa* and *badkan*, based on the quantity and quality of the three factors. There are also mixed types such as *rlung-mkhris pa*, *badkan-mkhris pa*, *rlung-badkan* and a type where all three factors exist. Altogether there are seven types in total.

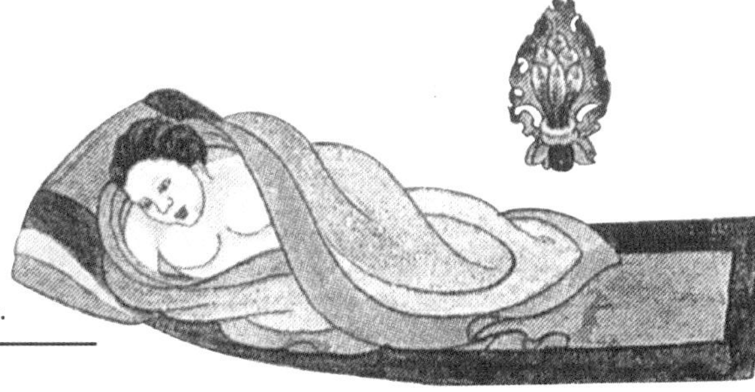

Fond of sleep with a long life.

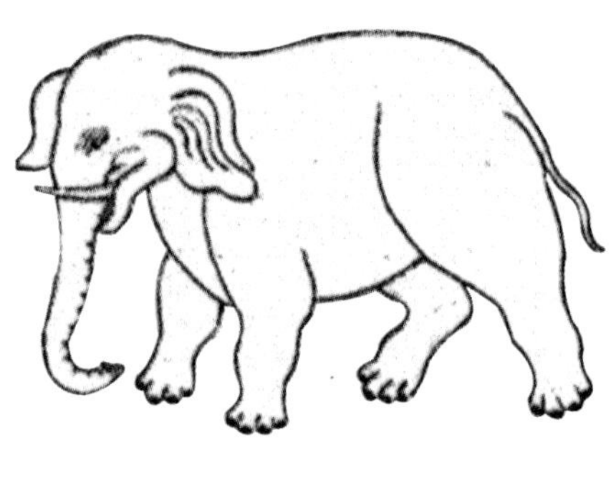

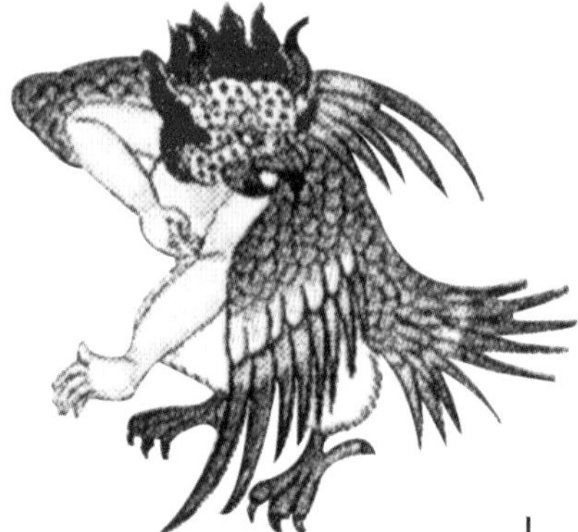

Resistant to drought, hunger, thirst and misery.

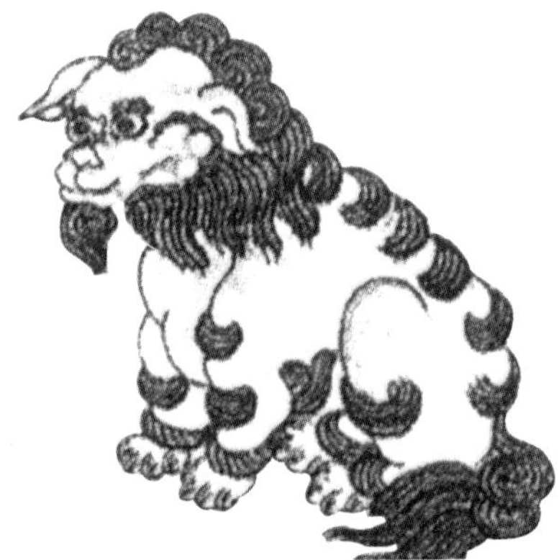

As strong and large as a lion.

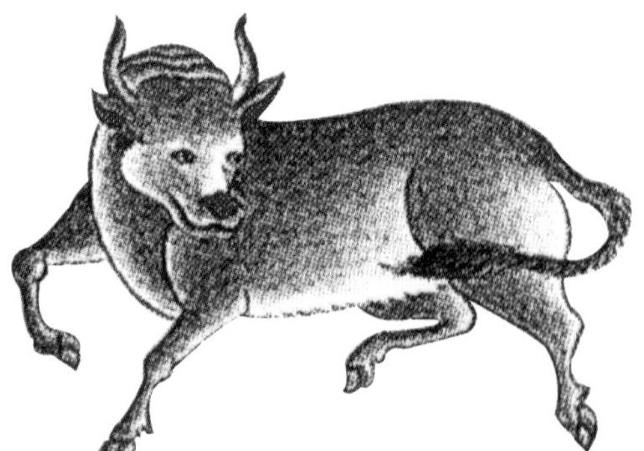

As powerful as an ox.

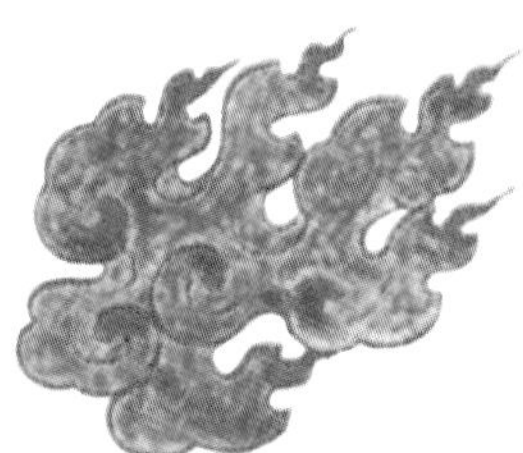

Understanding the truth of disease, mastering the principles of treatment.

In Tibetan medicine all disease occurs as a result of internal factors that are triggered by external causes. Under the influence of both internal and external factors the three factors, seven essences, and three excretions tend towards either predominance or debility. This is the basic mechanism of disease. Thus, the basic principles of treatment should be to prevent the external factors from causing illness and regulating the balance of life internally. In this aspect, Tibetan medicine has accumulated rich experience through long-term practice.

A bird can not separate from its shadow, no matter how far or how high it flies. So it is with humans and disease, they stick to people like shadows. For this reason Tibetan medicine stresses health cultivation. One must be able to recognize the diseases and problems that one's own unique constitution is susceptible to. With this understanding one can master methods that both prevent and treat such illnesses.

General Pathology

Under normal circumstances, the three factors, seven essences, the internal organs, the human body and its environment are all in a harmonious state. Diseases only occur when such harmony is broken. The causes of diseases include internal and external factors.

Internal causes

Tibetan medicine claims that the root cause of disease is the misunderstanding on the nature of *anattā* (the doctrine of non-self), which leads to craving, ill-will, ignorance and eventually to disharmony of the three factors and to disease. This is the internal cause of disease.

Legends involving disharmonies of the three factors

***Rlung* Legend**

It is said that a god named Dorji Pawa was responsible for qi (air). One day, he went to have a bath in the sea. While bathing, his eyes fell upon the beautiful goddess Norbu Drenpa. He approached her and courted her and soon fell in love with her. As they were playing by the sea he laid his bag full of qi aside. While he was frolicking about, some of the qi leaked out. Like the opening of Pandora's Box, *rlung* diseases spread throughout the world and have plagued humanity ever since.

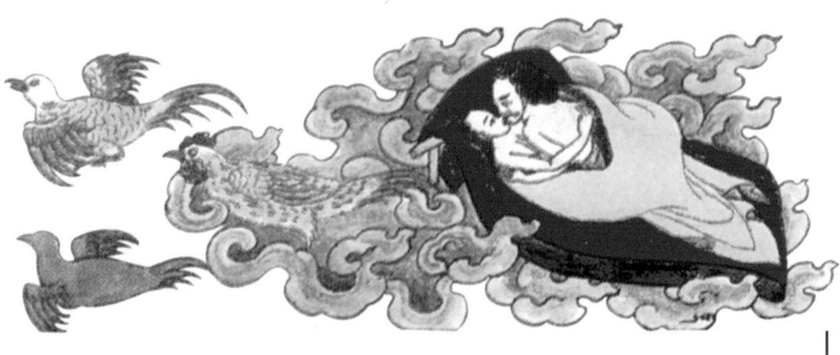

As greedy as a bird.

Mkhris pa Legend

It is said that Brahma invited Mahabharata to join an offertory ritual. Before the faces of all the assembled gods, Mahabharata was given the last seat. He was enraged and smashed all the ritual instruments. While he was smashing the alter, his third eye in the middle of his forehead became filled with enraged fire. Unable to contain it, Mahabharata sent it out into the world where to this day it is manifested as *mkhris pa* diseases.

Badkan Legend

Once upon a time, King Gyalbal Mintsan's queen Ramara had an affair with a minister. When the king found out, he was very angry and sentenced them to be thrown into the water to drown. The queen and the minister prayed and cursed frantically. From the strength of their prayers and curses the king fell ill with a *badkan* disease. The king was again furious and threw dirt at them. One tiny particle of this dirt was picked up and swallowed by a vulture. This tainted bird was later killed and eaten by man. Through the bird and then the man *badkan* diseases were spread throughout the land.

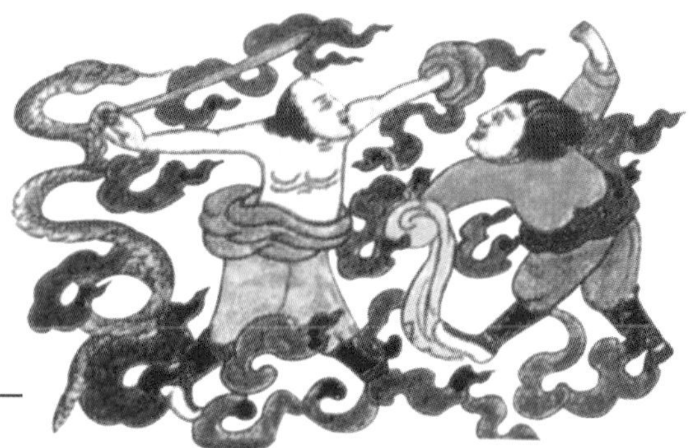

As angry as a snake.

Deciphering the legends

It can be seen from the above that craving, ill-will and ignorance are the sources of the three groups of diseases. Tibetan medicine goes further to explain that, "Craving is like the birds flying freely, ill-will is like the winding snake, and ignorance like an idle pig, knowing only eating, and unwilling to move." These three impurities then give rise to *rlung*, *mkhris pa*, and *badkan* diseases respectively. Under the influence of various external factors, functional disturbances increase or decrease, the original harmony is broken, and eventually health is jeopardized.

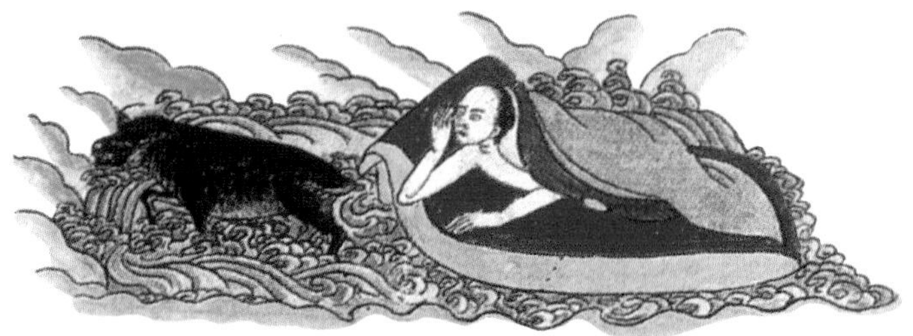

As ignorant as a pig.

External factors

This is an extensive category and includes seasons, weather, daily habits, diet, behavior, emotions and wounds. All of these can cause disturbances of the three factors.

External factors for *rlung* diseases include overeating of bitter, astringent (except chebule), light, rough, stable, active, and cold food or medicinals, over indulging in sex, going hungry or thirsty for a long time, eating too little, severe insomnia, overstrain, massive bleeding, and extreme emotional states.

External factors for *mkhris pa* diseases include overeating spicy foods, concentrated liquor, and foods of pungent, sharp, light, or foul nature, sudden overstrain, difficult labor, wounds, and over nutrition.

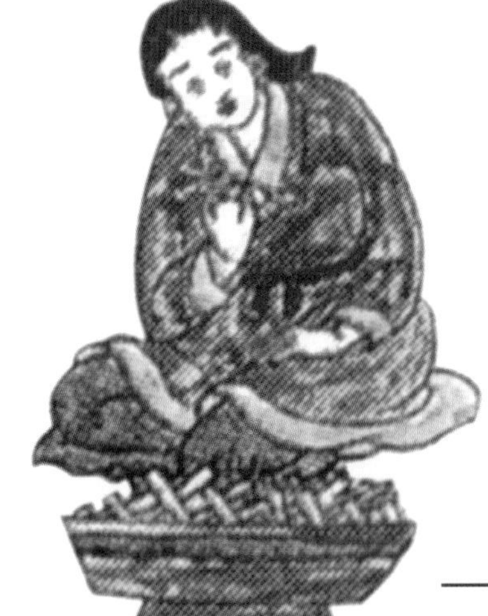

Diet

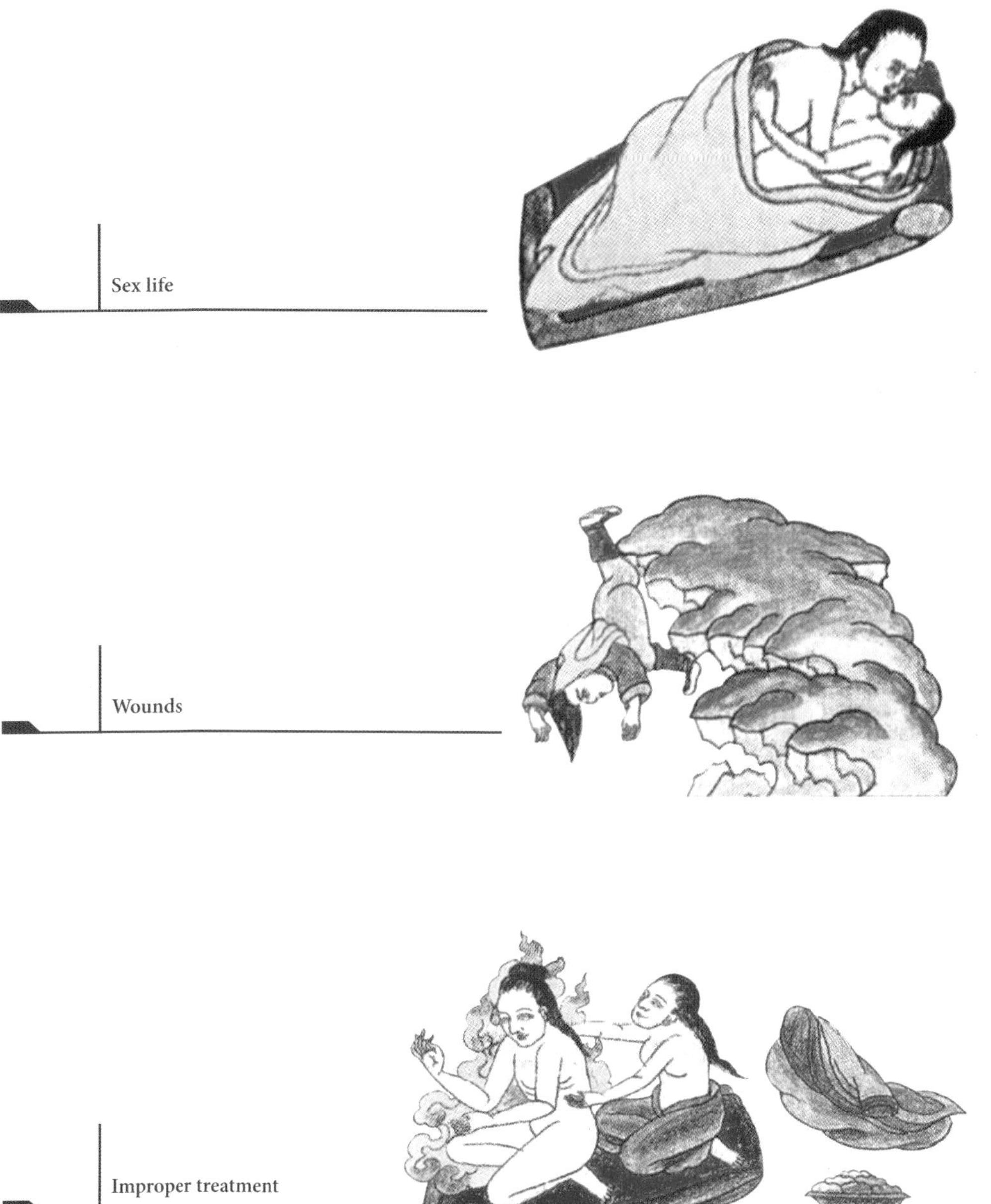

The external factors of *badkan* diseases include overeating food with bitter, sweet, heavy, cool, greasy, or stable nature, a lack of physical activity after meals, too much sleep, staying in a damp place and being invaded by cold pathogens.

External factors may combine to complicate the diseases mentioned above.

In summary, external factors may trigger an imbalance of the three factors. When this harmony is broken diseases occur. *Mkhris pa* leads to heat disease, and *badkan* to cold disease, and *rlung* diseases are light and mobile. Cold or hot diseases are also triggered by *rlung*.

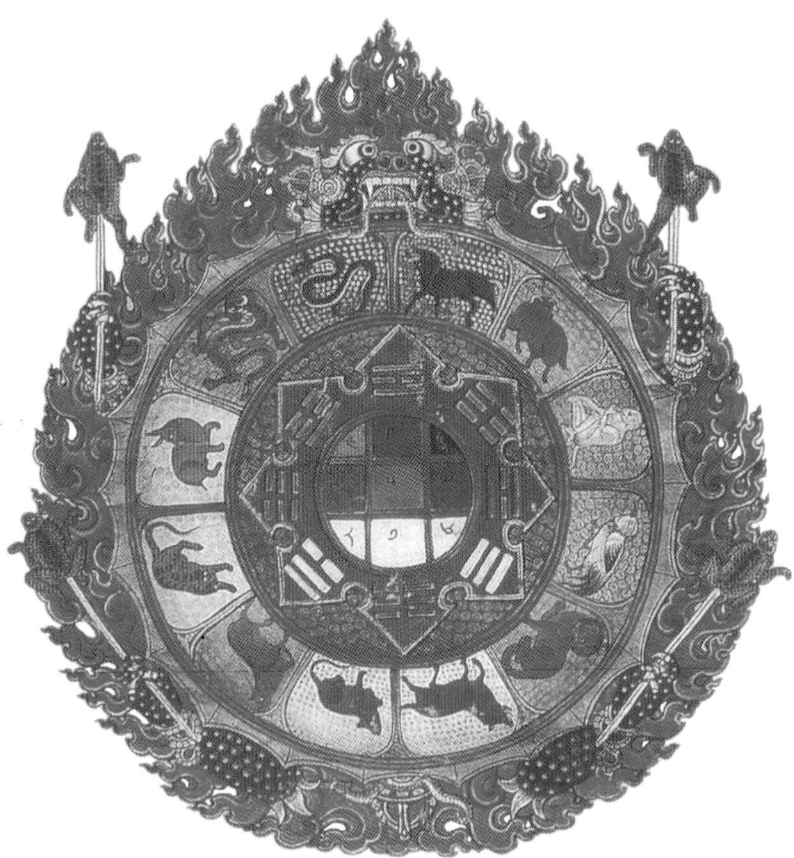

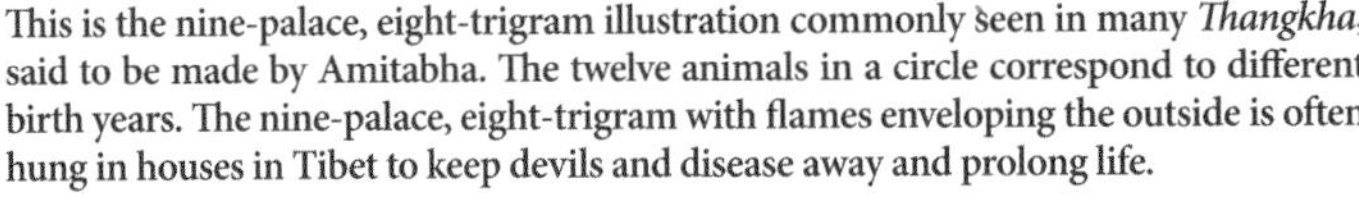

This is the nine-palace, eight-trigram illustration commonly seen in many *Thangkha*, said to be made by Amitabha. The twelve animals in a circle correspond to different birth years. The nine-palace, eight-trigram with flames enveloping the outside is often hung in houses in Tibet to keep devils and disease away and prolong life.

Beginning of Illness

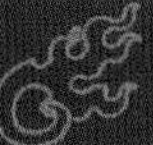

Tibetan medicine holds that, under normal conditions, the three factors, seven essences, and three excretions remain in a constant quantity. Under the influence of external and internal factors, the three factors might increase or decrease and both can result in disease. Predominance or debility of any of the three factors can disturb other factors. In short, increase, decrease, and disturbance are the basic mechanisms of disease.

The increase, decrease, and disturbance of the three factors

How increase and decrease take place

When the three factors are being produced, if one takes food one likes and does what one likes, *rlung*, *mkhris pa*, or *badkan* may increase. Likewise, when the three factors are being consumed, they might continue to be consumed when taking or doing what one likes. In other words, the increase or decrease is the outcome of one's desires.

Rlung diseases, for instance, in their early stages are marked by loss of desire to eat sweet food, and craving for bitter food, like taking large amounts of dandelion and tea. If the patient thinks that relaxed activities will not be helpful to his/her illness, and instead engages in light and rough activities, then *rlung* disease will increase.

When *rlung* is consumed, if the patient thinks that light, rough foods and activities are not helpful to his/her disease, tries to avoid them, and instead turns to heavy, greasy food and heavy activities which he/she thinks will be helpful to his/her disease *mkhris pa* will begin to be consumed. This is one way that *rlung* disease affects *mkhris pa* and *badkan*.

Manifestations of increase

Exuberance of *rlung*

Manifestations include emaciation, blackish skin, always staying in warm places, a trembling body, distension of the abdomen and gurgling sounds, constipation, dizziness, muttering, weakness, little sleep, decreased function of the sense organs.

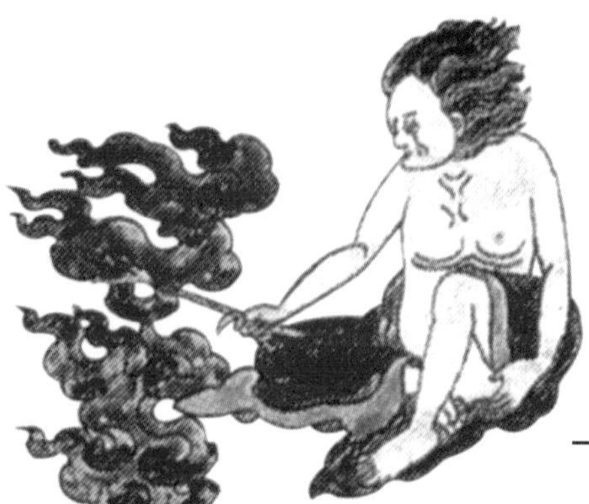

Exuberance of *rlung*

Exuberance of *mkhris pa*

Yellow urine and feces, yellow skin and cornea, always hungry and thirsty, high body temperature, poor and short sleep, diarrhea.

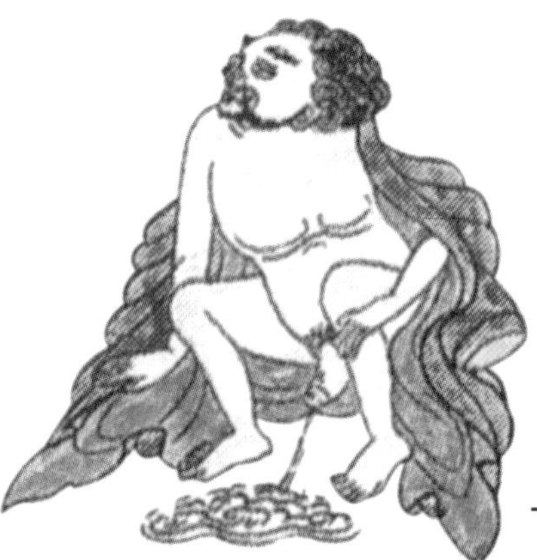

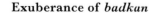

Exuberance of *mkhris pa*

Exuberance of *badkan*

Low body temperature, heavy body, difficult movements, greenish white urine and pallid facial complexion, indigestion, idle and averse to move, lots of sleep, weakness of the extremities, profuse sputum and saliva, difficult breathing.

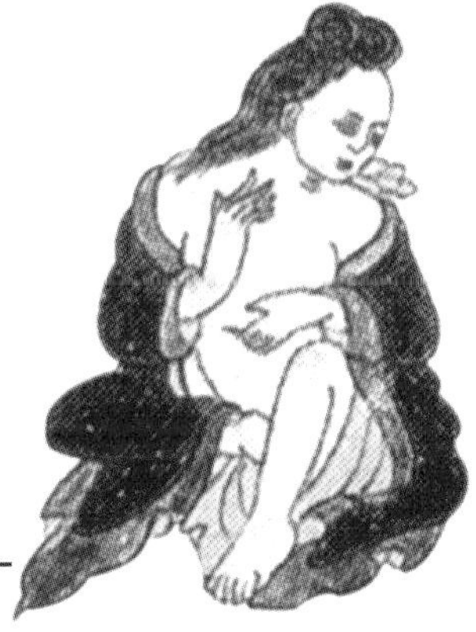

Exuberance of *badkan*

Manifestations of decrease

Decrease of *rlung*

Spiritless, reluctant to talk, weakness, decreased memory, may have manifestations of exuberant *badkan* such as low body temperature and indigestion.

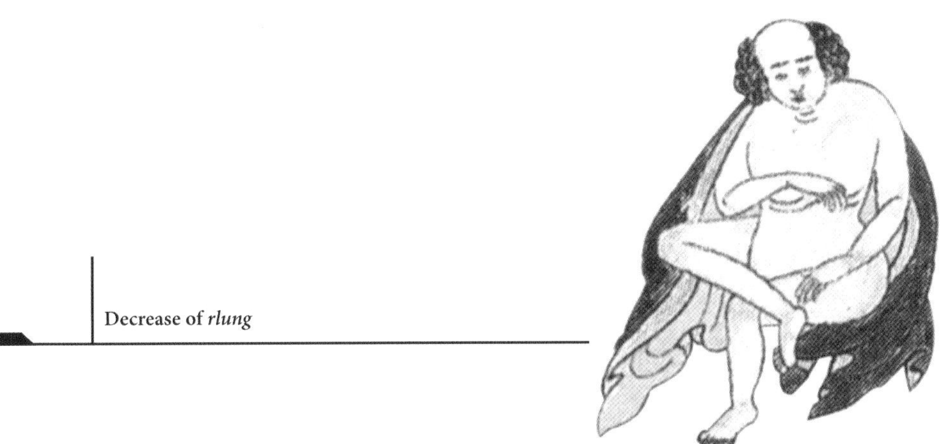

Decrease of *rlung*

Decrease of *mkhris pa*

The opposite of an exuberance of *mkhris pa*. Manifestations include low body temperature, cool skin and muscles, and blackish skin without luster.

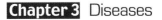

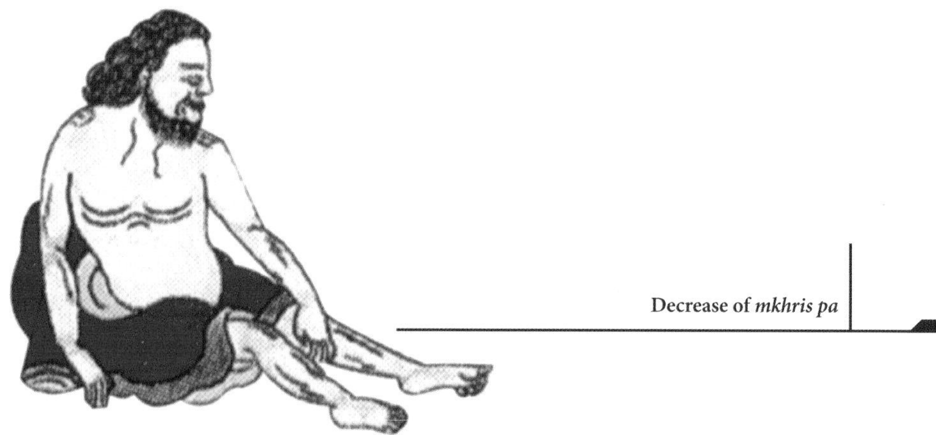

Decrease of *mkhris pa*

Decrease of *badkan*

Dizziness, heart palpations, soft joints. These symptoms are due to the brain being affected by a shortage of nutrition where *badkan* is located.

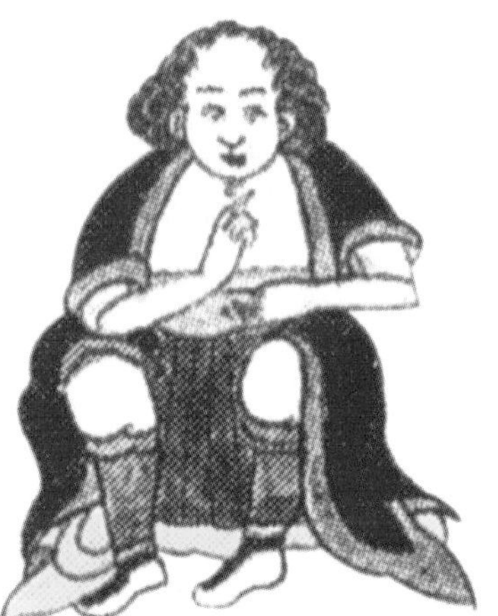

Decrease of *badkan*

The increase, decrease and disturbance of the three factors, seven essences, and three excretions are the internal basis of all diseases.

Disturbance

Disturbance of *rlung*

Manifestations include greenish and clear urine like water in a pool in the grasslands in summer. When cooled, the urine is still clear. The patient feels exhausted, is short of breath upon mild activity, absent minded, doesn't know what to do, feels dizzy, has headaches, faints, suffers from tinnitus, a dry red mouth, rough tongue surface, astringent sensations in the mouth, migrating body pain, feeling cold, body pain upon movement, joints that are difficult to flex and extend like they are bound, stiff limbs, feelings like skin is being separated from flesh, cracking pain in the bones, protruding eyes, itchy hair, unable to sleep but always yawning, irritable, always suspicious of others, pain in the waist like being beaten, pricking pain in the neck, cheeks and chest, severe pain when the vertex is pressed, nausea with the expulsion of foamy sputum in the morning, and a gurgling sound in the abdomen, especially after breakfast and dinner.

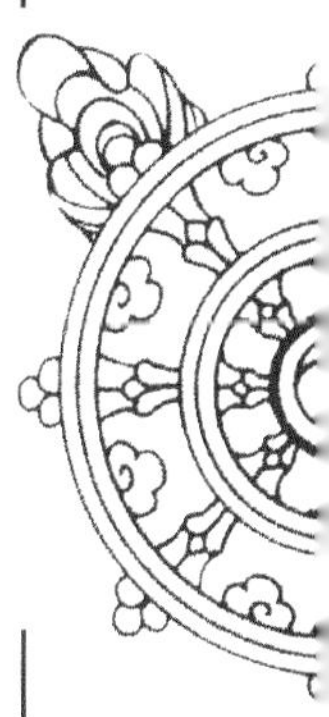

Disturbance of *mkhris pa*

Manifestations include a very tense, rapid, minute and fine pulse, or a rapid, rushing and large pulse, yellow or light-red urine, with a strong unpleasant smell. Since *mkhris pa* refers to the fire and flares upward, it can cause headache, burning pain in the flesh, sour and bitter tastes in the mouth, a thick grayish yellow tongue fur, dry nostrils, red-yellow cornea, fixed pain, poor sleep even in the daytime, craving to drink water, vomiting blood or bile, general sweating with a bad smell, red-yellow face and skin, and masses that rupture and diffuse to other parts of the body. All symptoms are worse after lunch or after eating in the middle of the night.

Disturbance of *badkan*

Manifestations include a pulse that can only be felt by forceful pressing, a feeble pulse, white urine with no odor, poor sense of smell, grey tongue fur and gums, whitish eyes, swollen face, profuse sputum and mucus, dizziness, exhausted and unwilling to move, no appetite, indigestion with undigested foods or mucus in the vomit or feces, lower back pain, general edema, swollen masses in the neck, poor memory, drowsy, aching pain in the legs, itching skin, stiff limbs with joints that feel like they are sticking together, a fat body, and slow movements. All manifestations are worse on overcast days and occur after the evening or morning meal. Since *badkan* is heavy and stable, its diseases are lingering and difficult to cure.

Increase and decrease of the seven essences

How increase and decrease take place

The internal factor involved in these changes is the digestive *mkhris pa*, which not only maintains normal body temperature but also deals with the food in the stomach that is between digested and not digested. It works with the fire accompanying *rlung* and transformation *badkan* to break down food. It distributes the nutrients in food and provides a warm environment for the seven essences to grow and transform.

Suppose the function of digestive *mkhris pa* fluctuates, this would result in the increase or decrease of the seven essences. When the absorption and digestion power of the stomach fire increases or decreases, the food in the stomach can't be digested, the body can't get enough nutrition, and the seven essences can't be nurtured. Conversely, when digestion is exaggerated the nutrients will be "overcooked" and essence will be consumed, leading to various diseases.

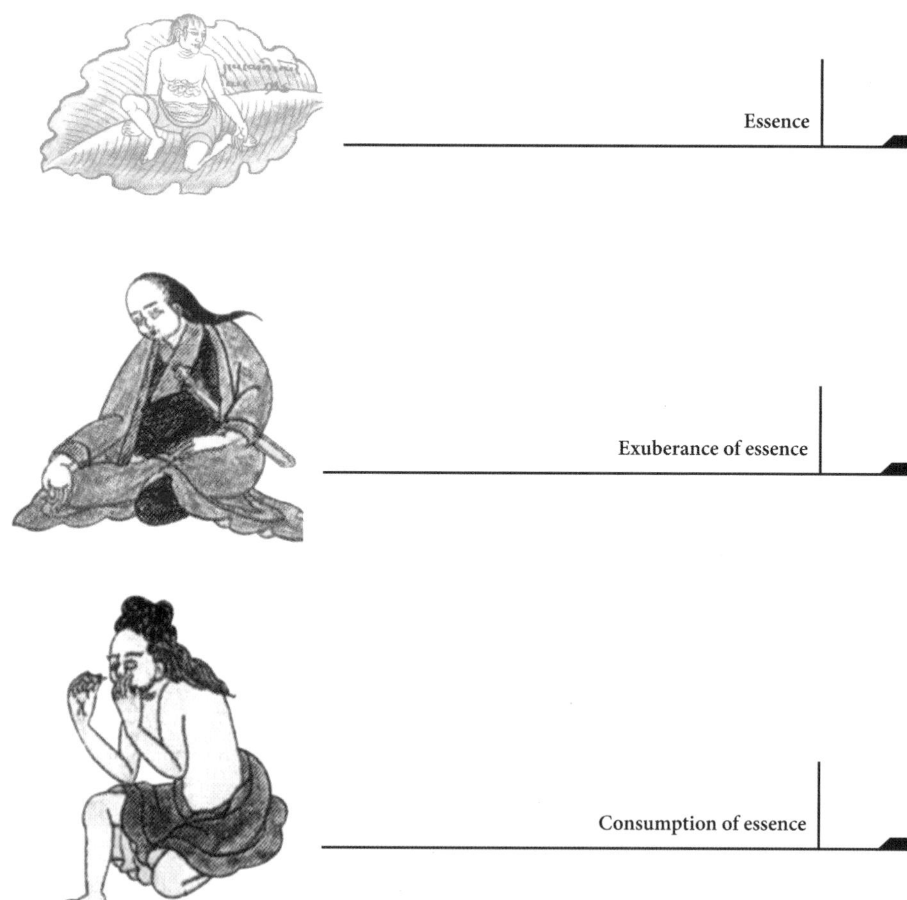

Manifestations of increase and decrease

Exuberance of essence yields symptoms similar to that of *badkan*, manifesting as a weakening of stomach function and a low body temperature. Symptoms of its consumption include emaciation, difficultly swallowing food, rough and hardened skin, averse to noise, and an increased likelihood to contract *rlung* diseases.

Exuberance of blood manifests red spots on the face, masses in the body cavity leading to pain in the organs, congestion and swelling of the spleen, leprosy, blood tumors, diseases due to congestion of the liver and gallbladder, yellow eyes, gingivitis, difficult movements, and red urine and skin. Blood consumption symptoms include an empty relaxed pulse like pressing on a green onion, rough skin, a preference for cold or cool places, and a fondness of sour foods.

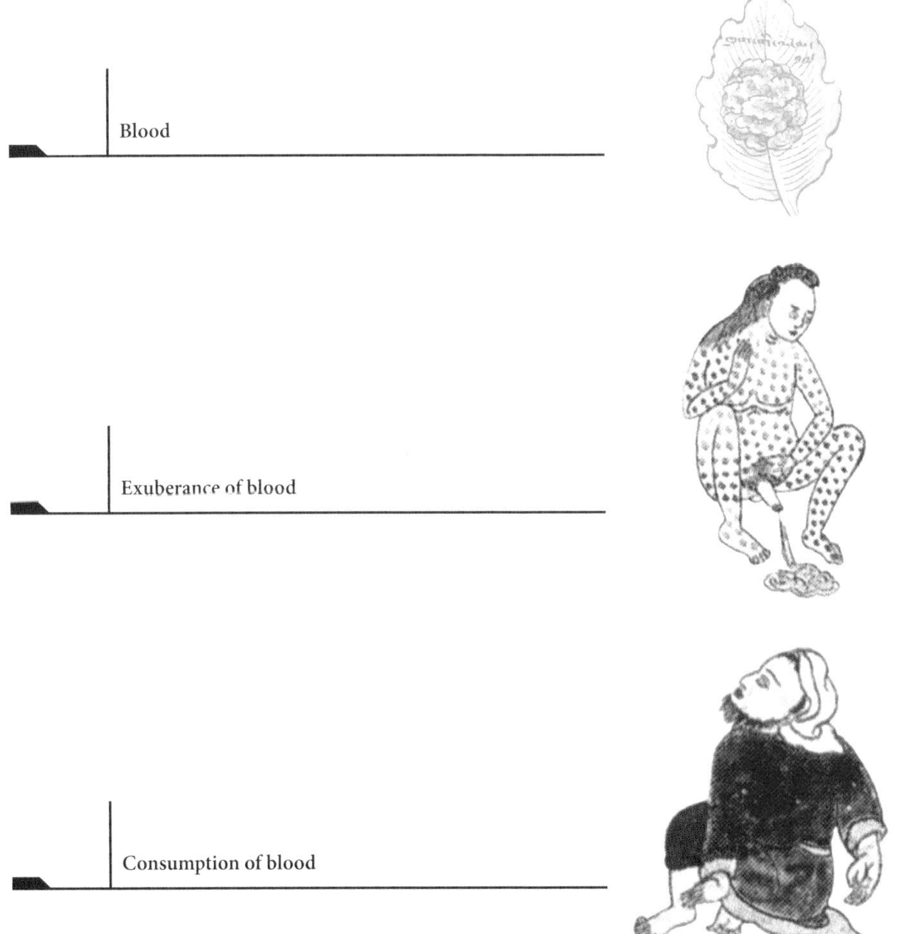

Exuberance of the muscles is evident in swelling of the lymph nodes and obesity, while consumption reveals pains in the joints and emaciation.

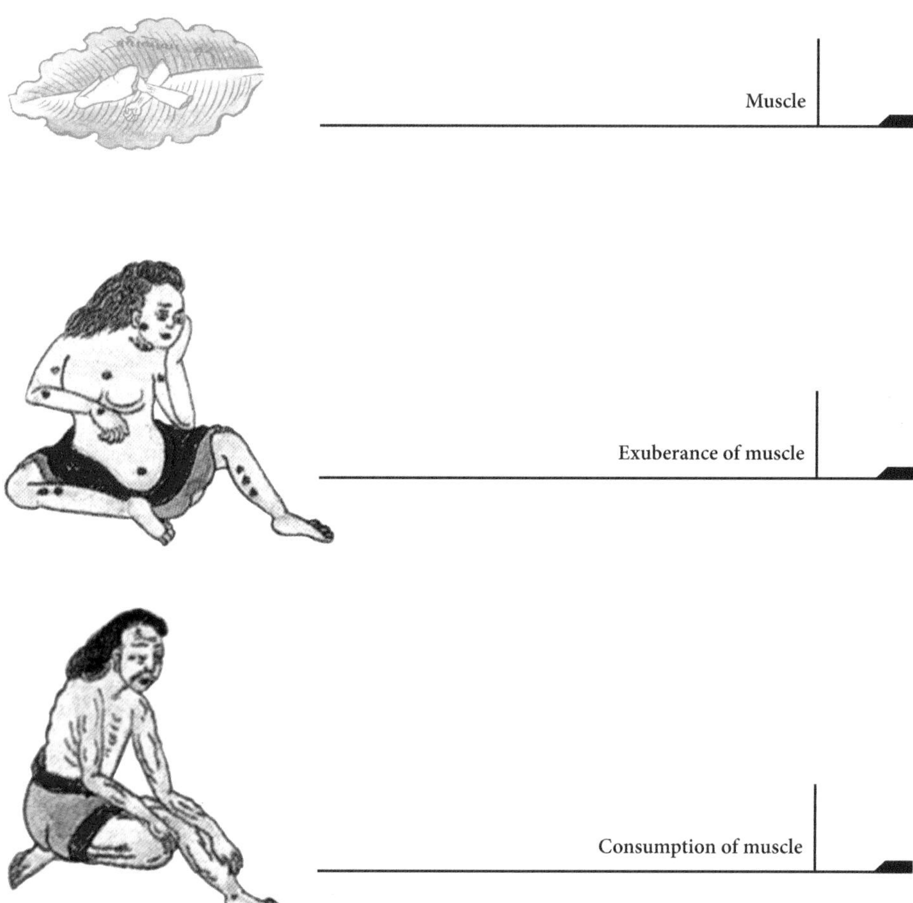

Those with exuberance of fat have fatigue, weakness, an inability to move vigorously, and fat accumulated in the chest and abdomen. In cases of consumption the patient will have poor sleep, emaciation, and grayish skin.

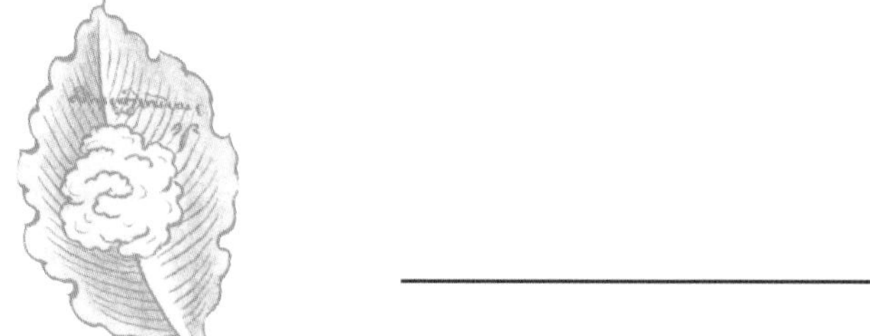

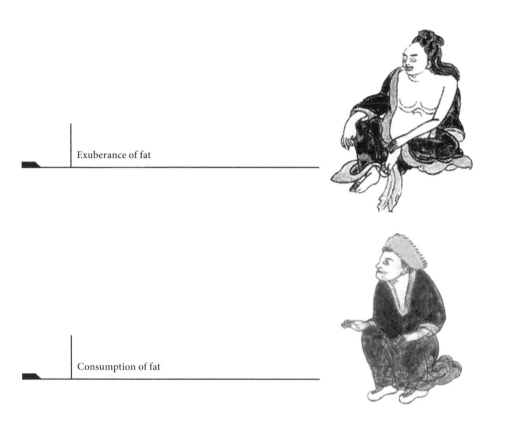

Exuberance of fat

Consumption of fat

Exuberance of bone is evident in bone spurs, excess growth of the teeth, while consumption will cause the teeth, hair, and nails to fall off.

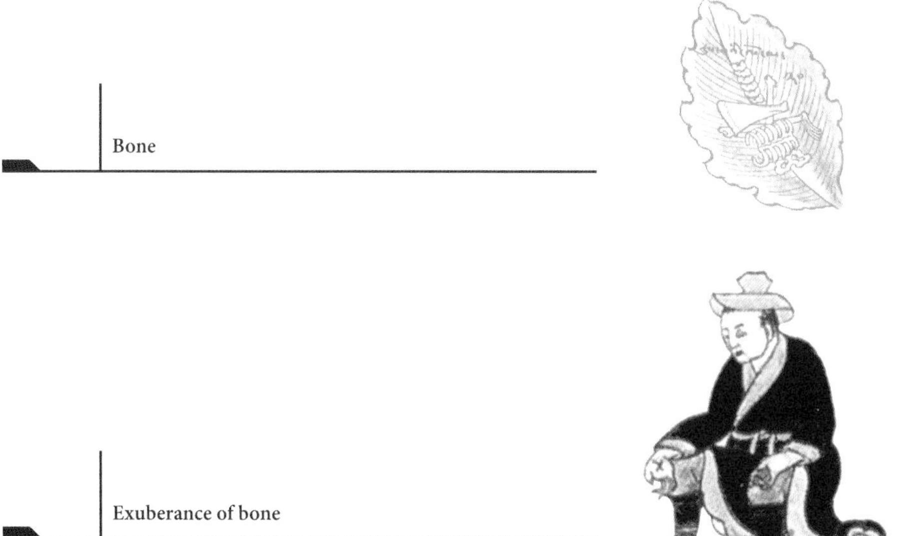

Bone

Exuberance of bone

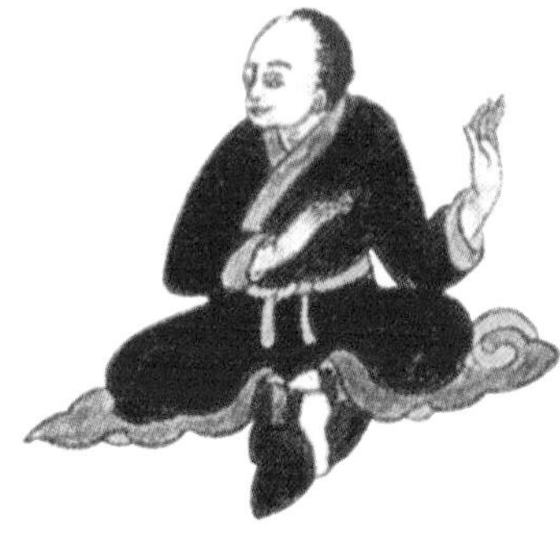

Consumption of bone

An exuberance of marrow is evident in a heavy body, difficult movements, loss of luster in the eyes, impaired vision, and swelling of the joints, while consumption reveals empty bones, headaches and dizziness.

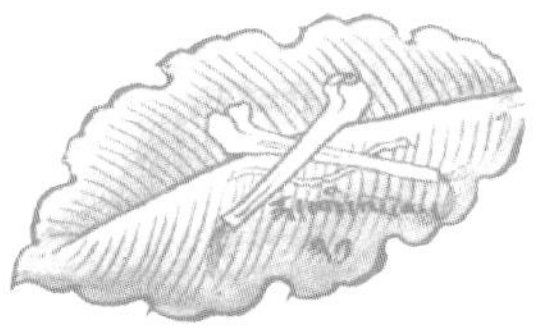

Marrow

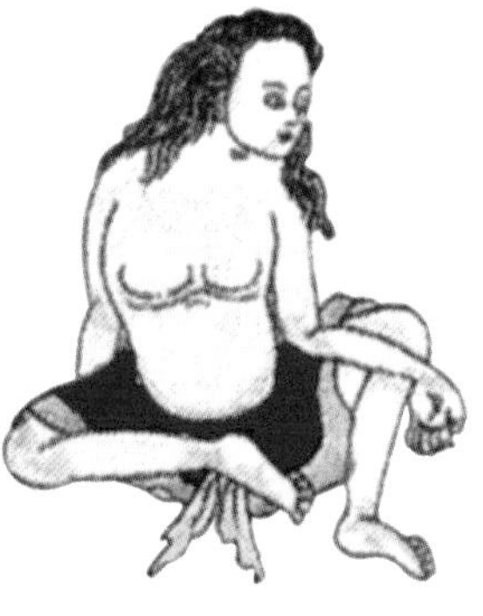

Exuberance of marrow

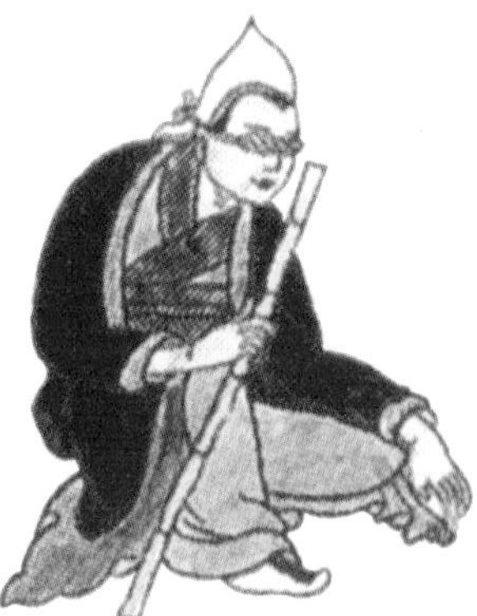

Consumption of marrow

An exuberance of semen reveals kidney stones and a strong sexual desire, while its consumption reveals genital bleeding, decreased sensation at orgasm, and a hot scrotum.

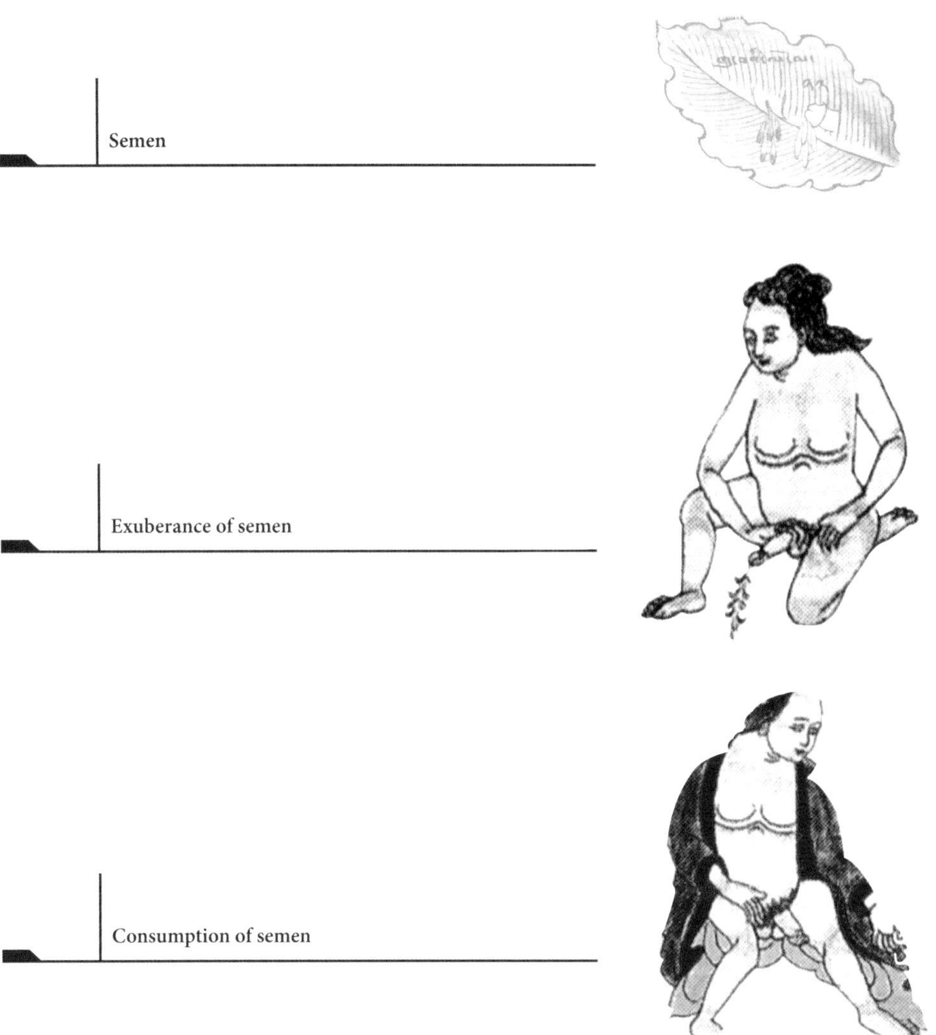

Exuberance and consumption of the three excretions

How exuberance and consumption take place

When the three factors and the seven essences become exuberant or are consumed, the three excretions will be affected, blocked, and instead of being excreted normally they may accumulate inside the body, or may even be excreted in surplus. Any of these imbalances can lead to illness.

Manifestations

Exuberance of feces manifests as a heavy and swollen body, lower abdominal pain with gurgling noises, and difficult movements. When consumption occurs it will manifest as a gurgling sound in the small intestine, farting, and occasional pain in the chest and rib-side.

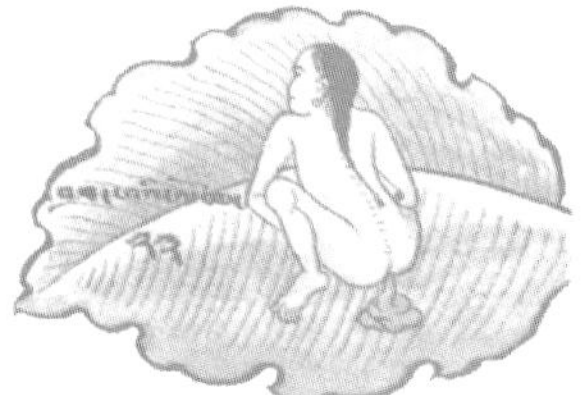

Feces

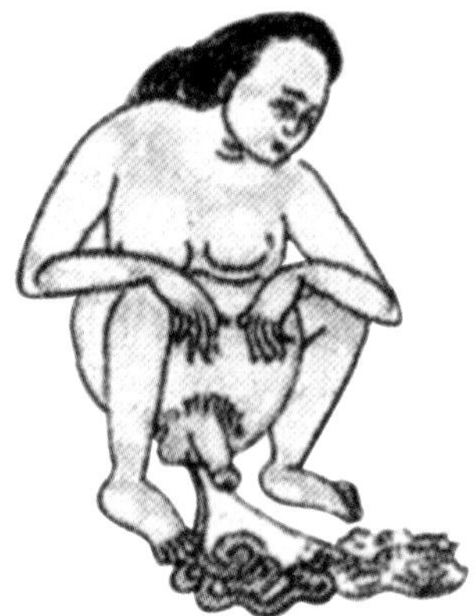

Exuberance of feces

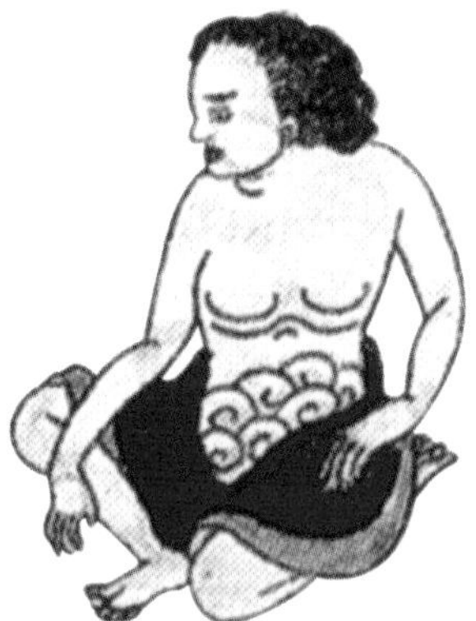

Consumption of feces

Exuberance of urine is evident when a person feels pricking pain in the urinary orifice, urgent and frequent urination, while consumption of urine reveals reddish yellow urine in a diminished quantity, and difficult urination.

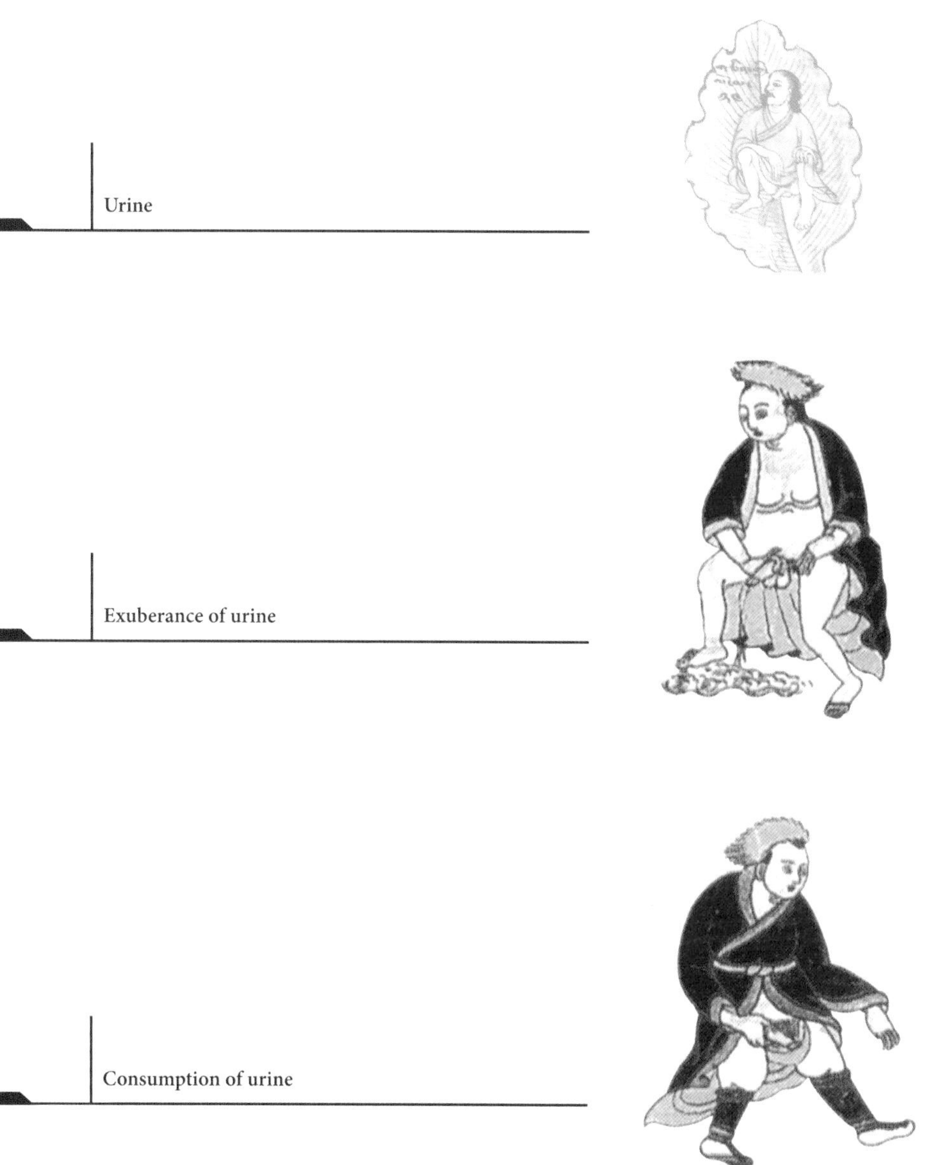
Urine

Exuberance of urine

Consumption of urine

Those with an exuberance will have profuse sweating with a strong odor and be vulnerable to skin diseases, while a consumption of sweat will result in dry skin, erect skin hairs, or possibly a loss of body hair.

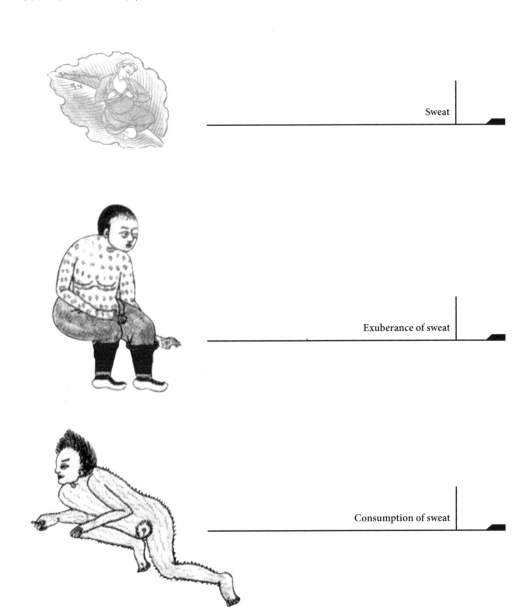

Sweat

Exuberance of sweat

Consumption of sweat

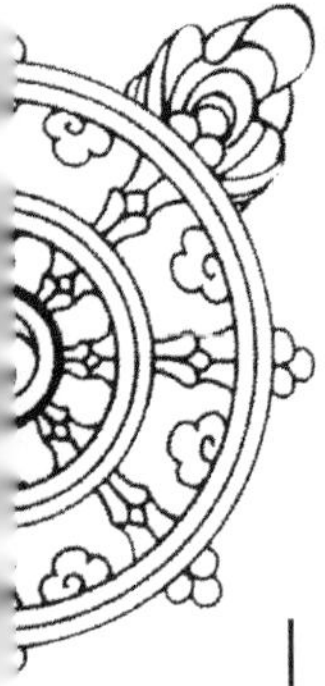

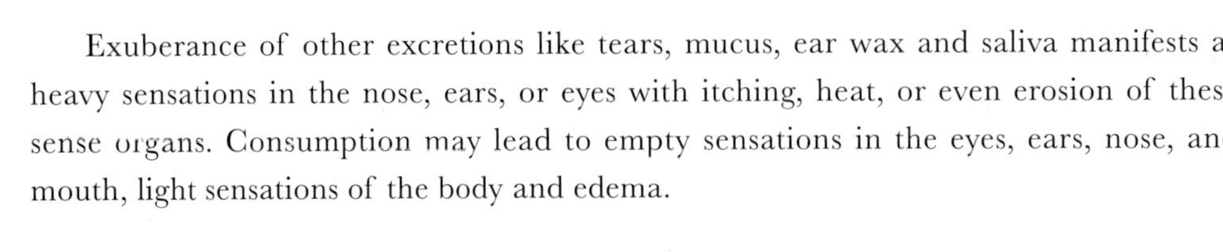

Exuberance of other excretions like tears, mucus, ear wax and saliva manifests as heavy sensations in the nose, ears, or eyes with itching, heat, or even erosion of these sense organs. Consumption may lead to empty sensations in the eyes, ears, nose, and mouth, light sensations of the body and edema.

In short, the seven essences are strongly connected to their dregs, which, when exuberant, may lead to disease, and when consumed will also seriously affect the essence of the whole body.

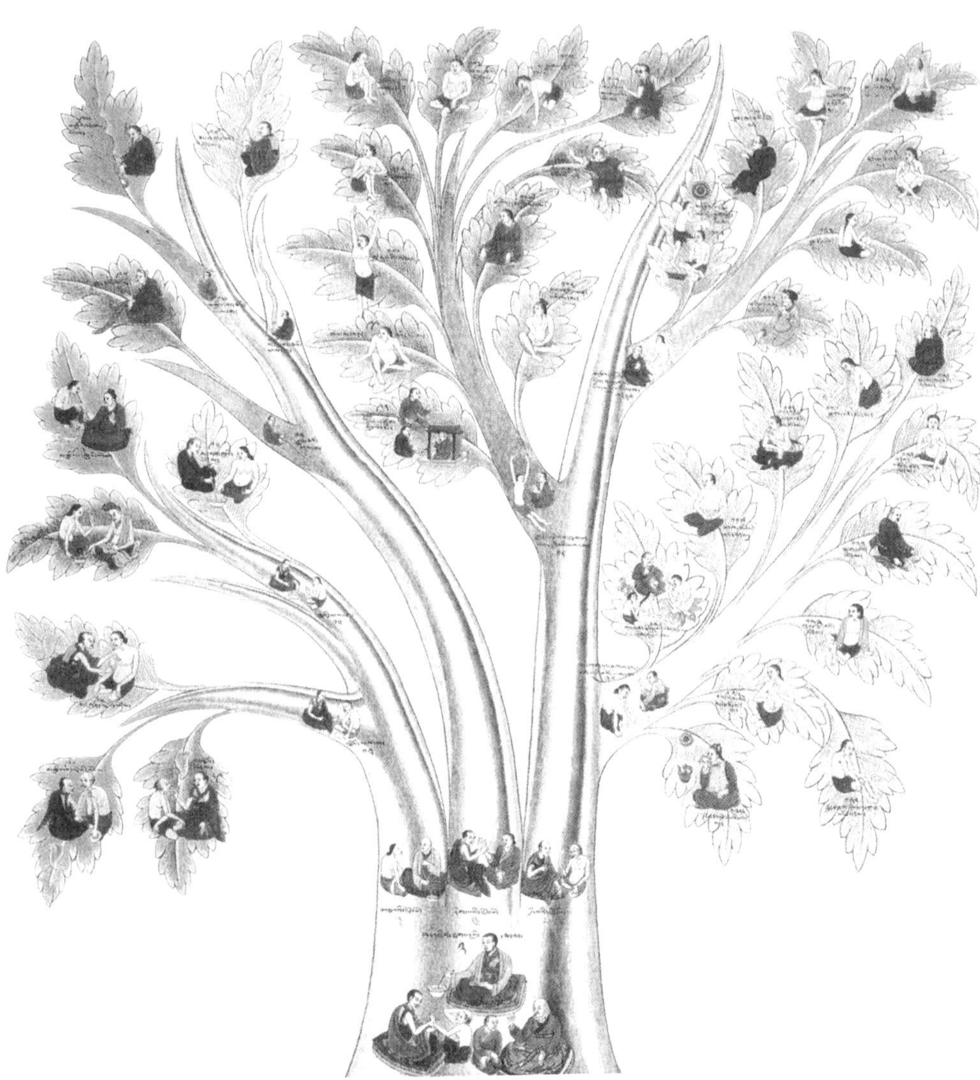

By understanding the inner changes of life and the various kinds of disease based on the external manifestations, Tibetan medicine has accumulated a rich field of knowledge. Using a tree with one root, three stems, eight branches, and thirty-eight leaves, the diagnostic methods of Tibetan medicine, including inspection, palpation and questioning are illustrated. (from *Thangkha* three in the *Sman thang* series of *The Four Medical Tantras*)

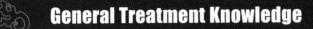

General Treatment Knowledge

The treatment of disease is an advanced art and can only be mastered through years of professional training. Nevertheless, when interpreted from the viewpoint of health cultivation, anyone can have some knowledge of treatment, and use it not only to effectively prevent disease, but also to adopt proper measures to tackle disease and expedite recovery. There are two sorts of treatments in Tibetan medicine, general and special. General treatment methods are reducing and nourishing. These methods can be administered without the help of a physician. Special treatment, on the other hand, can only be administered by a physician. Everyone should have an understanding of general treatment methods.

Nourishing methods

This approach includes nourishing medicinals, nutritious food, proper daily habits, and topical treatments that can nurture the seven essences, balance *rlung*, *mkhris pa* and *badkan*, strengthen the constitution, and promote resistance to disease. These are known as nourishing methods.

Those who should be nourished

Generally speaking, those with poor body constitutions and low resistance to illnesses, like *rlung* patients, women who bleed after delivery, people with serious lung diseases, those who indulge in too frequent sexual activity, the weak, the elderly, those with chronic insomnia, those in mourning, the depressed, those involved in ascetic practices, and people who are over worked should be nourished. During spring those who need to be nourished should make sure to receive it.

Nourishing measures

Nourishing measures cover four aspects: diet, daily habits, medicinals and external treatments.

In terms of diet, mutton, crude brown sugar, cane sugar, butter, cheese and wine are highly nutritious.

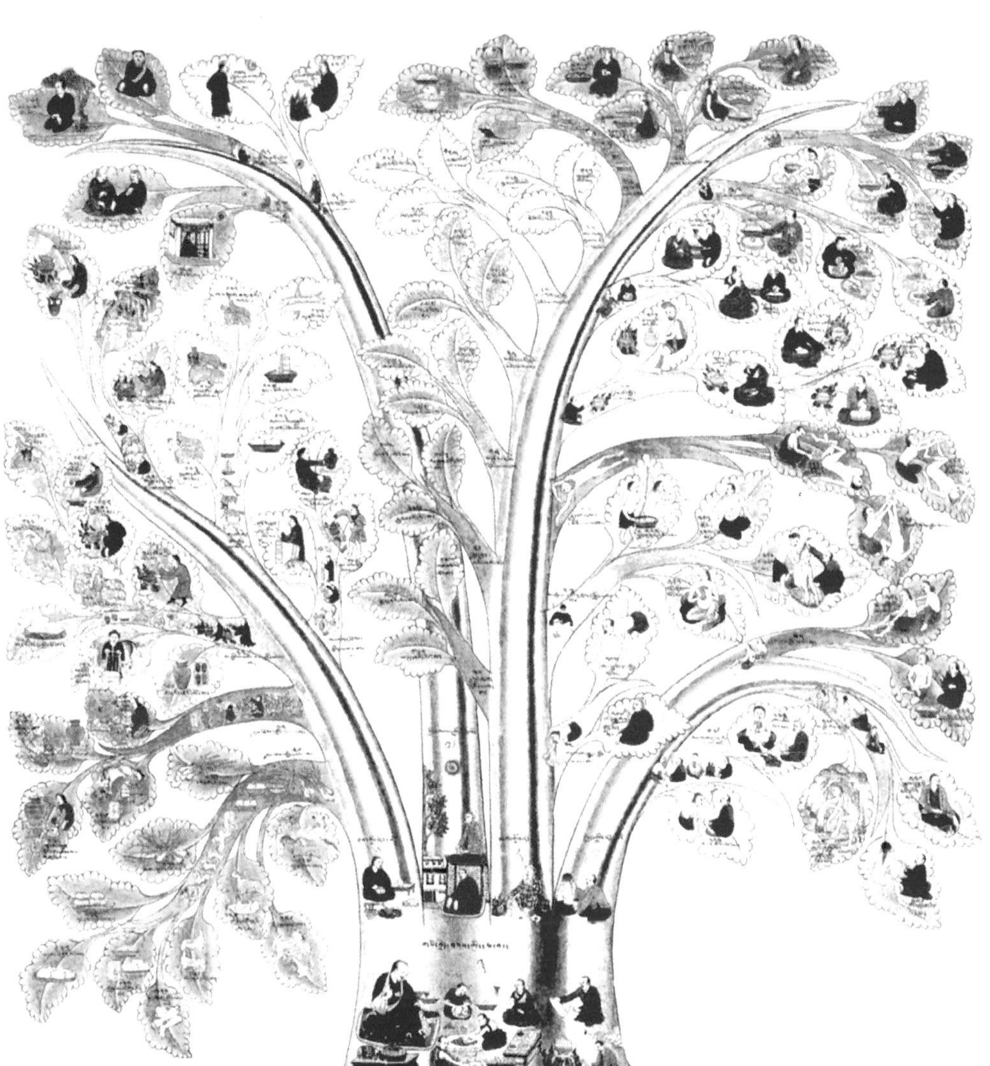

This painting uses a tree with four trunks to illustrate the four kinds of treatment: diet, daily habits, medicinals and external treatments. On the tree, there are twenty-seven stems and ninety-eight leaves to illustrate the various therapeutic techniques. (*Thangkha* four of the *Sman thang* series of *The Four Medical Tantras*)

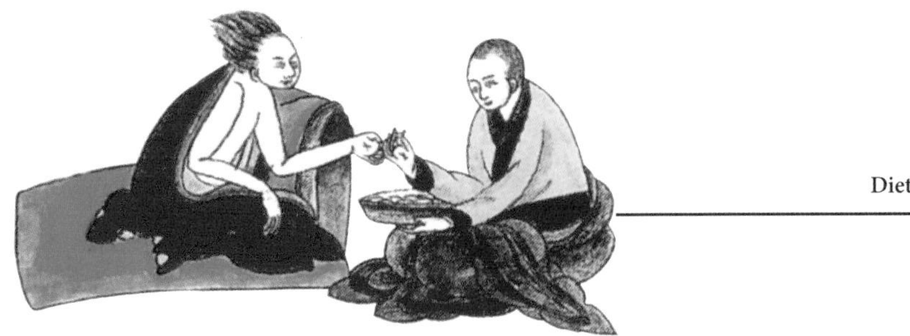

Diet therapy

In terms of medicinals: medicinal oil or pills suitable to the patient can be administered.

For external treatment, bathing, rest and relaxation, and an appropriate sexual life are recommended.

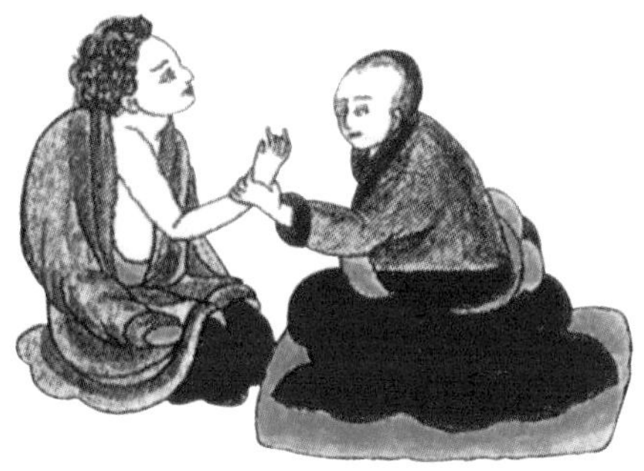

Medicinal therapy

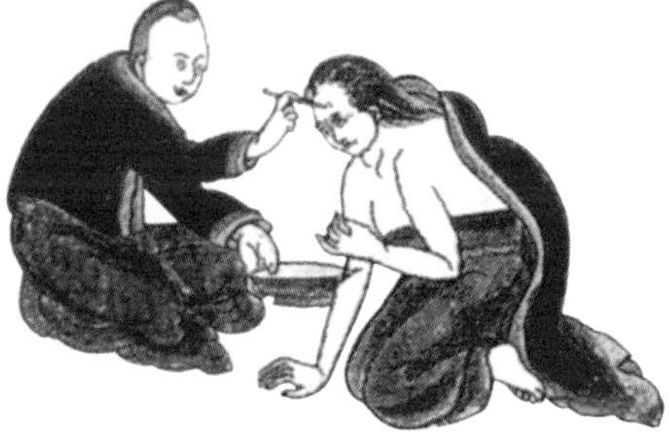

External therapy

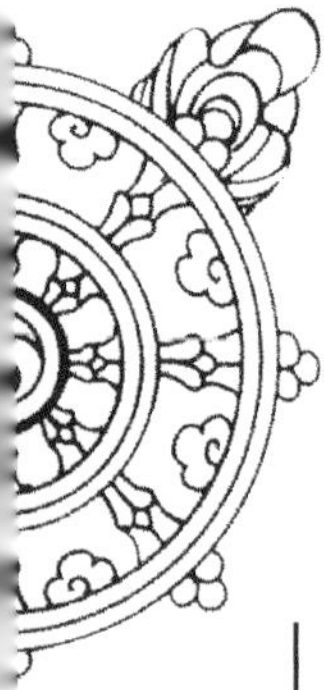

Appropriate application of nourishing methods can strengthen the body, promote internal harmony and prevent diseases of the three factors. Good nourishing treatment is like a weak person being rescued from his enemy by a strong man. Inappropriate nourishing methods are just the reverse; they may exaggerate disease and make it difficult to tackle. Hence, appropriate nourishing therapy is essential, neither too much nor too little.

Reducing methods

Also called dispersing methods, these include fasting, eating less, or taking medicinals with a reducing action in order to attack disease.

Those who should be reduced

People suffering from indigestion, those who consume too much greasy, sweet food, *rlung* patients with stiff legs, and cases of frequent urination, constipation, heat diarrhea, vomiting, a heavy body, loss of appetite, intestinal masses, obesity, jaundice, epidemics, diabetes, gout, rheumatic disease, spleen disease, lung disease, disease of the throat, heart disease, and when the body is still rather strong and energetic are all suitable cases for reducing methods. Reducing methods are best administered during the winter.

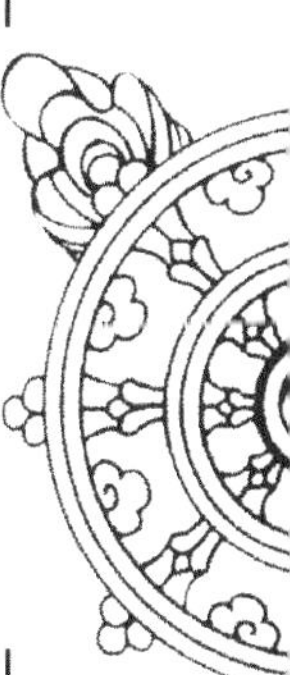

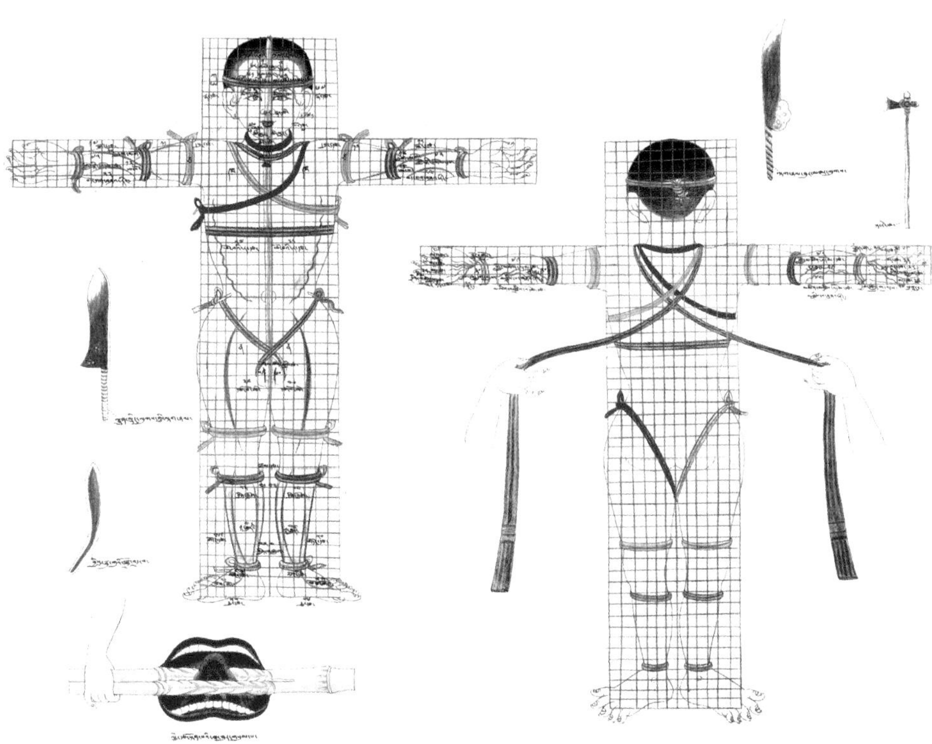

Bloodletting is a common reducing method, and is widely applied in Tibetan medicine. Here, the common points and binding locations for bloodletting are shown. The common bloodletting tools are also shown. (*Thangkha* seventy-two in the *Sman thang* series of *The Four Medical Tantras*)

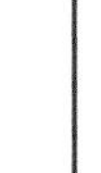

Reducing measures

These can also be administered through four aspects: diet, medicinals, daily habits and external therapies.

In terms of diet, reduction of the quantity of food eaten each meal with an increase in light and easily digestible foods is preferable. Food such as peas and highland barley flour is suitable. Diet therapy is frequently used in patients who are rather weak.

Medicinal therapy is indicated for patients with moderate body constitutions and poor digestion. *Sallucidum with Four Ingredients* and *Pomegranate Powder with Five Ingredients* are used to increase strength. For epidemic patients, medicines to accelerate the maturity of the fever can be used.

For patients with stronger constitutions, external therapy can be administered. Manual labor, taking medicinals or lying on a hot earth sleeping plateau (or sauna) to cause sweating, moxibustion (burning mugwort leaves over points or tender spots), hot compresses, medical baths, and bloodletting are all suitable methods.

For diseases of the stomach, emesis can be used, while for intestinal disease, drastic purging can be used, and for disease in the bladder or lower abdomen, enemas can be used. Diuretics and purging can also be used.

Appropriate use of reducing methods will render the sense organs sensitive, the body energetic, improve the appetite, strengthen the constitution, regulate the diet, and ensure normal digestion and excretion. However, inappropriate use will bring side effects.

The five solid organs preserve and transform the five sources, while the six hollow organs accept and transform the five sources. Through the three factors, the vessels, orifices, and organs establish connections with the body surface that forms an organic whole, offering the background for recognizing and treating diseases.

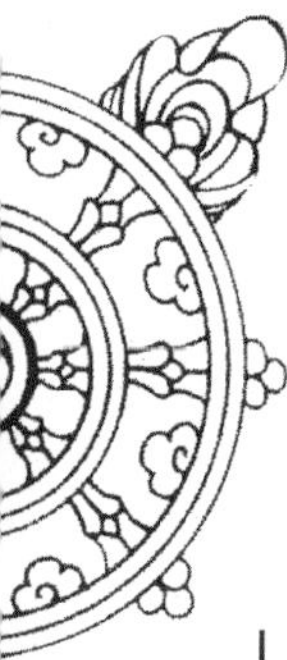

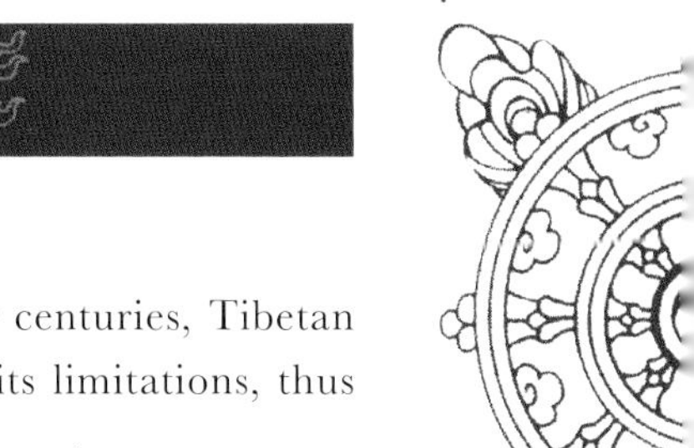

Treatment Principles

To what degree does medicine contribute to our health? Over centuries, Tibetan medicine has recognized the effectiveness of medicine as well as its limitations, thus differentiating those diseases that can be cured and those that can't.

Important questions

During the long process of fighting against disease, people have explored many different therapeutic techniques, and have also pondered on the role of medicine. Is it better to exaggerate the role of medicine, or to negate its role? Eventually, people reached a reasonable balance. In *The Four Medical Tantras*, the problem of treatment is summarized in three aspects:

First problem: Why, even when a patient receives timely treatment, does the condition still develop and the medication doesn't work?

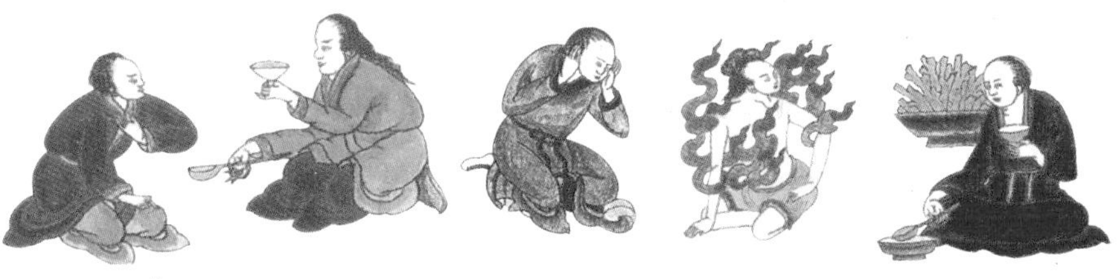

Why does the treatment yield no effect even when treated in time?

Second problem: Why, when a patient frequents an excellent physician and leads a comfortable healthy life, does the patient ultimately die?

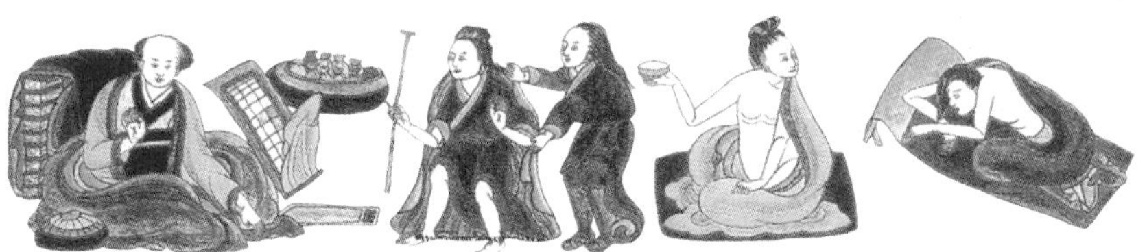

Why can't excellent physicians and excellent medicines prevent death?

Third problem: Why do some diseases heal without receiving any treatment, are recoveries seen even with maltreatment, or are healing possible even with poor doctors and in situations where medicine is not available?

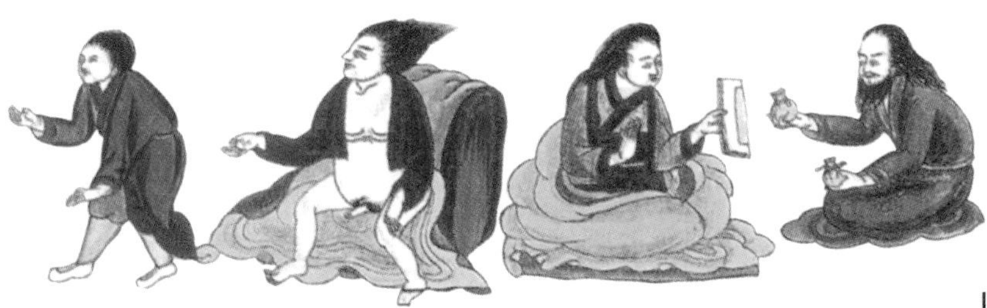

Why do diseases heal even if the treatment is not satisfactory?

Answers to the questions

Tibetan medicine claims that there are altogether 404 diseases. Among them, 101 are temporary with pseudo-manifestations, and can be healed without treatment, or are readily cured when treated properly. This is like how a man who falls can stand up again alone, or even more easily when assisted by other people, or a cloudy sky clearing naturally.

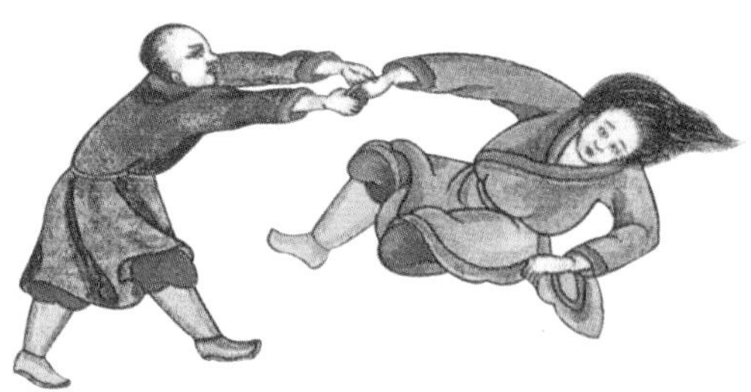

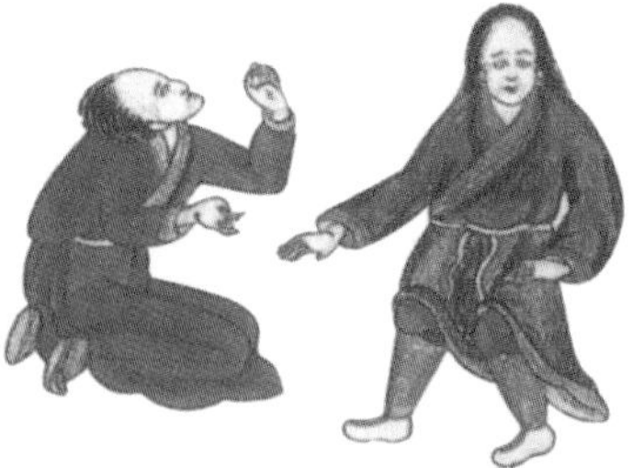

There are 404 diseases, 101 of them are temporary and will heal without being treated, just like someone who stands up again after falling down.

Like the sun shining again after the rain.

Another 101 diseases belong to mental diseases and can only be cured by psychological treatments and not by medication. This is like a prisoner that can only be set free by someone bribing the guard.

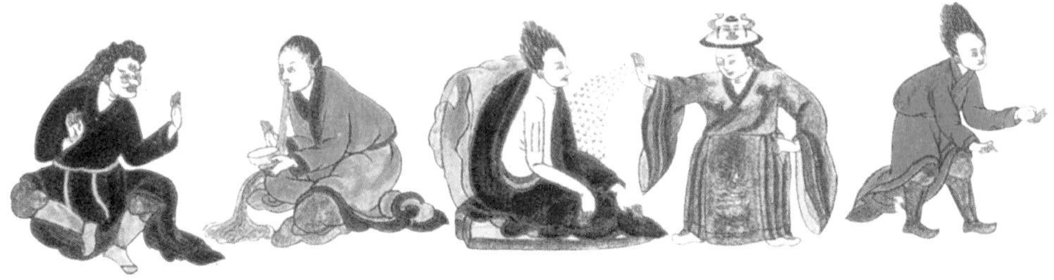

101 diseases are mental disease, which can only be cured by psychological approaches and not by of medication.

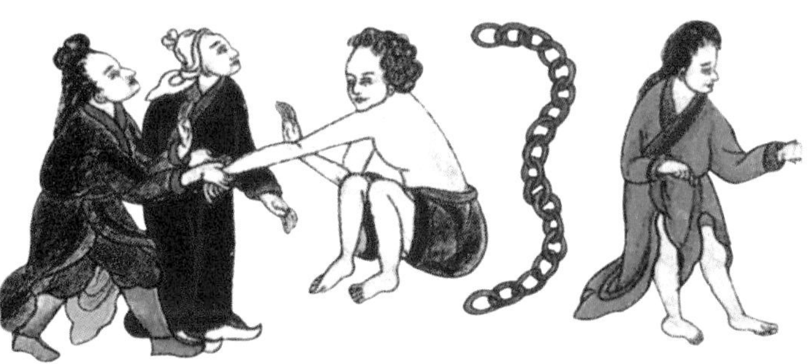

With bribes to the jail keeper, a prisoner can be set free.

Still another 101 diseases occur naturally and will cause death without treatment. Only with correct treatment and the right medicinals can the patient survive. However, when the medication given is inappropriate, death is unavoidable.

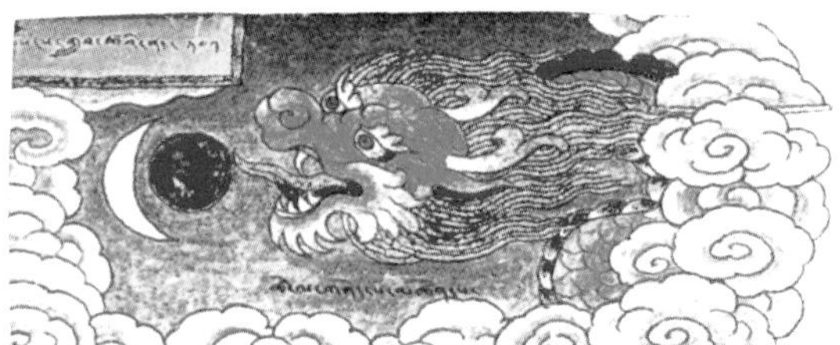

Like eclipses of the sun and moon, 101 kinds of diseases happen naturally.

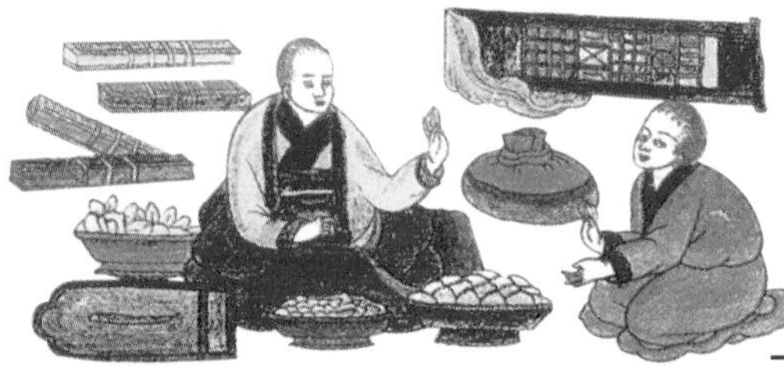

Disease can be healed with the right treatment.

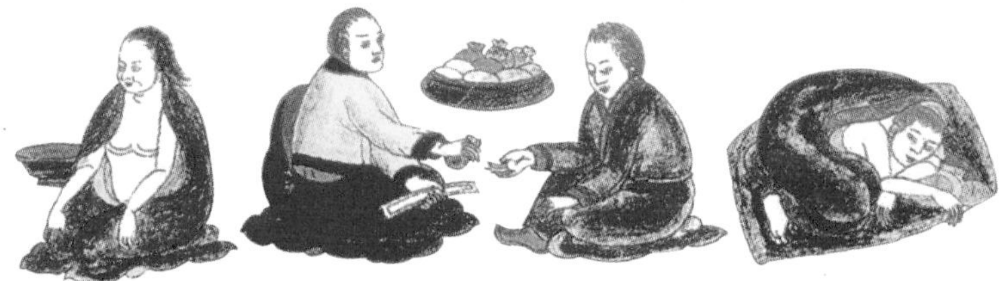

Only proper medicinals can cure, wrong medication causes death.

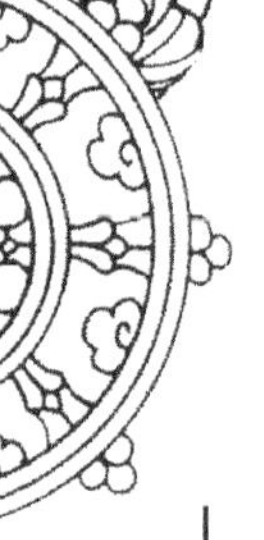

The course of treatment is divided into three stages, primary, intermediate and final. Diseases that involve fevers, for instance, generally are not able to heal without treatment. Proper and timely medication can prevent complications. At the initial stage of a fever, anti-heat medicinals can cure it. When a high fever appears in the intermediate stage,

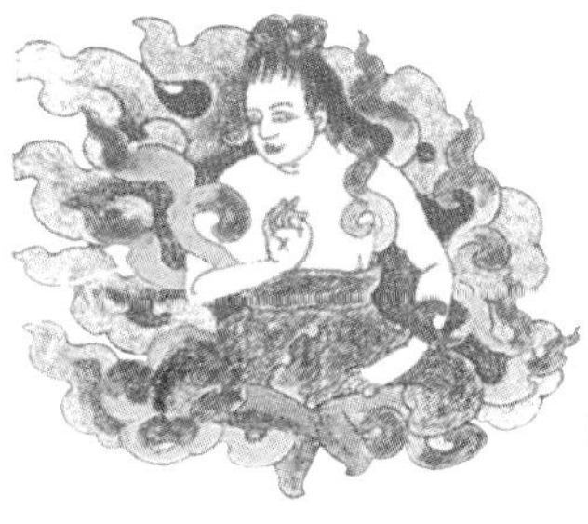
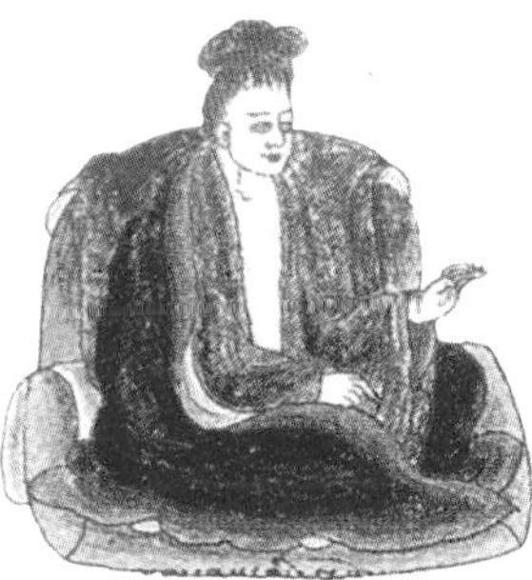
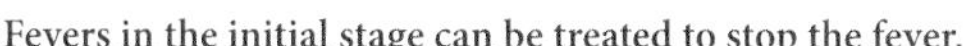

Fevers in the initial stage can be treated to stop the fever.

medication must be used to arrest the fever, as a dam can only be built when the current is mild. When the disease advances to a severe condition, active medication with heavy dosage should be given to cure it, just like a guard is necessary to protect merchandise and ensure it reaches its destination safely.

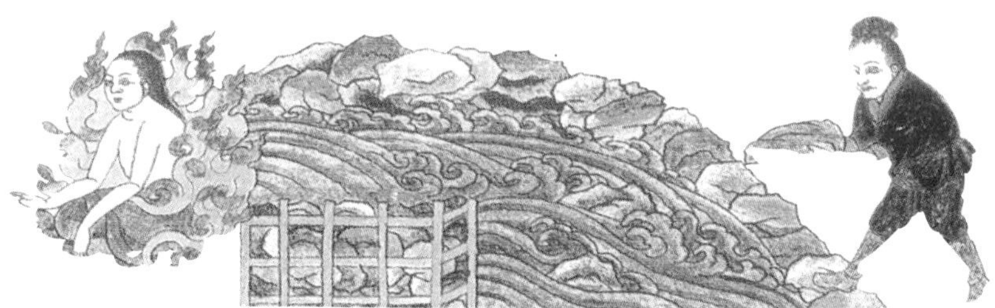

High fevers should be stopped by giving continuous medication, like continuously working to build a dam and prevent a flood.

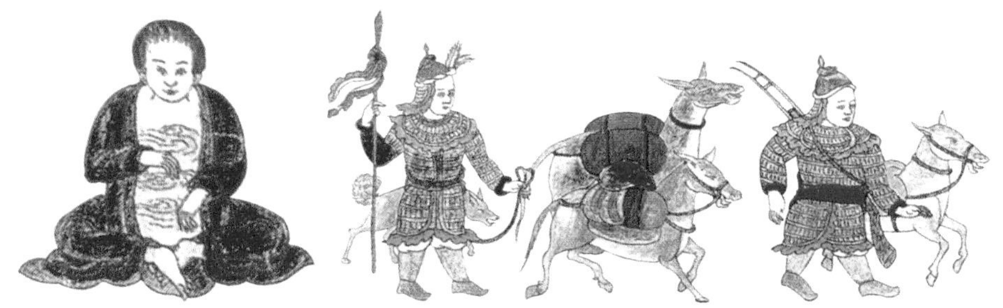

Severe diseases can only be cured by heavy doses of medication, like a valuable shipment being protected with armed guards to ensure its safety.

Finally, there are 101 kinds of diseases which are doomed to death. Even if treatment is given, it will be of no use.

Obviously, physicians are not almighty. Based on the quality and type of the disease, the kind of treatment will naturally differ.

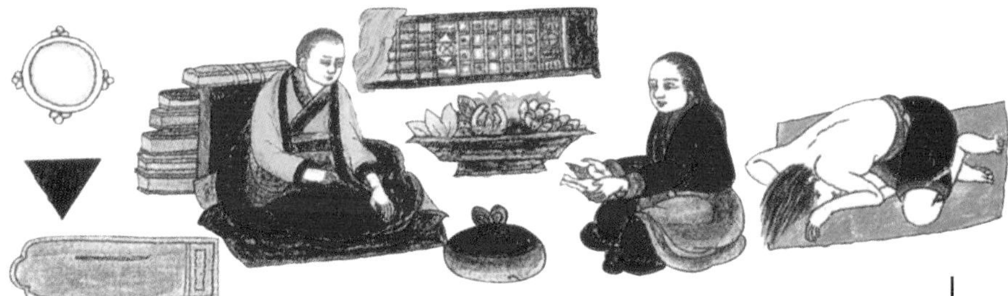

Still another 101 diseases are doomed to death and can't be cured.

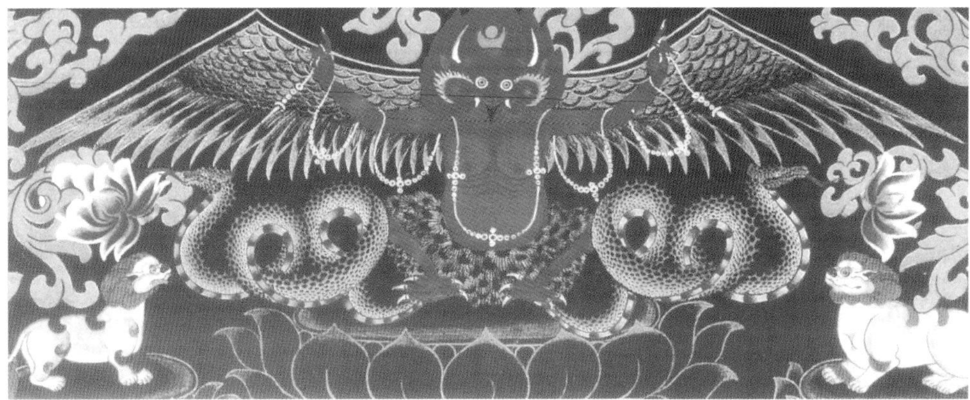

A roc has a red body with golden wings and wide-open round eyes. Tibetan people always put its picture on the door to guard against plagues. (part of a *Thangkhu*)

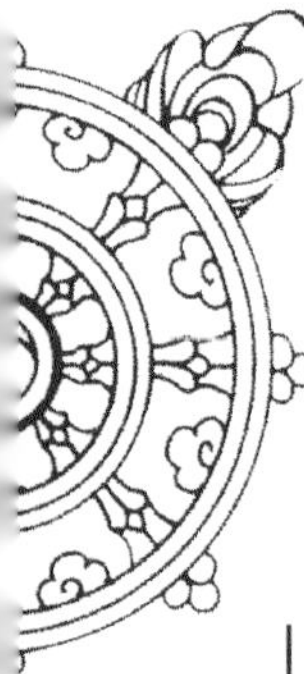

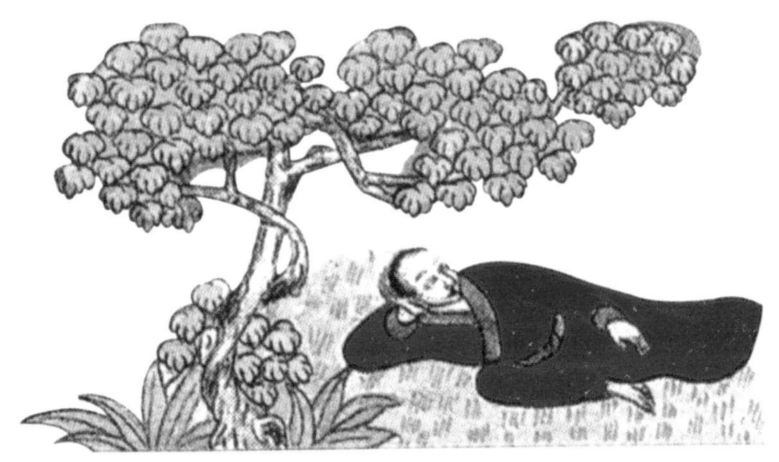

སྤྱོད་ལམ་གྱི་ལུས་བླངས་གསོ་བ།

CHAPTER 4 HEALTH CULTIVATION HABITS

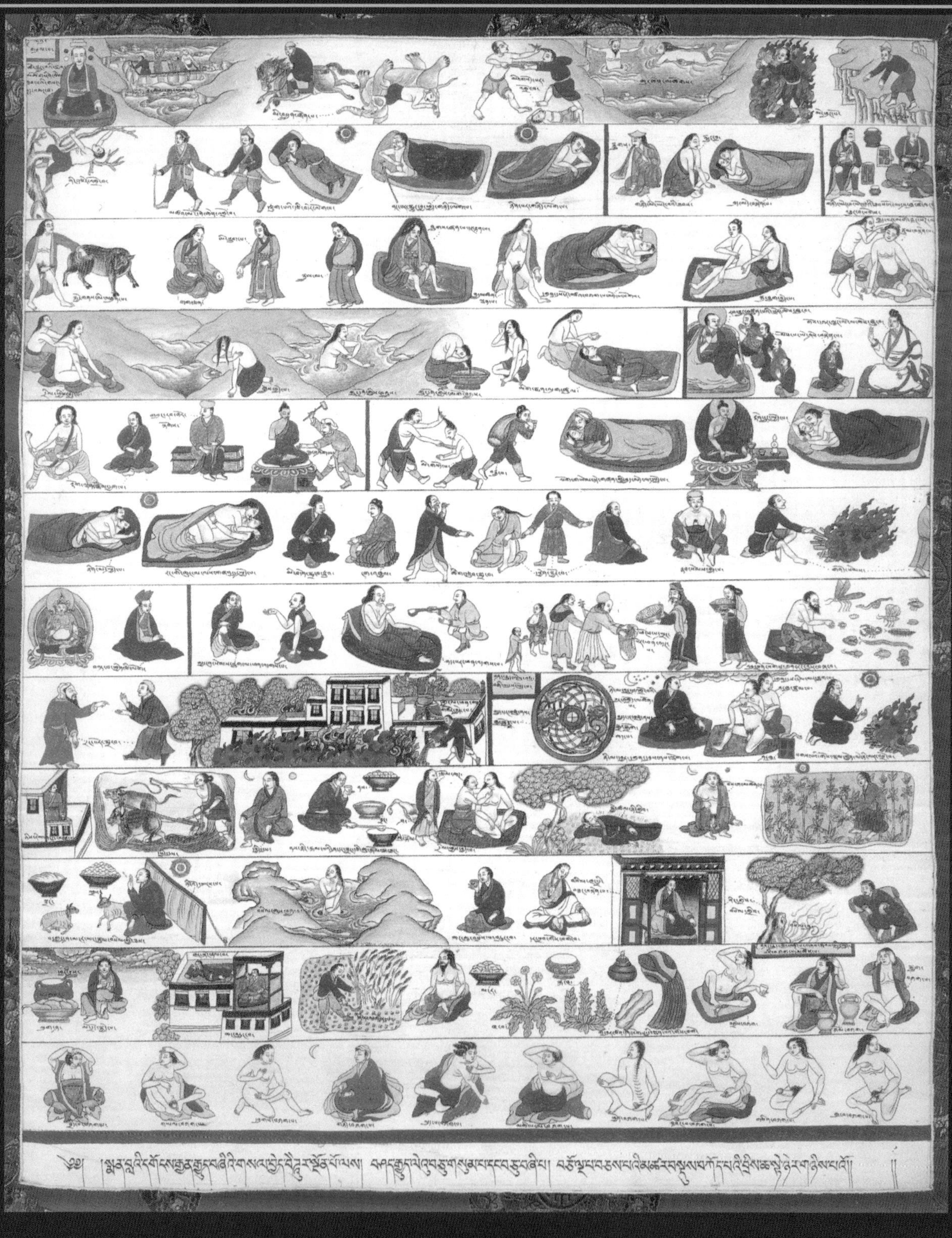

Daily life, *Thangkha* twenty-two in the *Sman thang* series of *The Four Medical Tantras.*

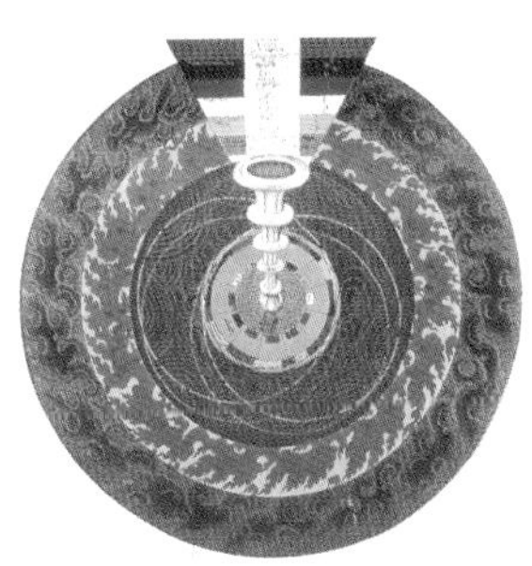

Daily life includes three aspects, body, speech, and mind.

Everyone wishes to live a long life. To reach this end, one must begin from body, speech and mind so as to develop the factors beneficial to life, and decrease or prevent those that jeopardize it. This is also the basic principle of health. Good habits for health cultivation are divided into seasonal and daily behavior.

Being the basis of all behavior, correct daily habits prevent disease and also help rapid recovery when one happens to fall ill. In Tibetan medicine, this is an important aspect of health cultivation.

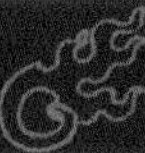

Seasonal Health Cultivation

There are six seasons in the Tibetan calendar: early winter, winter, spring, summer-heat, summer and autumn. Each season is two months long. Recommendations for health cultivation in each season are different.

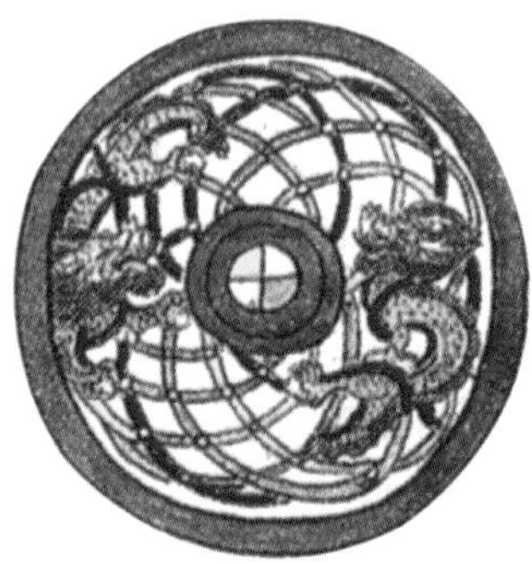

In the Tibetan calendar, there are six seasons in each year: early winter, winter, spring, summer-heat, summer and autumn.

Daily life in early winter

This season covers the 10th and 11th months, during which the weather is cold and the hair follicles are closed, so heat is accumulated inside the body. Hence, people have high heat energy, and the fire-accompanying *rlung* strengthens the body temperature further. If one takes too little food, the blood and fluid will be affected and the essence will decrease or even dry up. One should take plenty of sweet, sour, and salty food. Furthermore, since

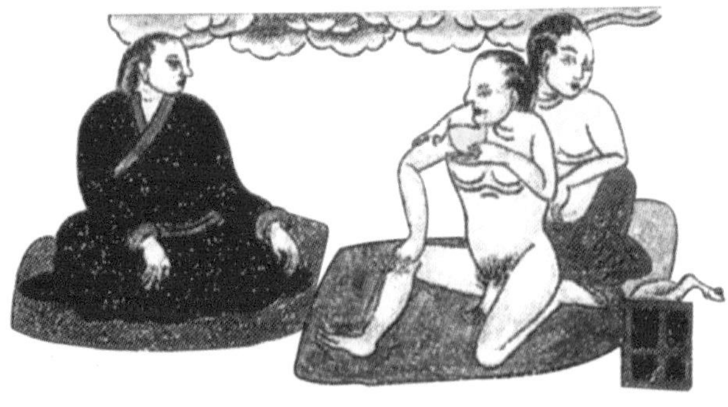

In early winter, rub the body with sesame oil, wear enough clothes and eat plenty of sweet, sour and salty food.

the night is longer than the day, one may feel hungry before dawn. Remaining hungry will decrease heat energy and weaken the essence. Having broth made from mutton or beef is encouraged, plus butter, crude sugar, wine, dairy, and oily products. Use vegetables and sesame oil to rub the body.

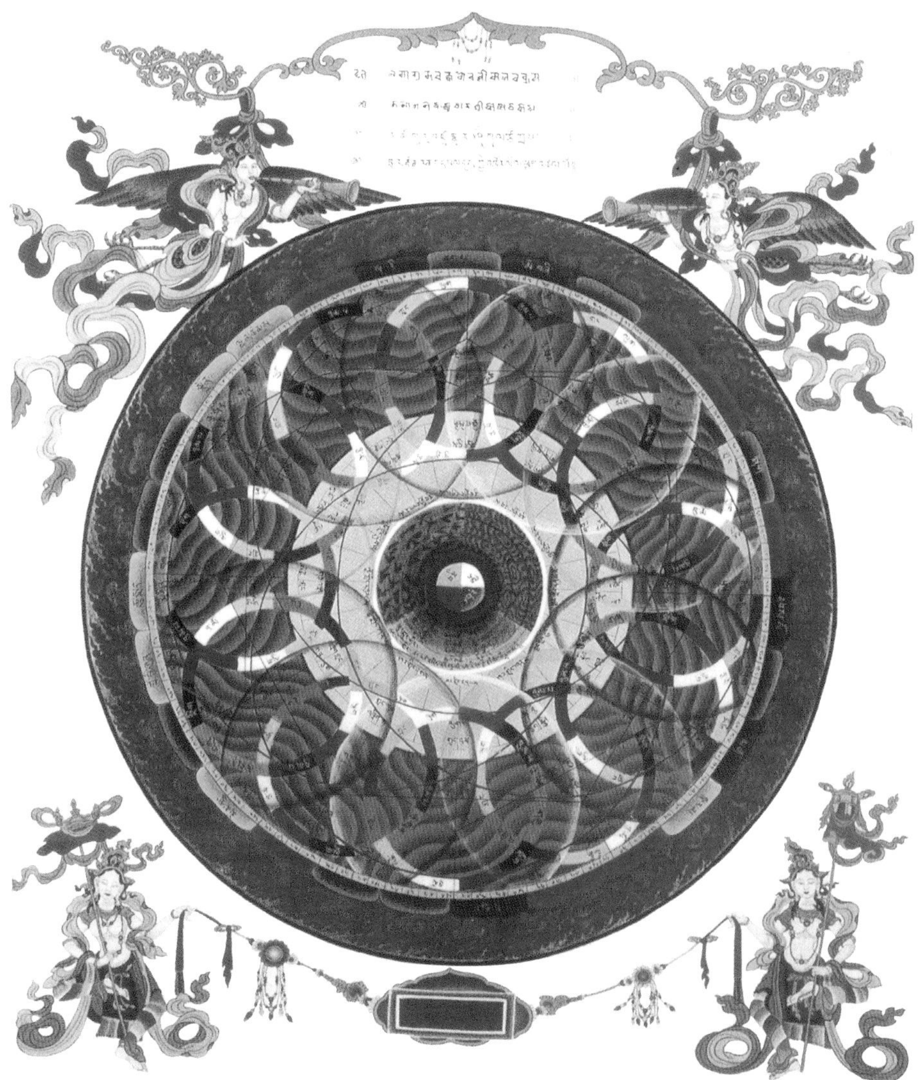

A picture of the movements of the sun and the moon in Tibetan astronomy (part of a *thangkha*).

To resist cold, one must wear wool clothes or fur-lined jackets and cotton boots. Hot compresses, staying in the sun, warming oneself by the fire, and residing in a room with sufficient sunshine will help increase one's heat energy.

Daily life in winter

This includes the 12th and 1st months, and is even colder than early winter. The diet should be basically the same as in early winter. Thick clothes must be worn to resist cold. In terms of diet, oily or fatty food is encouraged, such as cooked meats, mutton broth, and beef broth. Since green leafy vegetables are in short supply, poor nutrition may result through relying only on fatty food. One should strive to eat as many vegetables as possible.

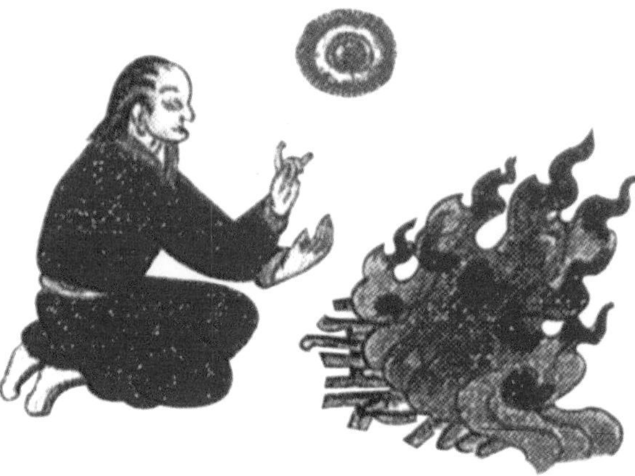

In winter, wearing woolen clothes, boots, staying warm by the fire, staying in the sun, and residing upstairs are all helpful.

Daily life in spring

Spring includes the 2nd and 3rd months, when the weather begins to warm. Though warm yang-qi* has begun to sprout, weather is still cold and snow may appear with strong wind. Spring approaches only sluggishly.

* Yang-qi is a Chinese concept. In this case it can be loosely translated as "warm, moving energy." Yang is the warming, growing, active aspect of the universe. This term is used several times in this book.

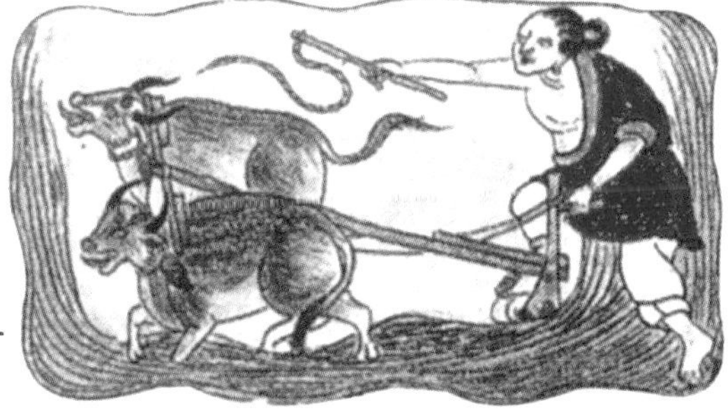

Spring time

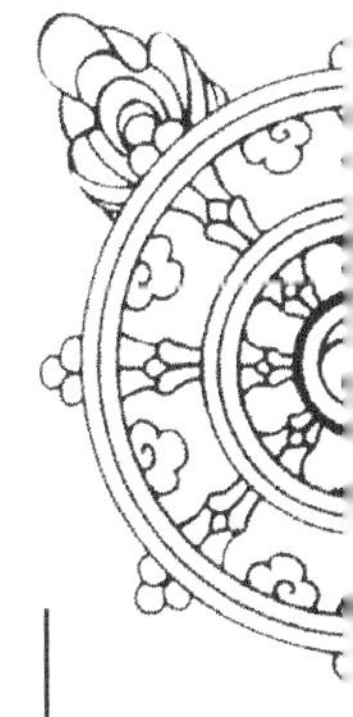

During the cold winter, the accumulated *badkan* in the body does not easily attack. However, when the sun shines and the weather becomes warmer, the hair follicles begin to open a bit, the yang qi within the body begins to disperse, and the stomach fire begins to weaken. At this time *Badkan* begins to attack. To prevail, one must eat of the three bad tastes, which are bitter, pungent and astringent, as well as old highland barley flour, birds and wild animals from dry land, bee honey, hot boiling water, ginger soup and light, rough foods. Walk in warm places, relax the bones and tendons. Rub the body with dry pea powder to remove *badkan* disease. Spend time in places full of flowers and trees with fragrant and cool gardens.

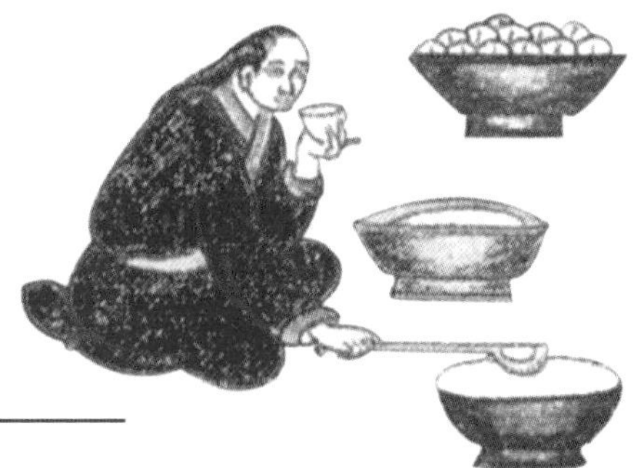

Take bitter, pungent, and astringent foods such as bee honey and ginger soup.

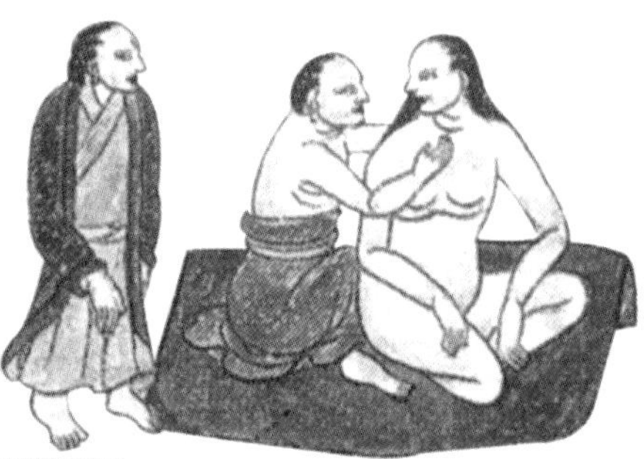

Rub the body with pea powder.

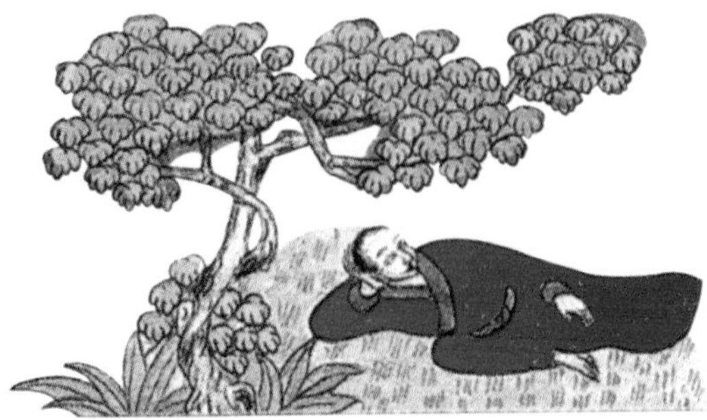

Stay in a fragrant cool garden.

Daily life during summer-heat

This season includes the 4th and 5th months, when the sun moves north towards the Tropic of Cancer. During this time the sun shines strongly and body's strength is weakened. The body's qi and blood tend to disperse outward, as well as any heat accumulated inside.

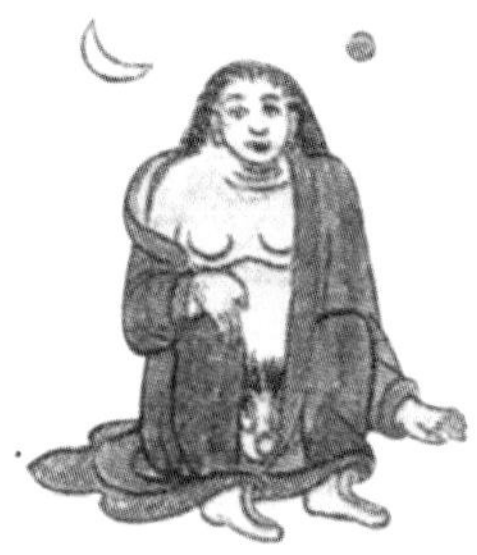

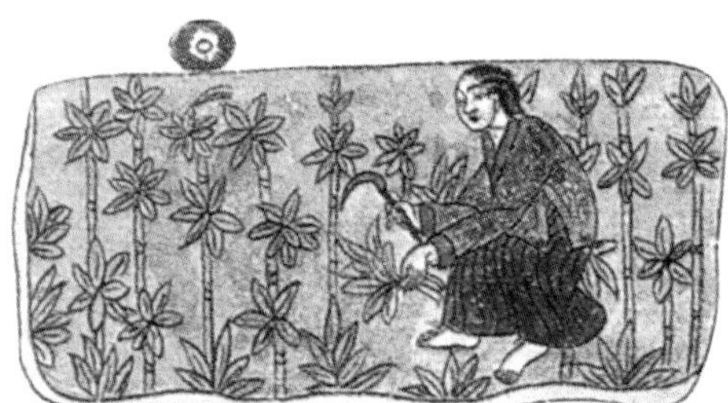

Summer-heat season.

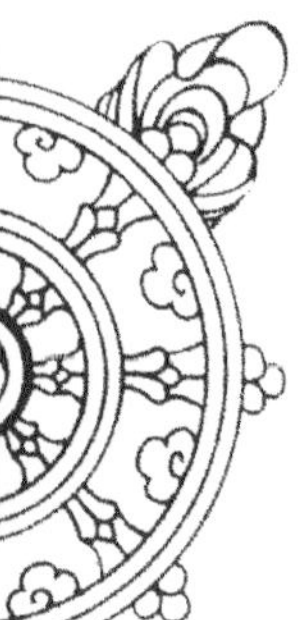

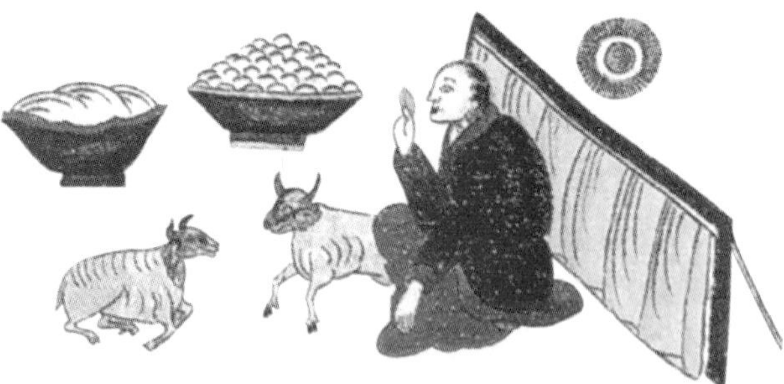

Taking light, moist, cool foods such as rice, beef and bee honey.

The diet should change from fatty to plain and warm with plenty of light, cool, and moist food. If salty, spicy, or sour food is eaten, *rlung* pathogens will be increased. Eat as much green leafy vegetables, like spinach and celery, as possible, and very little fatty food. Wine diluted with water is acceptable, but pure wine should be avoided.

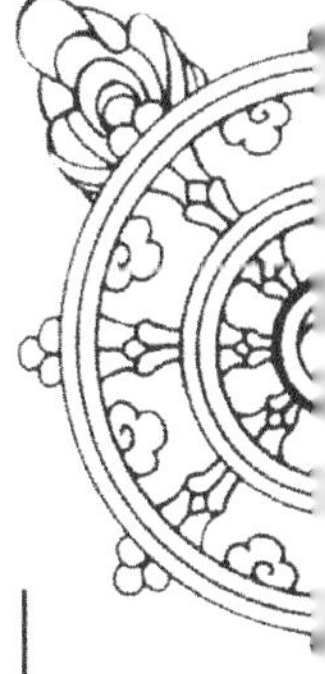

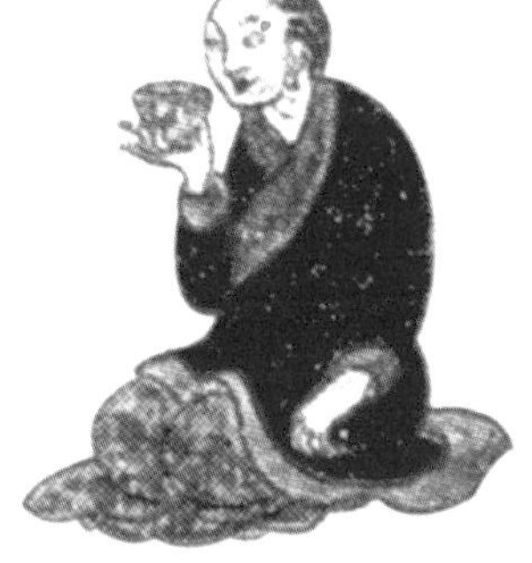

Mix water with wine for drinking.

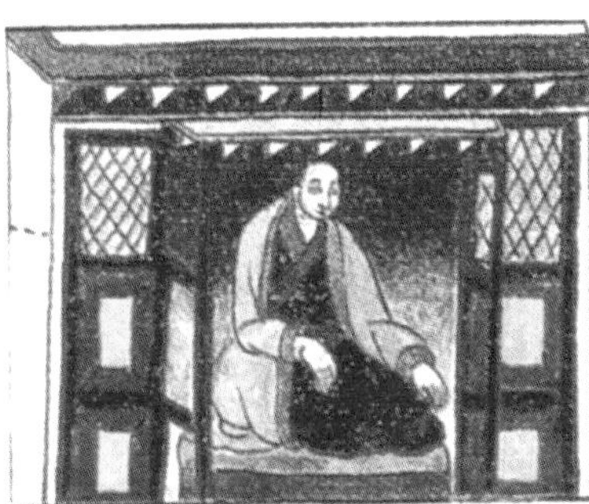

Reside in a cool place.

One should wear thin silk clothes, increase the amount of outdoor activity, stay in a cool room, and spray water with borneol, sandalwood and perfume on the floor. The room should be ventilated and clean, with flowers and plants outside, a nice breeze, and without direct sunshine.

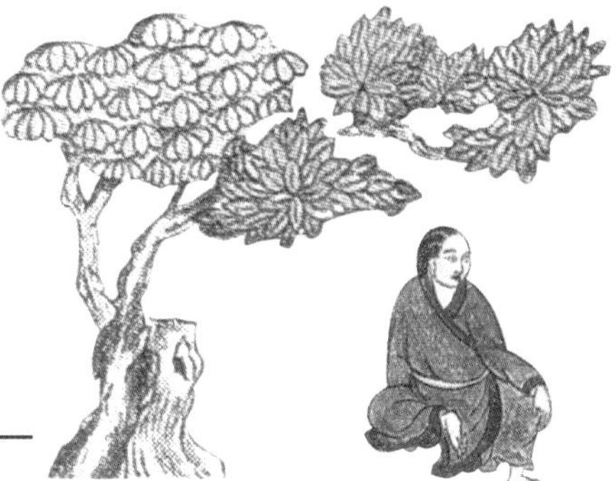

Stay under a tree to enjoy the cool shade.

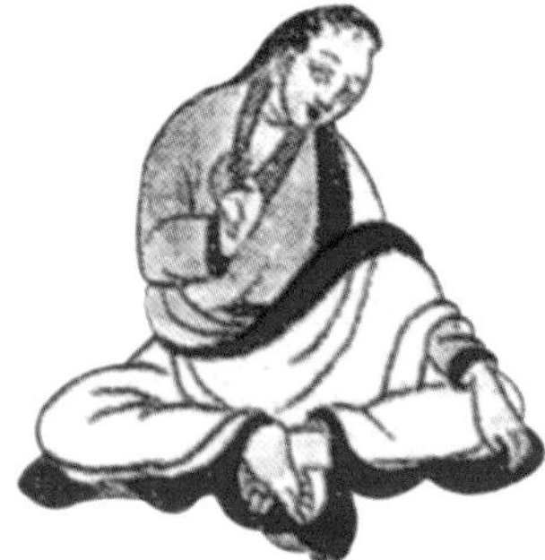

Wear thin clothes

Daily life in summer

Summer includes the 6th and 7th months when the rains are heavy and the earth is wet, the breeze is humid, water in the ground evaporates and the rivers are turbid. All of the above conditions are harmful to the stomach fire, and may cause poor digestion. Daily habits should help the stomach fire by eating sweet, sour, and salty foods such as wine prepared with bee honey from a dry climate and broth. Generally speaking, the amount of meat taken should be less and the amount of cheese, fresh vegetables and fruits should be more. Cool dishes can be prepared with mustard and garlic added to kill bacteria and promote the appetite. However, cold and raw food should be limited, as well as iced drinks. This is especially true for children and the elderly. Do not reside in the top floor of a house or rooms that are too breezy.

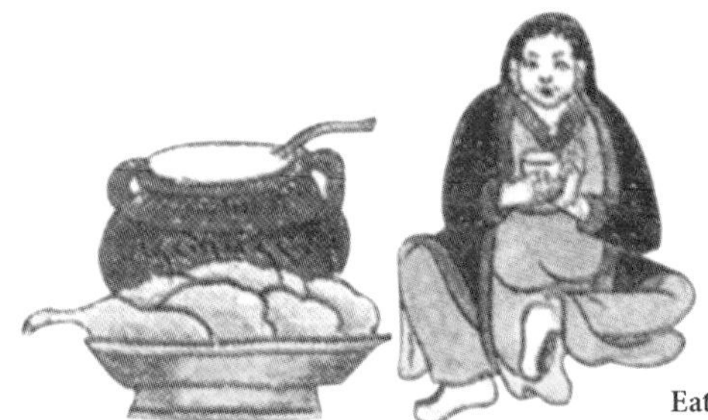

Eat mutton, milk and other easily digested foods.

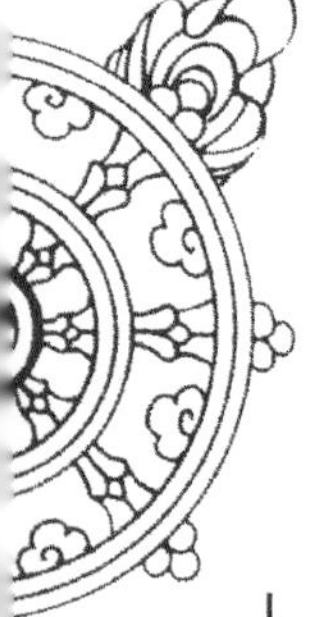

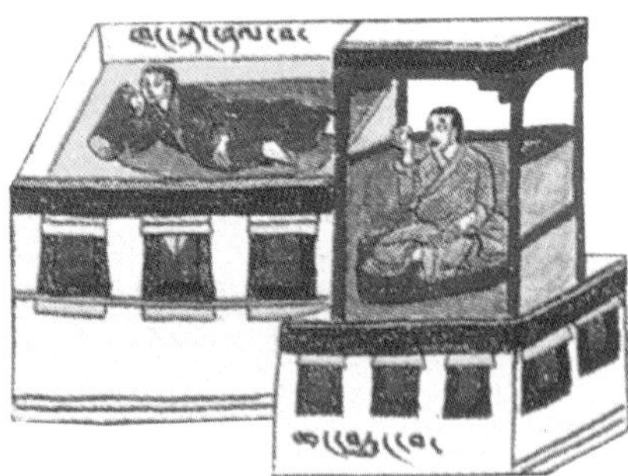

Rest on the roof

Daily life in autumn

Autumn includes the 8th and 9th months when the cool wind and rain suppress the *mkhris pa* which has been accumulated. In autumn, when sunlight is strong *mkhris pa* disease may occur. To avoid this potential threat, sweet, bitter, and astringent food should be eaten. Since a great variety of foods such as vegetables, fruits, meat, eggs, and cheese are available, the menu should varied to avoid eating too much of any certain thing. Spread some borneol, white sandalwood and other aromatic materials on the clothes and spray the rooms with fragrant materials. This will increase happiness as well as longevity.

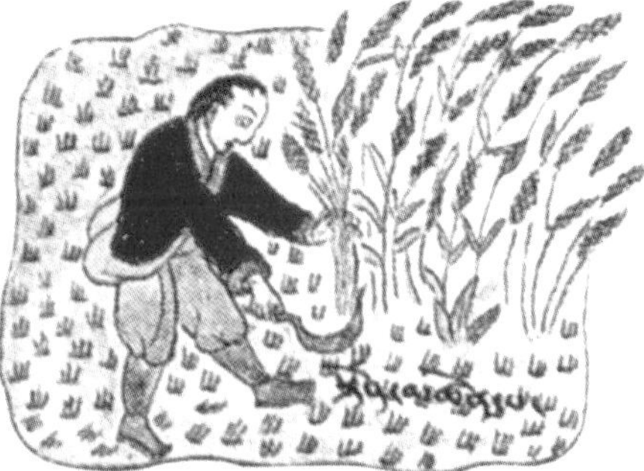

Autumn

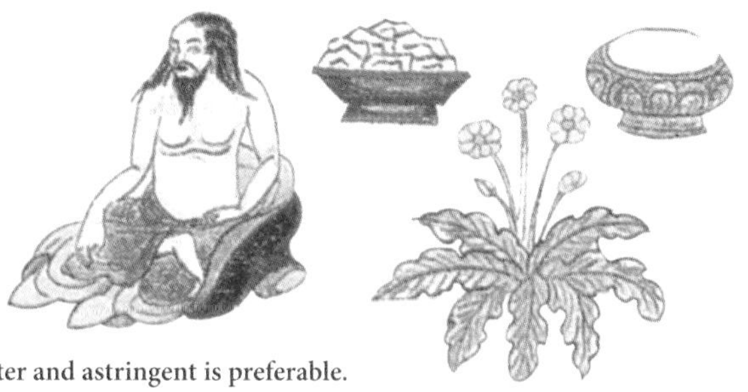

In autumn, food that is sweet, bitter and astringent is preferable.

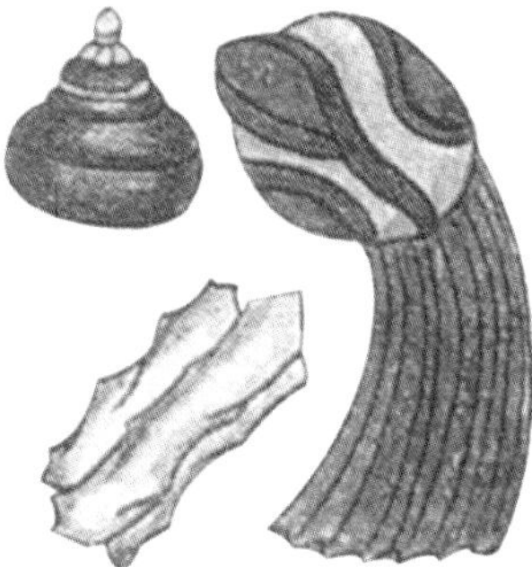

Fumigate the clothes with camphor or sandalwood.

In summary, in spring, rough foods are recommended; in summer and winter hot food and activities of a hot nature are preferable; in summer-heat and autumn cool foods and cool natured behavior is best. In treatment of disease, various strategies can be adopted, some that vary on the season. To treat *mkhris pa* disease, purging can be used. To eliminate *badkan* disease in the spring, vomiting can be induced. If *rlung* disease occurs in the summer, mild purging is appropriate. Although therapy should correspond with the six seasons, exuberance or insufficiency should be well recognized and the condition of the patient and their living environment should be given importance as well. Understanding how the seasons affect *rlung*, *mkhris pa* and *badkan* is the way to mastery of health.

People are more energetic in winter, and less energetic during summer-heat and summer. Activity is usually moderate during spring. Daily habits should be adjusted accordingly to adapt to the changes of environment so as to maintain one's health.

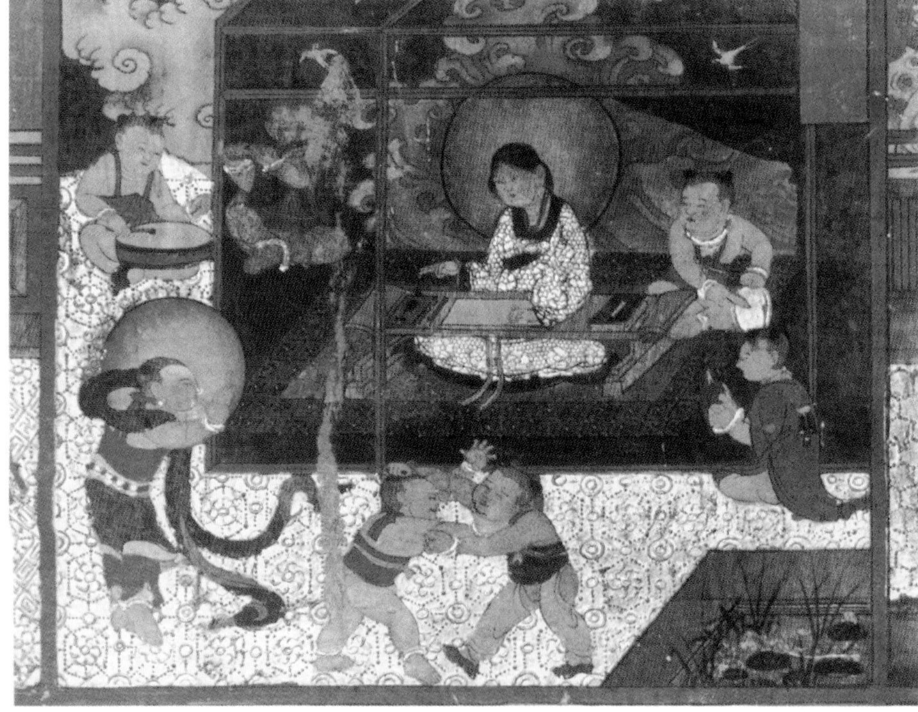

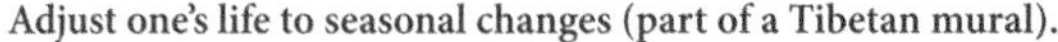

Adjust one's life to seasonal changes (part of a Tibetan mural).

Daily Health Cultivation

This refers to concrete measures taken in everyday life for cultivating health. This includes obeying the natural laws, keeping safe and avoiding danger.

Healthcare knowledge

Sleep

Enough sleep is essential. Working the whole night through should be avoided. Tibetan medicine claims that working the whole night through makes people rough and triggers *rlung* diseases, which will lead to uncomfortable feelings and great misery. If overwork

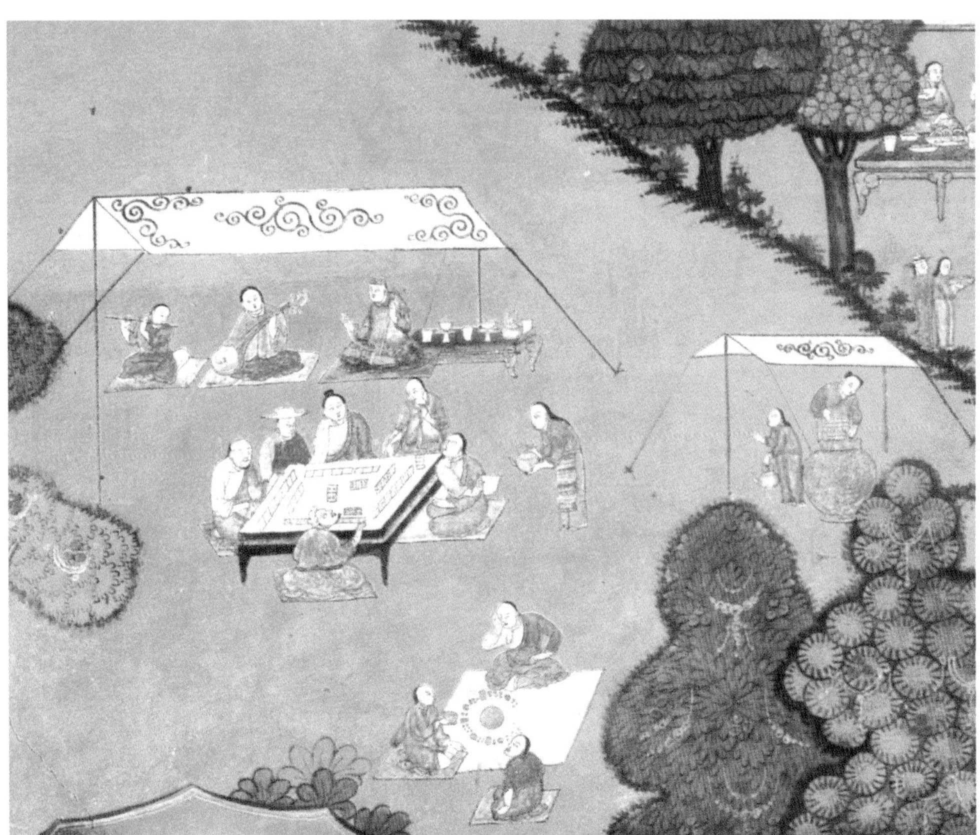

Healthy and rich daily life entertains one's body and mind (a chess party from a mural).

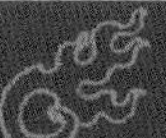

happens at night, to avoid an exuberance of *badkan*, fasting is necessary the next morning as is sleeping for half the total time worked during the night. Only by this method can fatigue and the occurrence of *badkan* diseases be avoided.

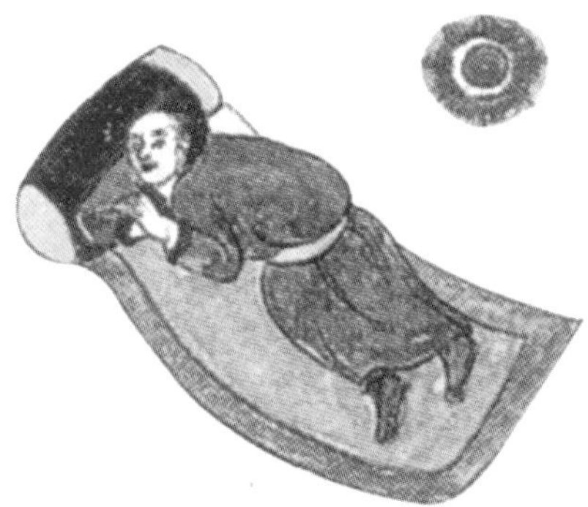

Enough sleep

During the summer-heat season, daytime is longer and nighttime is shorter. The nature of all creatures becomes rough, and the human spirit is reduced, as is the strength and complexion of all beings. These factors lead to the exuberance of *rlung*, and as a result *rlung* diseases occur. For people with chronic disease, those who are debilitated and weak, the elderly, drunks, those easily frightened, people who perform heavy manual labor, or those that work with their mind should take a nap after lunch. Even a short rest is very helpful. By doing so, the moist, heavy calming nature of the body can be restored, *rlung* diseases eliminated, and the body's strength reinforced.

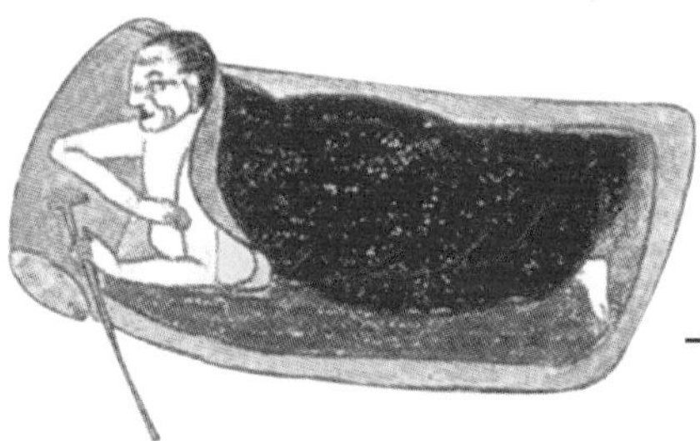

If you didn't sleep well, fasting the next morning and a nap is essential.

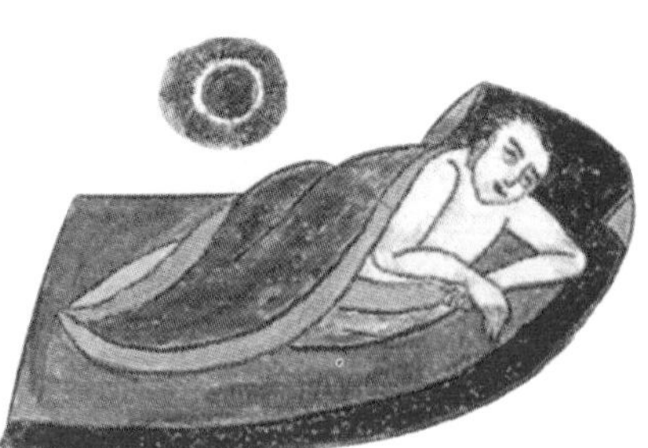

For the drunk, those with low spirits, depressed, people who must speak a lot and the elderly, a nap in a dry location during summer-heat season is crucial.

When one has had too much sleep, the drowsy *badkan* must be eliminated. For this, vomiting can be induced after awakening (tickling the throat with the finger or feather is effective). Eating and sexual activity should be reduced. When one has had too much sleep, can't fall asleep, or is easily awakened, one should eat cheese, wine and broth, or rub the face and head with sesame oil so as regulate sleeping habits.

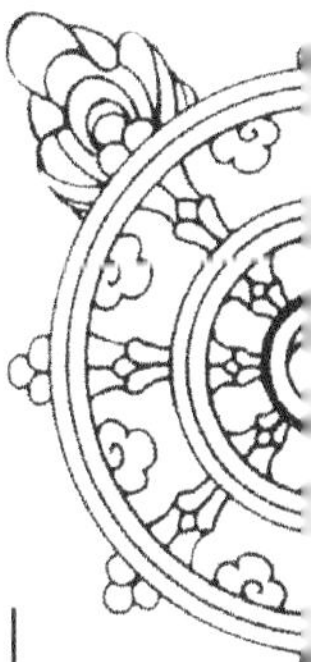

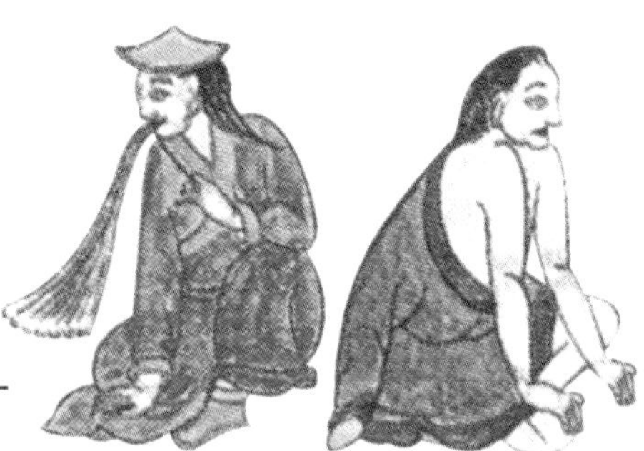

Too much sleep can be checked by inducing vomiting or fasting.

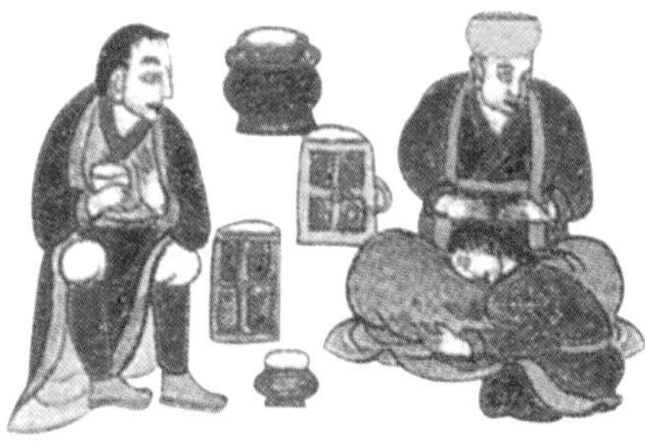

Too little sleep can be remedied by eating milk, cheese, or broth.

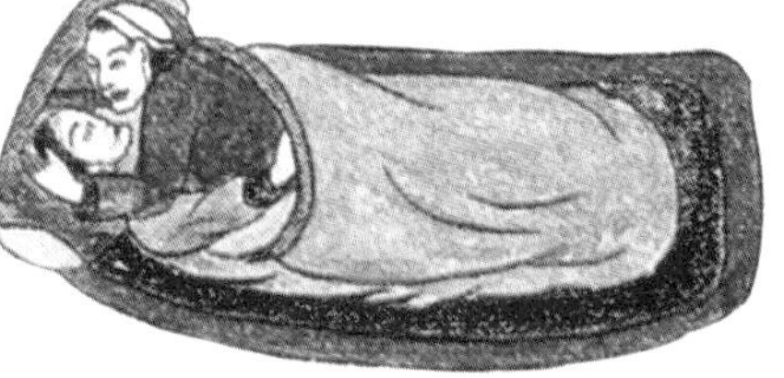

Sexual activity is one of the measures to reduce sleep.

Sexual life

Sexual desire is a normal necessity. Appropriate sexual activity is very helpful to one's health and in prolonging life. One should be neither an ascetic nor overindulgent in sexual activities.

Winter is the season when *badkan* accumulates. When *badkan* is exuberant, its diseases will be prevalent in the spring. Sexual activities will decrease *badkan*. If one has plenty of energy, sexual activities can be somewhat frequent. *Rlung* diseases occur frequently in hot summer, and too frequent sex can cause *rlung* to be exuberant and disease to occur. Thus, intercourse once in two weeks is appropriate during this season.

For an energetic youth, frequent sex is fine in winter, while in spring and autumn, once in two days is appropriate. In summer, *rlung* pathogens are likely to be exuberant, so once in half a month is suitable. For the weak and the elderly, the frequency of sex should be decreased. For a patient with an active disease, or during recovery, no sex is allowed, or the condition will become worse. In summary, the frequency of sex should vary with one's constitution, age, interest, present condition and amount of endurance. It is unwise to consume at the same time one is nourishing.

By leading one's life by the principles of health cultivation, disease and misery can be avoided.

Key points for daily health care

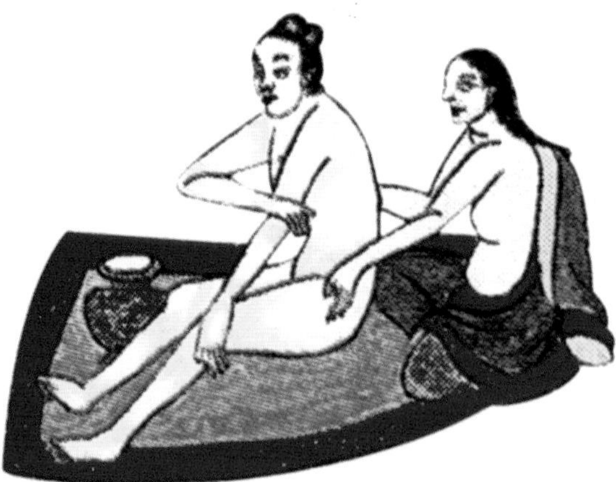

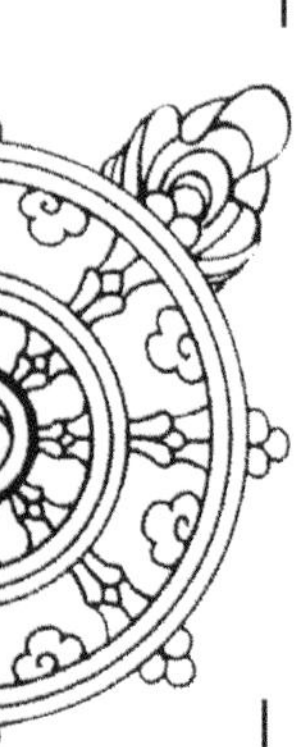

Frequently rubbing the body with oil prolongs life and expels wind.

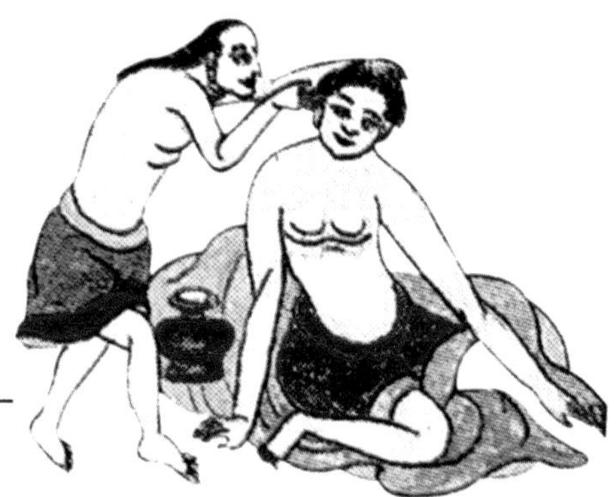

Rubbing oil on the head, limbs and ears eases one's body and mind.

Health massage: rub or massage the body with sesame oil, concentrating on the head, face, limbs, and ears. If frequently practiced, this can eliminate fatigue, ease the body and mind, promote the muscles and delay aging.

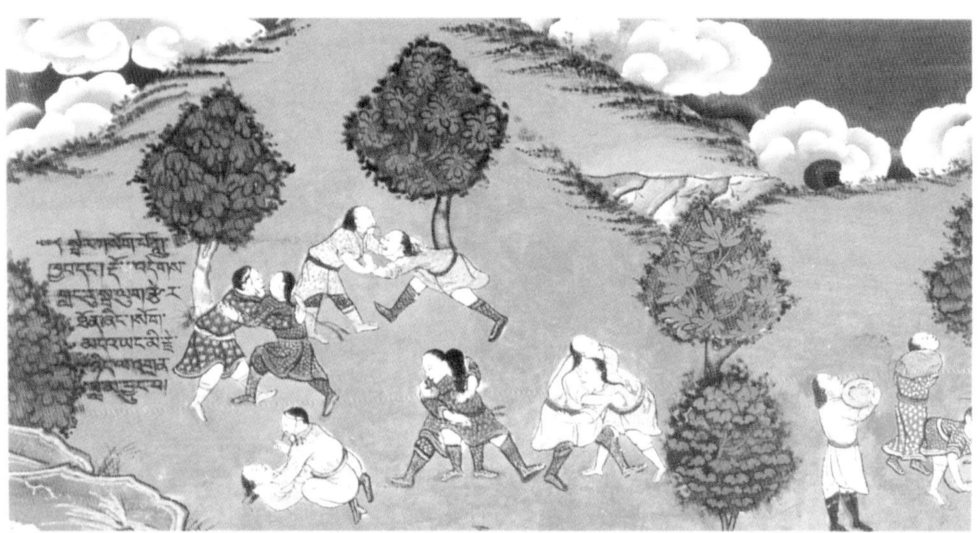

Wrestling is a common activity among the Tibetan people (part of a Tibetan mural).

Healthy sports: frequent and appropriate movement is very helpful. One must choose sports that are appropriate to one's own condition, and practice so that sweating is not profuse. Long-term training makes one feel relaxed, decreases body fat, and promotes growth in children. But overstrain gives the opposite result and should be avoided in the elderly and those with weak constitutions.

After training, scrubbing and rubbing the body with oil followed by rubbing the body repeatedly with dry flour should be performed. This will strengthen the muscles and make the skin lustrous. With strong muscles *badkan* disease need not be feared.

Bathing: bathing the body in cold water, such as a stream or river in the 7th and 8th months, is helpful in strengthening yang, helping the body look healthy, eliminating bad odors, and prolonging life. For patients with ear diseases, or just after meals, do not wash the head or bathe with hot water.

Protection of the eyes: the eyes belong to the fire nature. Since *badkan* belongs to the water and earth natures, diseases of *badkan* are harmful to the vision. The eyes will become inflamed and tears will flow. In this one can see the fire nature of the eyes and the water nature of *badkan* interacting. To strengthen and nurture the eyes, use barberry ointment drops in the eyes once a week.

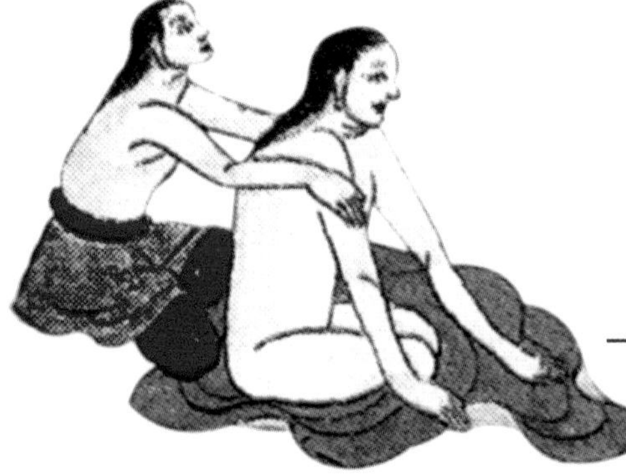

Scrubbing is beneficial to eliminate fat, moisten the skin, and strengthen the limbs.

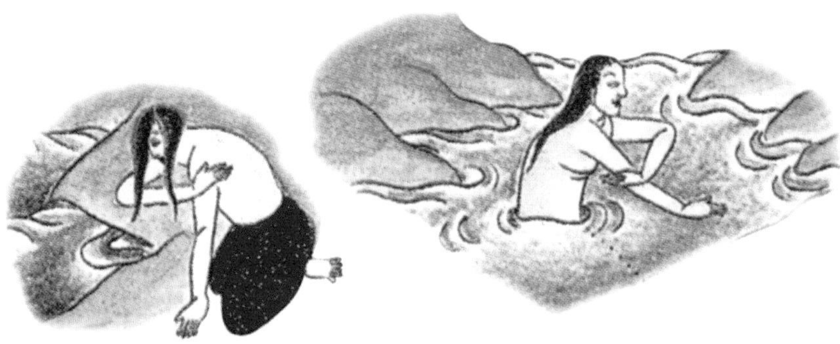

Frequent baths and swimming in hot springs can increase energy, nourish the complexion, and remove filth.

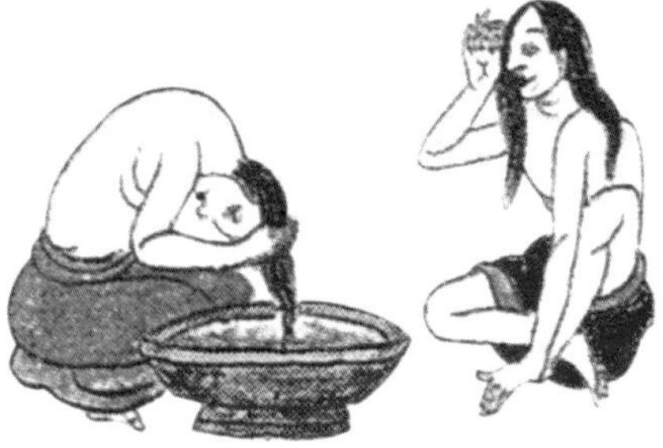

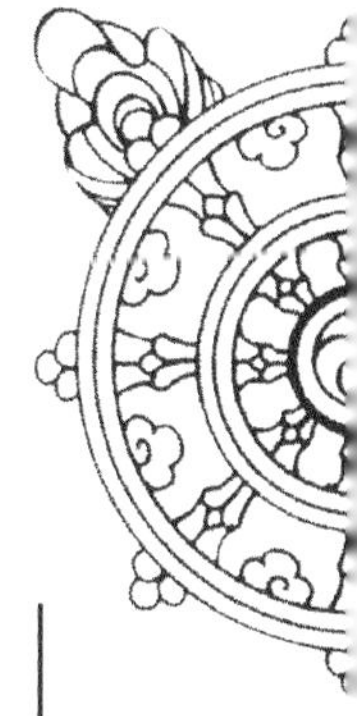

Wash the hair with warm water.
Hot water is harmful to the eyes and hair.

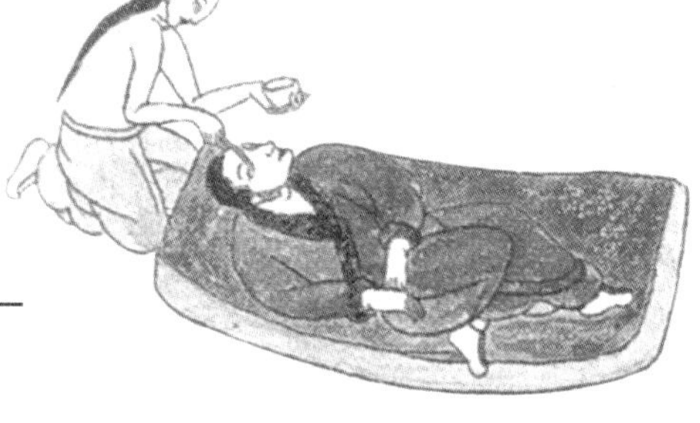

The eyes belong to the fire nature,
use medicinal drops once a week.

Tibetan medicine tells us that the best treatment is prevention. Therefore, one must master the basics of health cultivation. Naturally, all measures require consistent practice to achieve a satisfactory effect.

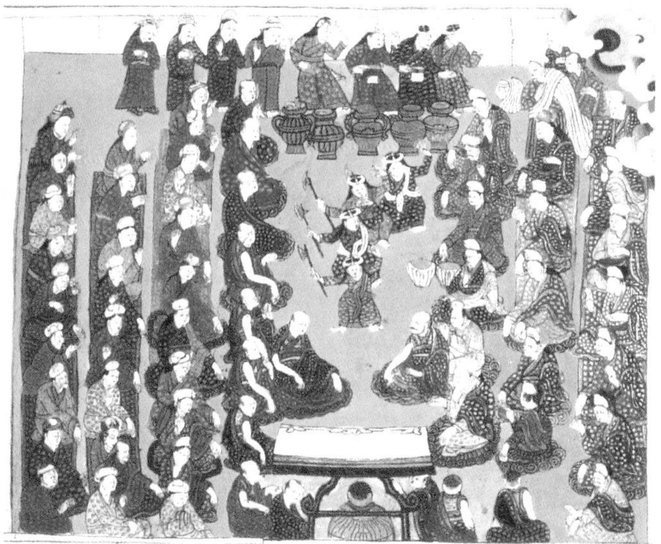

Dancing activates the body and improves the mood, being an important part of daily life for the Tibetan people part of a Tibetan mural.

Living according to nature

In order to enjoy the satisfaction when hunger and thirst are relieved by eating and drinking, the demands of the body should be guided by natural conditions so as to maintain health. In Tibetan medicine, compliance with physiological demands is highly stressed.

Hunger

When one feels hungry, if one does not eat in time, the body will be weakened. If, after a long time without food, one eats suddenly the appetite will be harmed, swallowing will become difficult, and dizziness or even fainting may occur. At this time, clear, dilute and easily digestible food that is low in calories should be eaten, such as porridge, wheat gruel or rice paste. After the appetite is recovered, food with more fat and dishes of a warm nature, such as broth, can be given in order to regain health. However, the best way is to avoid this situation by cultivating good and regular eating habits.

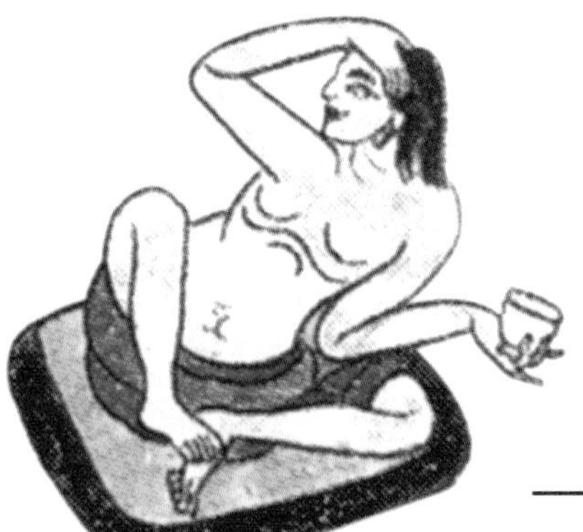

Suppressing hunger causes dizziness.

Thirst

Thirst and a dry mouth indicate that the body is in need of water. An adequate amount of water or other drinks should be taken. Suppressing desires to drink may lead to a shortage of water in the body, manifesting as thirst, dizziness, heart palpations, fever, or in severe cases even coma and loss of memory. If someone becomes ill due to thirst, move the patient to a cool ventilated place, and spray cool water on their face to resuscitate them. Then have them drink buttermilk diluted with wine and other cool drinks. Do not suppress the desire of thirst. Apply cooling treatment methods to cure illnesses due to the suppression of thirst.

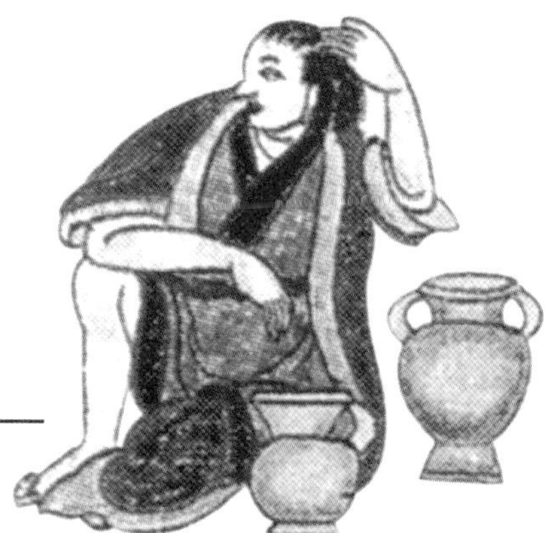

Suppressing thirst may result in dizziness and dry mouth.

Vomiting

Vomiting usually occurs after bad food is eaten or if stimulated by something in the environment (bad smells, etc.). Due to the mess that vomiting makes, people always try to prevent vomiting. This is harmful to health because if the filth is not expelled and is instead retained inside the body, the result will be loss of appetite, food blocking the esophagus, rough breathing and a predisposal to epidemics, edema, dermatitis and plagues. If any of these illnesses occur, one should fast, burn sandalwood, eaglewood and other aromatic materials to fumigate the nostrils, or boil them and keep the decoction in the mouth for a bit before swallowing. The aromatic properties can expel the filthy qi from the patient's body.

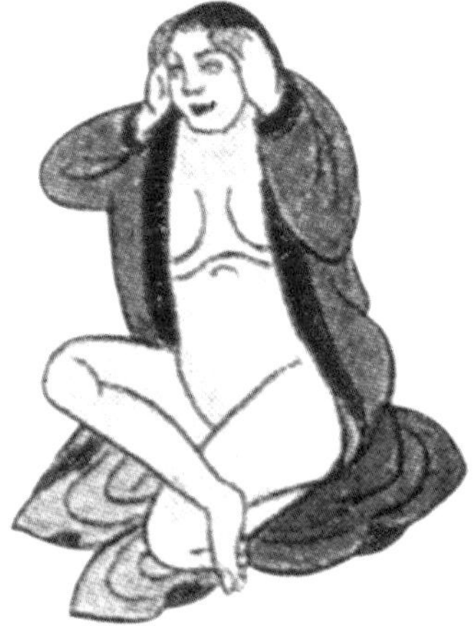

Suppressing vomiting may lead to a blocked sensation in the chest, edema and eye diseases.

Sneezing

Sneezing is a normal reaction of the body to expel pathogens. Suppression of sneezing may lead to a decline in the sensitivity of the sense organs, especially the eyes. Headache, hindered movements of the neck, a deviated mouth and face, and difficultly chewing may also occur. Use sandalwood and eaglewood to fumigate the nose and mouth, mix asafetida and nutmeg mixed with butter and drip into the nose, or look into the sunlight to cause sneezing. Of course, the best way is to sneeze freely and naturally when the desire comes.

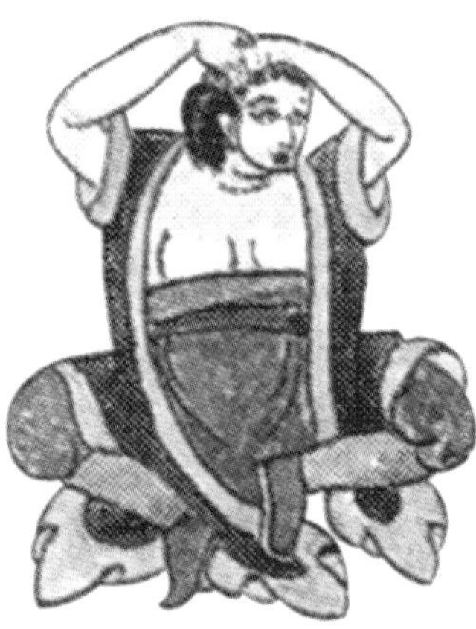

Suppressing sneezing may lead to blurred vision and headache.

Yawning

Yawning occurs when the body desires sleep and is a normal physiological reaction that shouldn't be suppressed. Suppressing yawning intentionally may lead to similar problems as suppressing sneezing. The treatment is also the same. All these illness are related to *rlung*. To treat, food or medicinals that eliminate wind can be taken, such as nutmeg powder, or *Asafetida Powder with Twenty-five Ingredients.*

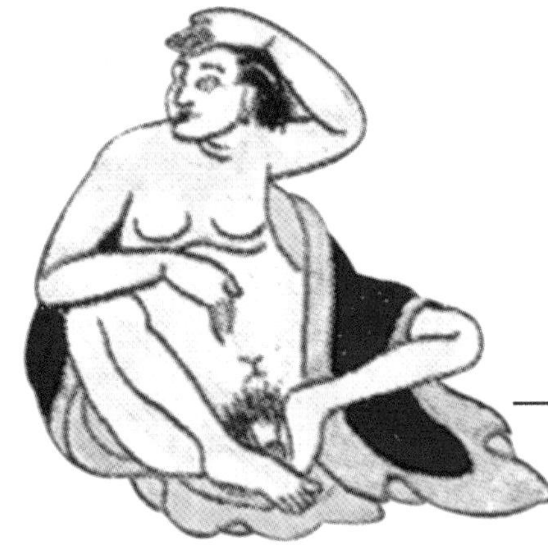

Suppressing yawning may lead to blurred vision and headache.

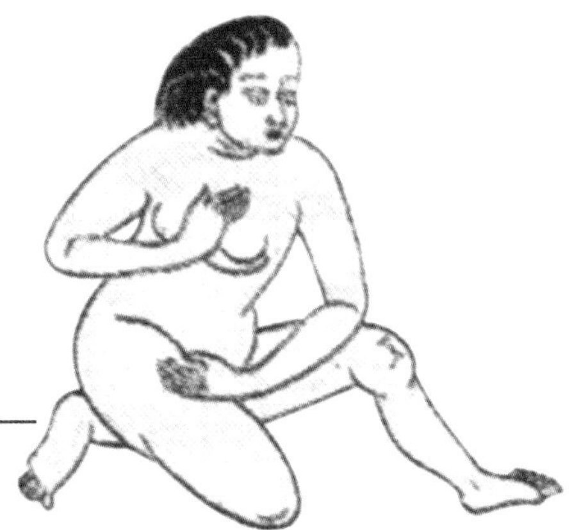

Rough breathing due to fatigue is likely to cause hard lumps and heart disease.

Wheezing

Overstrain may cause wheezing or difficulty breathing. Suppression of these may lead to internal blockages that result in lumps, heart disease, coma, loss of memory, or fainting. Proper treatment includes rest, and food or medicinals for eliminating wind are indicated. Habits that eliminate wind such as not wearing thin clothes on cold days, avoiding windy places or receiving topical therapies that eliminate wind are recommended.

Sleeping

Working late into the night or not sleeping at all is common nowadays. These are very harmful to health. Tibetan medicine claims that sleep is the main way the body combats fatigue. Lack of sleep or no sleep at all may lead to disturbances like frequent yawning, drowsiness, a heavy brain, blurred vision, and indigestion. Treatments include eating mutton or broth, rubbing the body with sesame oil, and restoring regular sleeping habits.

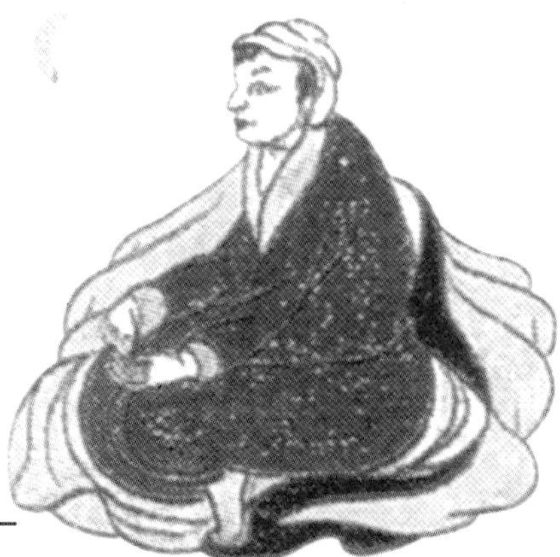

Suppressing sleeping may lead to yawning, fatigue, a heavy brain and indigestion.

Sputum

Profuse sputum often occurs in external diseases. As it is a pathological product, sputum should be excreted. Swallowing of sputum is very harmful. The breathing passages might become blocked causing difficulty breathing. Habitually swallowing sputum may cause emaciation, hiccough, heart disease, or loss of appetite. Treatment includes taking ginger, brown sugar, and long pepper which can effectively expel sputum. However, the best treatment is to avoid catching colds.

Crying

Crying is a way of pouring out one's sorrow. Suppressing tears is harmful to the body and may cause heart disease, dizziness, headache, runny nose, and loss of appetite. Treatment includes sleeping to supplement energy, and drinking and chatting with good friends to relieve vexation. However, natural crying is good for health.

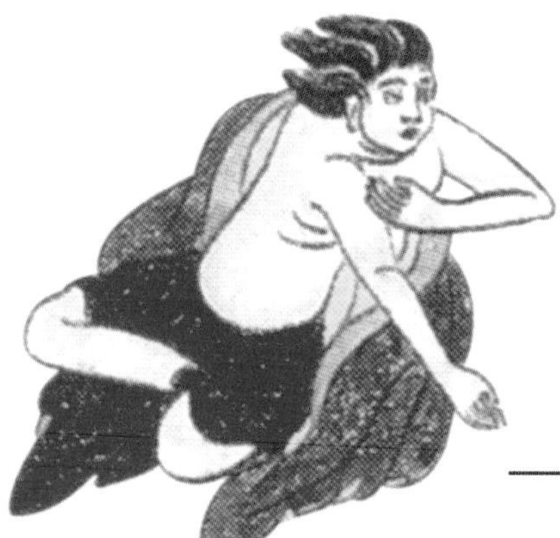

Swallowing sputum may cause sputum to increase, rough breathing, and hiccough.

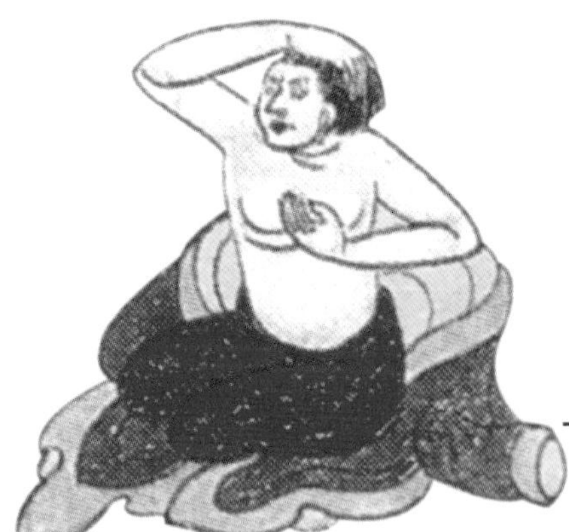

Suppressing crying may cause heart pain, headache, runny nose, and loss of appetite.

Defecation and farting

Both are important ways the body expels toxins. Normal defecation and farting promotes the metabolism. Holding back of farts may cause constipation, tumors and masses, distended organs, blurred vision, poor digestion and heart disease. Suppressing defecation may cause counterflow of air, leading to a bad smell in the mouth, headache, convulsion of the limbs, and catching colds. Treatment includes normal defecation habits and not holding back farts. Proper flow is very important to health.

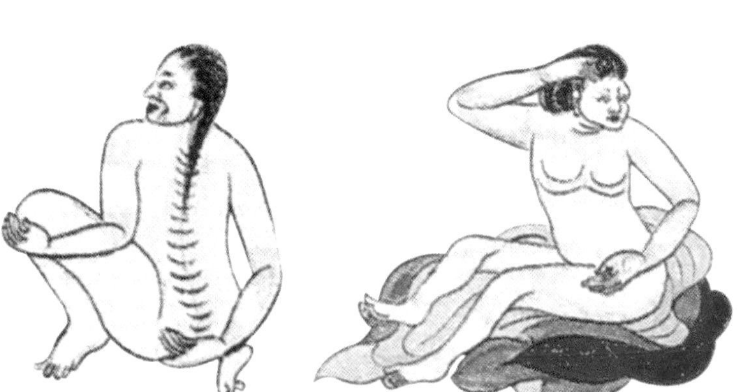

Suppressing defecation and farting may lead to constipation, the formation of masses, and colicky pain.

Urination and ejaculation

Being metabolic products, urine and semen shouldn't be prevented from being excreted. Suppressing urination is likely to cause kidney stones and diseases of the penis or the urethral opening. Harm to the descending *rlung* can be caused by suppressing defecation, farting or urination. To avoid this, mild or drastic purgatives can be administered as enemas, or one can wash in a hot spring or with *Five Ingredient Nectar*. Rubbing the lower body with sesame oil, or using a hot compress or fur dipped in wine is also effective. Nourishing medication should be used.

Suppressing ejaculation can cause dripping of semen, pain in the penis, inability to urinate, kidney stones, impotence and a decrease in sexual desire. Treatment includes draining the urethra and hot compresses. Intercourse is also necessary to expel the semen that is retained in the body. Drinking of vegetable oil, milk, wine and poultry can serve to nourish and strengthen yang.

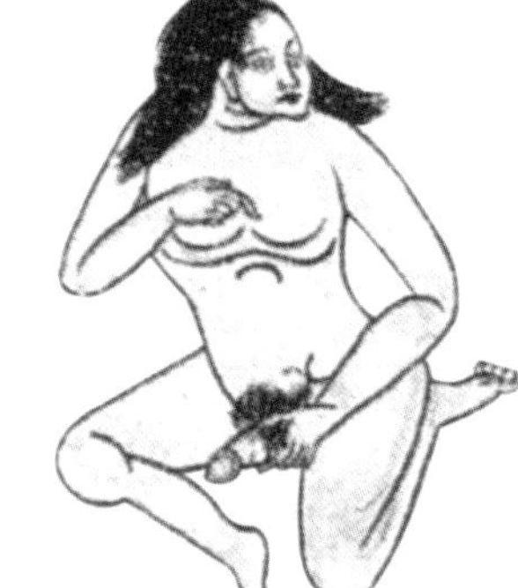

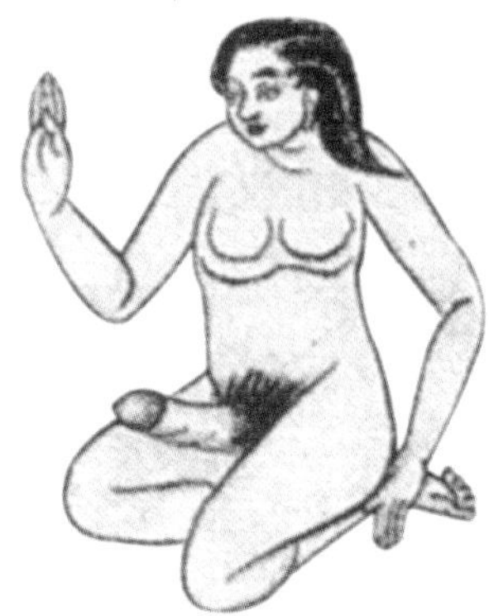

Suppressing urination and ejaculation may cause kidney stones, inflammation of the urethra and impotence.

All of the above actions of the body should be allowed to happen naturally. Prevention is necessary when no disease is present. One must understand cause and effect and the advantages and disadvantages of all actions. Let all behavior comply with the natural processes of the body. This is the basic tenet of health cultivation.

Just like hunger demands eating and thirst demands drinking, to ensure health, the natural functions of the body should be guided by natural desire, instead of suppression.

Avoiding danger

In addition to disease, sudden attacks or accidents may also seriously threaten one' s health. Tibetan medicine also stresses proper daily behavior so danger can be avoided. One must avoid activities that threaten health. *The Four Medical Tantras* lists a variety of conditions that endanger health and life. By examining these activities one can understand what one should do to cultivate health.

Crossing a river

Before crossing, the speed of running water should be tested. Do not cross a river by wading or swimming when the depth of the stream is not clear. Torrential streams or circumstances where there is nobody to help in case of an accident should be avoided.

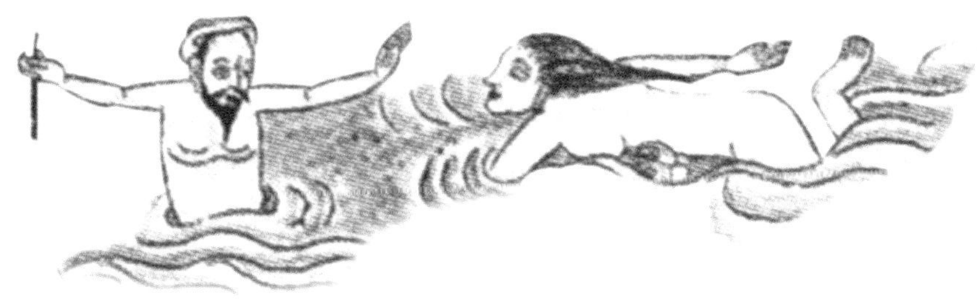

Do not force a river crossing.

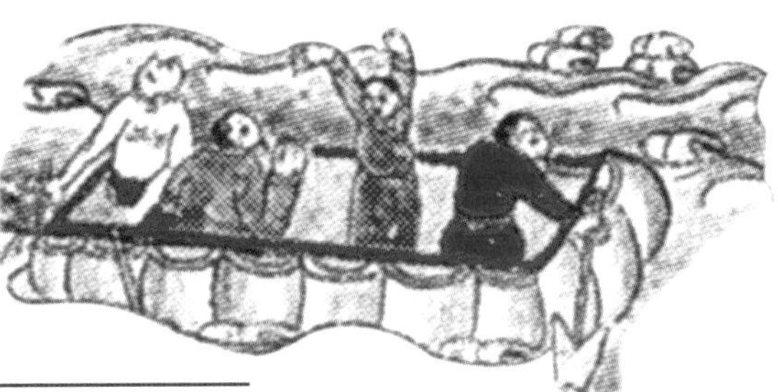

Do not travel on a dangerous boat.

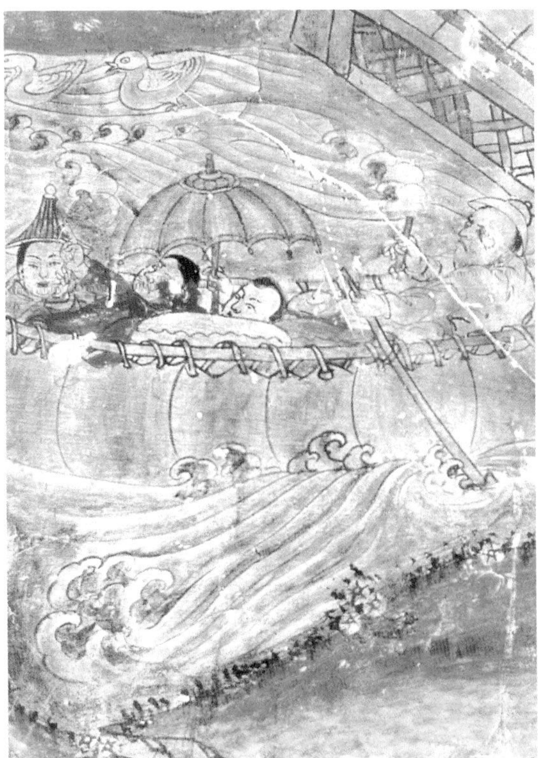

Cowhide rafts are common in Tibet part of a Tibetan mural.

Traveling instruments

When traveling by boat, do not ride on boats with broken sails or broken bottoms. Cattle should be tamed or inherently mild. Careful selection of good traveling instruments is essential.

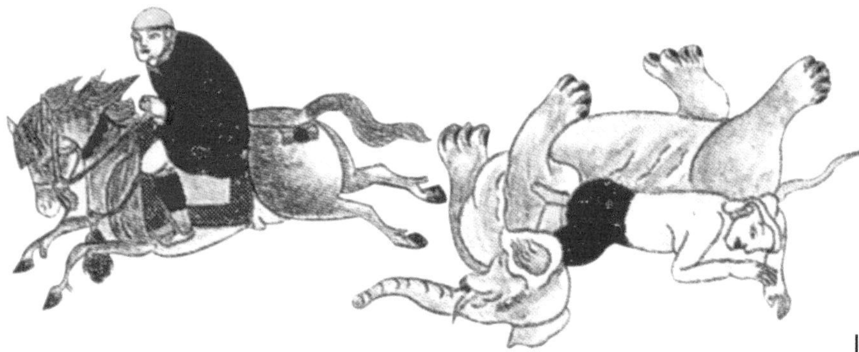

Do not ride on an inferior horse.

Traveling

When traveling, pay attention to the security of places along the way. Avoid places known for robbers and fierce animals. Choose a secure route for traveling. Forests or grasslands that have recently been on fire but are not completely extinguished should be avoided.

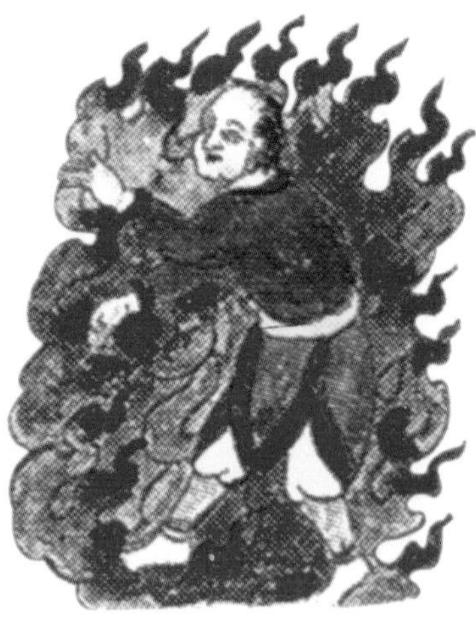

Keep distance from fire.

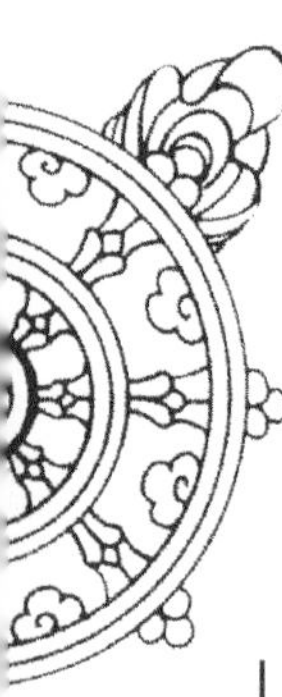

Avoiding danger in summer

In summer roads and trails may be covered with dense plants and the way can not be seen clearly. Care should be taken so that one does not fall off a cliff or down a steep slope. Insufficient care while walking could lead to life-threatening falls.

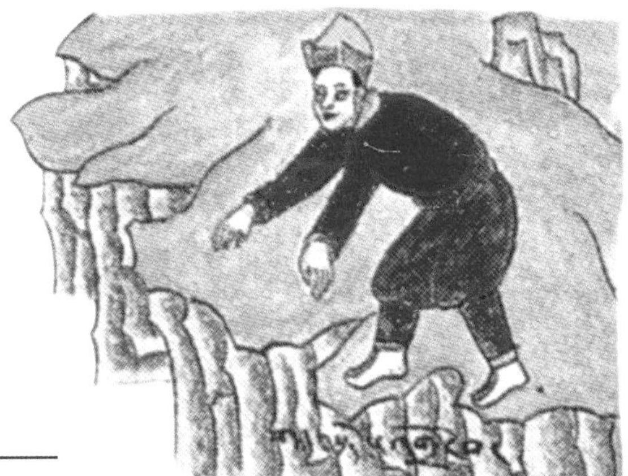

In summer stay away from cliffs.

Avoiding danger in winter

In winter, leaves fall down and a tree's water and nutrients flow to its roots, causing the branches to become fragile. Do not climb trees as it is easy to fall because of broken branches.

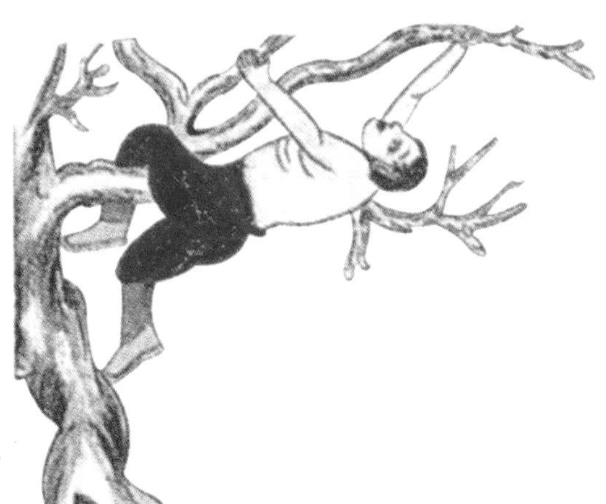

Do not climb trees in winter.

Avoiding danger at night

Do not travel late at night because fierce beasts and robbers may be hiding and waiting. If travel is unavoidable, bring a big stick, weapon or travel with strong friends.

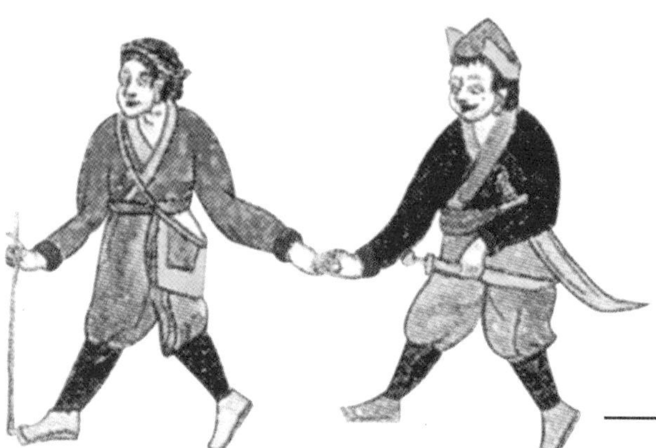

Travel in groups at night.

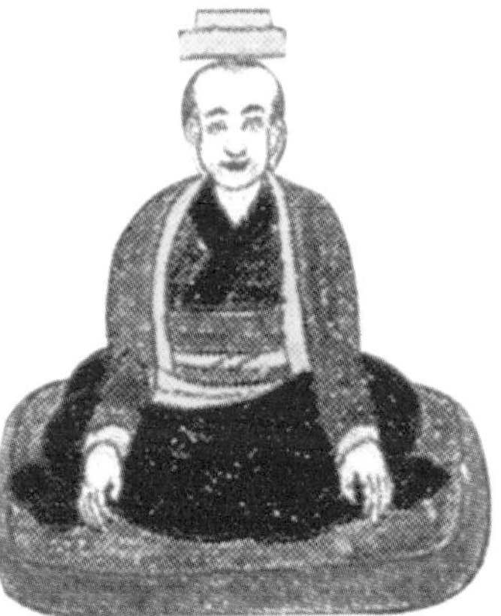

Bring excellent medicine.

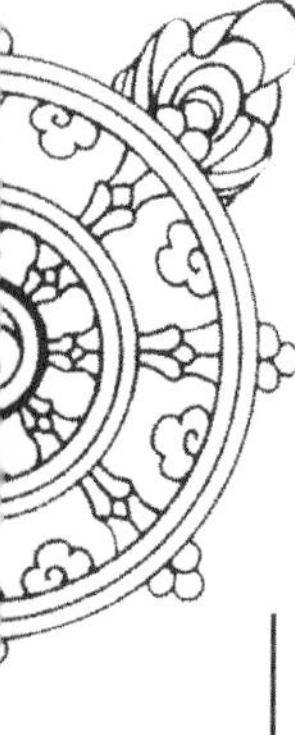

Avoiding danger as a patient

Patients with heart disease or that have had a stroke should avoid long trips and big movements which may cause their condition to get worse. Good medicine should be carried at all times for emergency use.

Keeping distance from trouble

While traveling, do not try to stop people who are quarreling when the situation is unclear. Quickly leave and don't stay around and watch, avoiding unnecessary trouble.

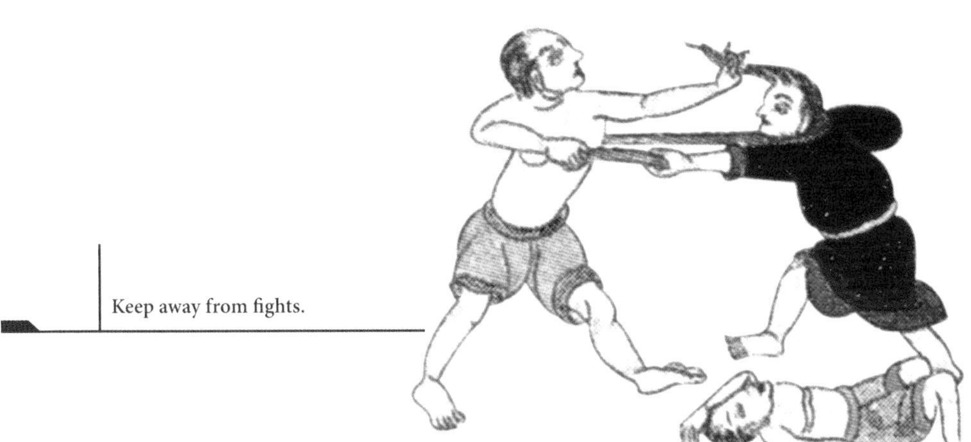

Keep away from fights.

In short, plan carefully before traveling. Examine the places one chooses to rest. Careful planning will ensure safety and help avoid danger.

Internally, avoid fatigue in body, speech and mind. Externally, fight against all outside causes of disease. By so doing, longevity and a naturally long life is possible.

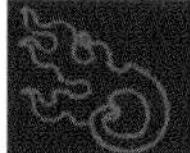

Behavior in Accordance with Buddhist Teachings

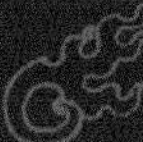

Under the influence of Buddhism, the principles of health cultivation in Tibetan medicine have adopted Buddhist ideas that are beneficial to the moral norms of body and mind. Wellbeing and happiness in life can only be achieved at the root through behavior in accordance with Buddhist teachings. *The Four Medical Tantras* says, "For the happiness of all creatures endeavoring in the affairs of the world, happiness may become the source of all miseries if there are no Buddhist teachings." The eulogy of *Sutra of Preserving Life* says, "A man over fifty-five years of age who has accumulated merits by selfless efforts based on the true teachings can achieve happiness and wellbeing without any disasters." Here, the true teachings refer to the teachings of the Buddha, which play a very prominent role in Tibetan health cultivation.

Doing good deeds

Helping others

Trying to help others attain happiness is the highest concern in Tibetan medicine.

Helping others to avoid irritation and vexation

Vexation and irritation is a shadow on daily life, which can come at any time and can not be driven away. When someone is irritable and vexed it is good to chat quietly with them, listening to their complaints and helping to solve their problems so that they can live happily. If a person's friends are free from irritation and vexation then he will feel happy as well. Helping others to be free from irritation and vexation is a good deed that one should be happy to do.

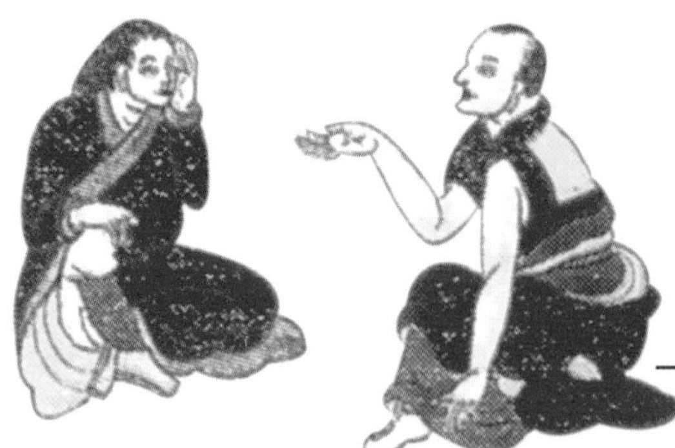

Enthusiastically help others to be free from irritation and vexation.

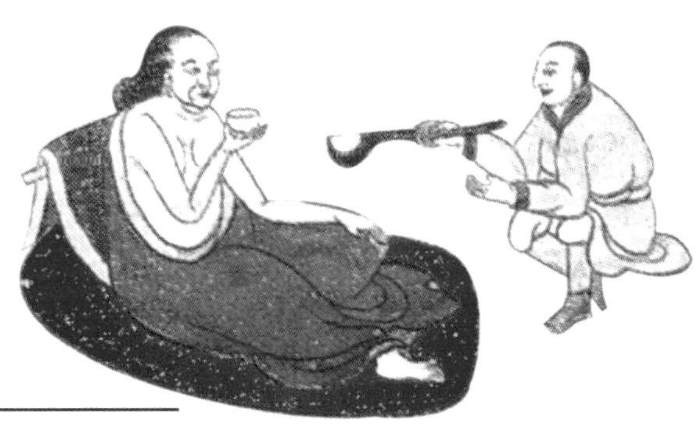

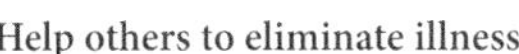

Help others to eliminate illness.

Helping others to eliminate illness

Diseases come with life. They jeopardize not only one's health, but one's happiness as well. All sick people hope for a state of beautiful health after recovery. We must help them. Doctors should help with their know-how. Those who do not know medicine can donate money or other materials, give sympathy, or pray for their health. In short, do anything that will help them escape from the misery of disease.

Helping others to escape from poverty

Whatever your condition is, there will be someone poorer than yourself. They have met with difficulties in their life. For those following the true Buddhist teachings, it is a duty to help the less fortunate escape from poverty. Donating money or other things, or simply visiting them are good deeds. Show warmth to the less fortunate! With high morals help others live well.

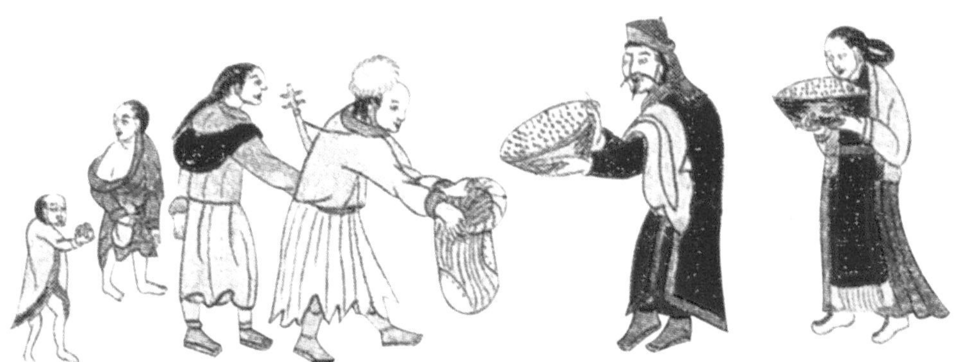

Helping others to escape from poverty.

Treating others well

All beings are equal! To treat others well is to treat oneself well!

Respecting Buddhist monks

Buddhist monks are ardently pursuing the teachings of Buddha. They are people who lead us on the road of Buddhism, and are models for our speech and behavior. We must respect them; respect their morals and their practices. Do not blame them, insult them, or cheat them in any way.

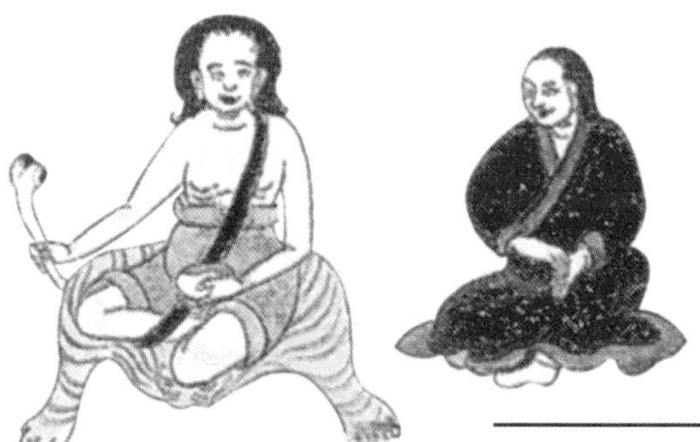

Respecting Buddhist monks.

Respecting those who give donations

One must respect those who give anything, especially tutors who teach you knowledge. We must never forget their favors. Your parents, uncles and aunts, sisters and brothers teach you how to live, they are people who have given great favors and have high morality. You must be filial to and respect them. Obey the elderly! Do not abandon them, or become estranged from them.

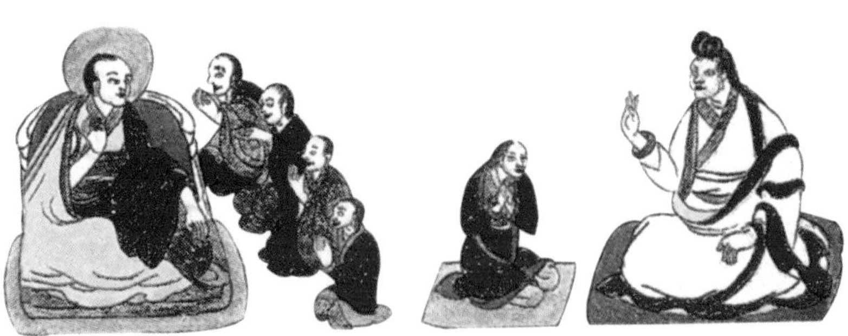

Respect your tutors, benefactors and the elderly.

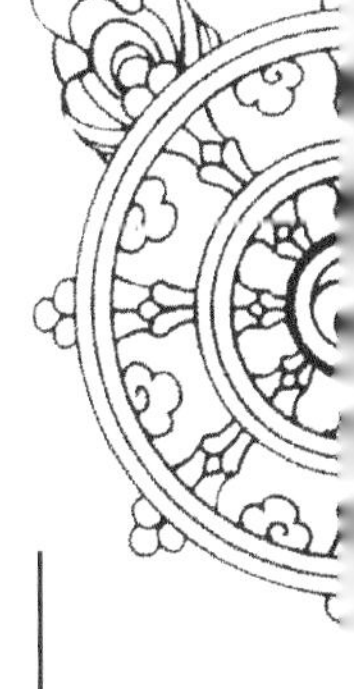

Treating other with sincerity and faith

To promote communication with others, you must treat them with sincerity and faith. Without sincerity, people won't trust you. Whatever the conditions, and whoever you are facing, sincerity is important. Only sincerity and faith will lead to progress on the path of Buddhist teachings.

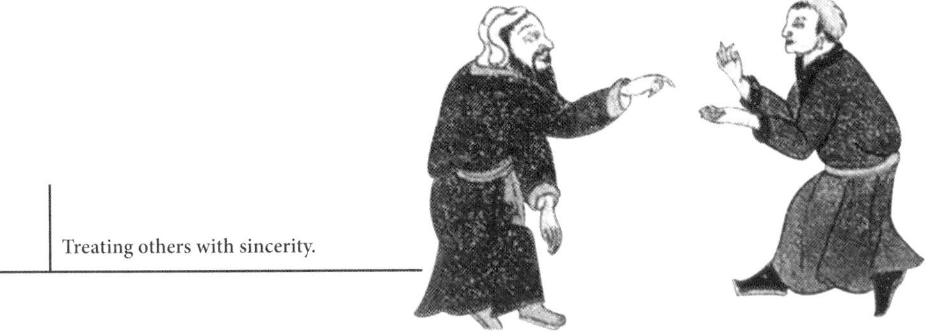

Treating others with sincerity.

Treating all creatures well

All people are equal. Thus, one must treat others like treating oneself. Do not abuse or beat other people. Do not lie, cheat, or con others. Comfort others with kind words when they need help. One must be peaceful and kind in one's body, speech, and mind to show loving care towards others.

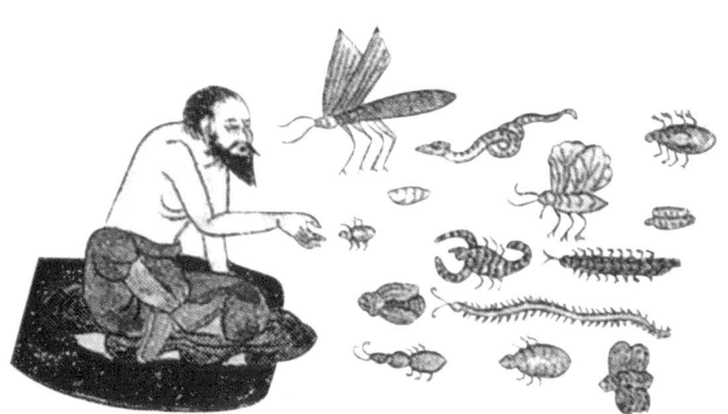

Love all creatures like you love yourself.

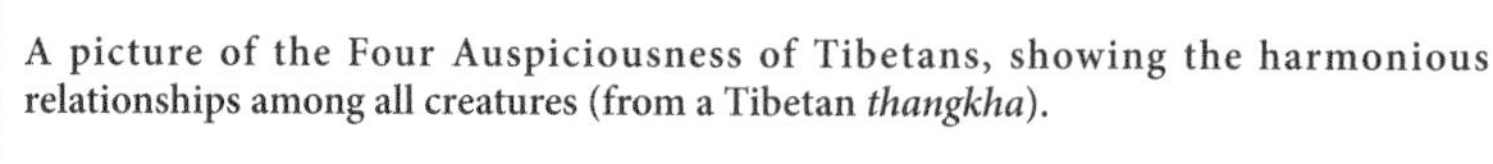

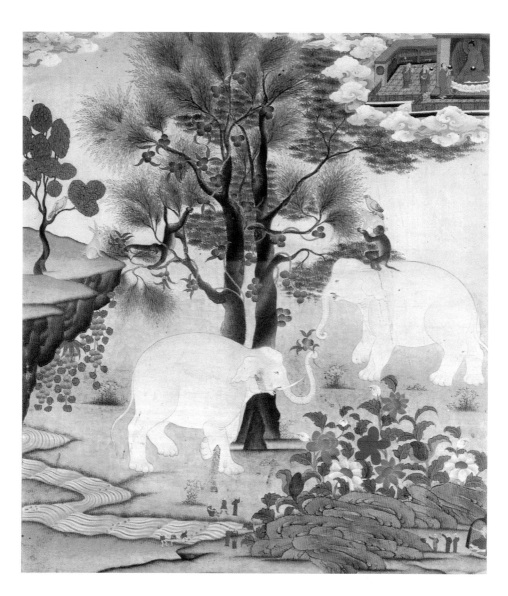

A picture of the Four Auspiciousness of Tibetans, showing the harmonious relationships among all creatures (from a Tibetan *thangkha*).

Forgiving others

One must be big-hearted towards those who have committed mistakes and repented. To those who are hostile, you should not ignore them, but you should avoid their rash behavior. You should conquer them with kindness like a spring breeze. To evil doers, you must convince them with words, principles and emotions so that they can understand their mistakes and eventually become your friends. Progress in the true teachings of Buddha is possible only by accomplishing these deeds.

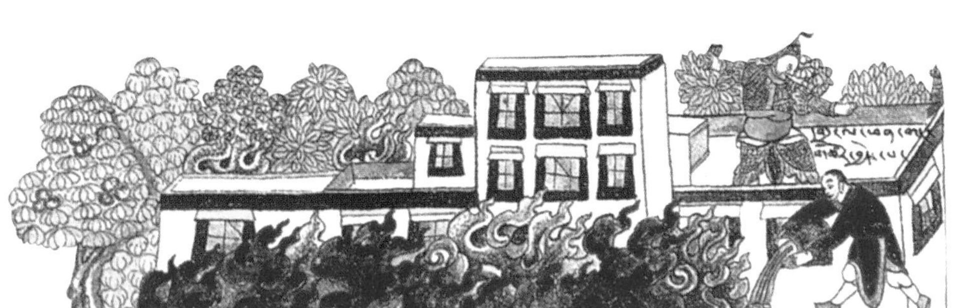

Be big-hearted to others, and return a good deed for an evil one.

Treating oneself well

To achieve longevity by following pure Buddhist behaviors, one must not only treat others well and help others, but one must treat oneself well also.

Be diligent in work

Do not neglect your career. You must be loyal to your own path so as to create and accumulate wealth and not to waste it. Of course, one must not be stingy either. At the same time work hard to cultivate high morals.

Be peaceful

No matter what a person does, one must do it bravely. Be kind to others. Whenever you are victorious do not become proud. Even if you are skilled in worldly affairs and culture do not become proud. Instead, be honest, careful, and avoid arrogance. When one is poor, do not be greedy or try to take other's wealth.

Other proper actions

Do not seduce or slander. Do not scold others with a lower social position than yours when they commit wrongs. Do not envy other people with a higher social position than you. Do not harm the Buddha, Dharma, or community of monks. Treat monks and lay people equally well.

Carefully ponder before starting something, and once you decide to do it, do it well without delay. Do not regret even if the outcome is not satisfactory, this will only cause trouble for yourself.

In short, good behavior includes treating others well, treating yourself well, and being happy to help others. Practicing these three principles conscientiously leads to smooth progress on the path of pure Buddhist teachings. By doing so, you will not be cheated even if you are alone, instead, you will be respected by all.

> One must endeavor to walk on the path of true Buddhist teachings, for the wellbeing and happiness of all creatures. Without this, happiness will become misery.

Taboos

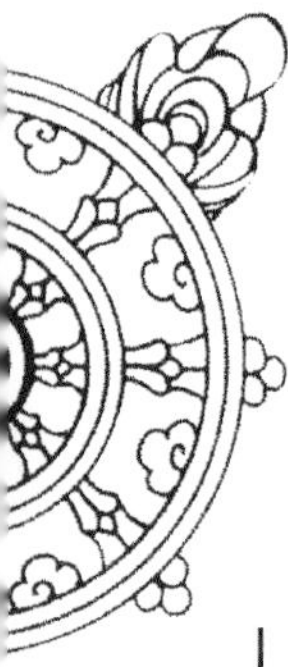

Taboo against disdaining the Buddha

This means disrespecting the Buddha. In the eyes of the Tibetans, Buddha occupies a holy position, and this is the reason why the Tibetan people include respecting Buddha as an essential part of health cultivation. Specifically this includes not sitting on Buddhist statues or sutras, and not having intercourse in front of a Buddha statue. A pure mind is the basis of longevity.

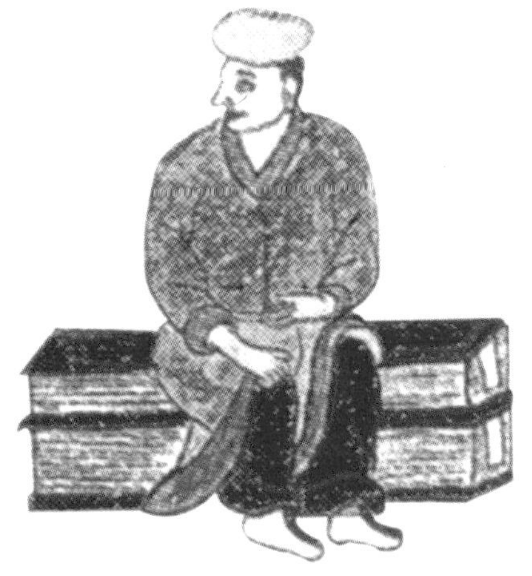

Do not sit on Buddhist sutras.

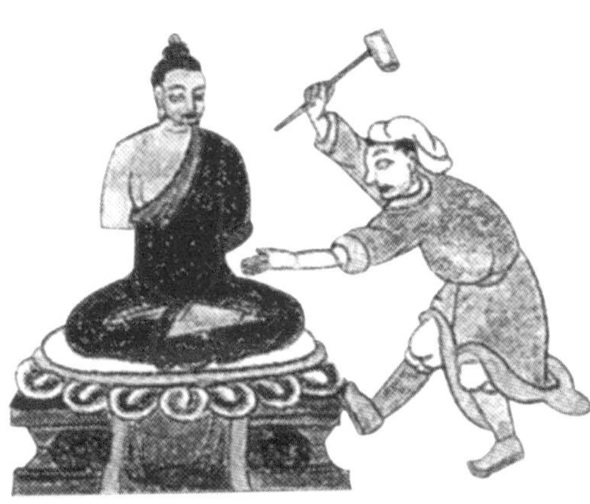

Do not destroy Buddhist statues.

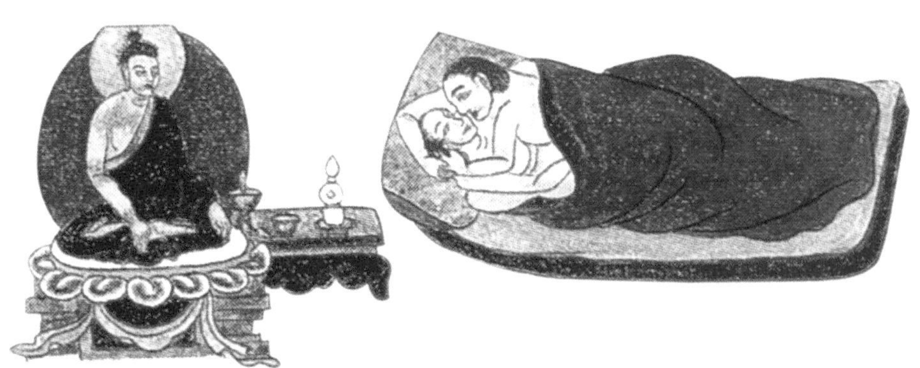

Avoid intercourse in front of a Buddhist statue.

Taboo against violence

Violence will not eliminate divisions between people, rather it deepens the differences and increases feelings of enmity, causing an endless cycle of retaliation. When someone offends you, no matter how serious it injures you, never choose murder to solve the problem. Use the law and morality to regulate your attitude and solve the disagreement.

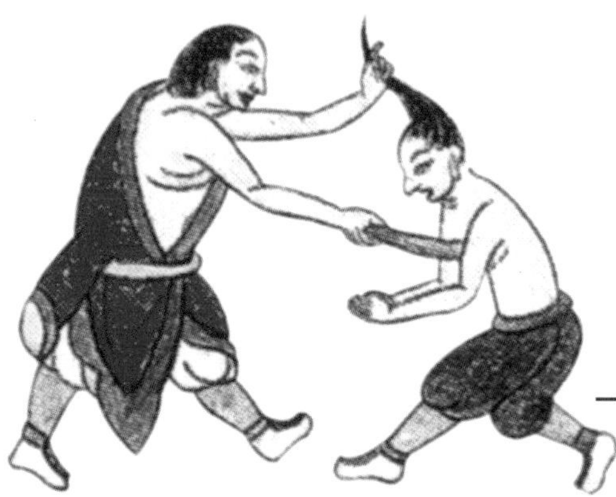

Taboo against murder.

Taboo against stealing

Legally or illegally, stealing is an obscene and base behavior. It is a shameful thing to obtain wealth unlawfully. It shows an unhealthy and deceitful mind. Never try to steal anything from other people, even a tiny object. Such action will leave a shadow on your heart forever. If one happens to steal, quickly correct the wrong and stop this malicious behavior. Stealing goes against true Buddhist teachings and will destroy your life.

Those practicing pure Buddhist teachings will not be limited by other people even if he himself is a servant. Instead, he will be respected by other people. For eternal happiness, practice diligently.

Taboo against obscenity

Sexual intercourse is moral and natural. *The Four Medical Tantras* says, "Among all the desires, sexual desire is the loftiest." However, abnormal sexual practices are contemptible. It destroys the will, disturbs Buddhist practices, and injures both mind

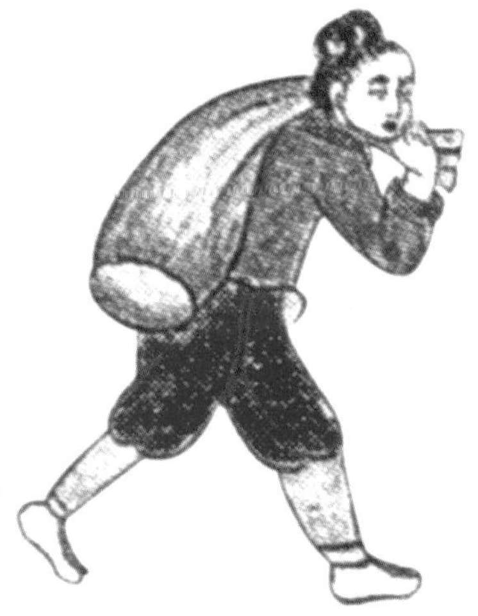

Taboo against stealing.

and body. Tibetan medicine objects to adultery, rape, and intercourse in the daytime. Avoiding all such distractions gives purity to the mind, and creates a strong foundation for practicing Buddhism and cultivating health.

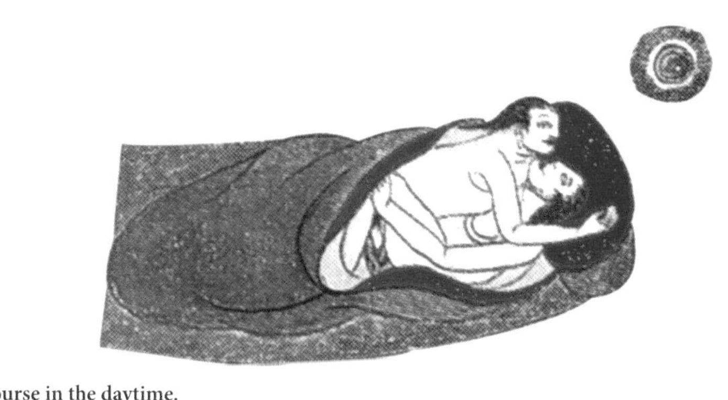

Do not have intercourse in the daytime.

Taboo against lying and talking nonsense

One should not lie, talk nonsense or distort the facts. In Buddhism, refraining from talking nonsense is the most important of the Five Taboos. Following this rule is essential to those that practice health cultivation. Honesty is the most important quality in making friends. Never deceive! Do not hurt others with malicious words. Be especially careful not to talk nonsense to those who are sensitive or have fragile minds. Pray for close friends to have eternal friendship. Never start discord between people. This will hurt both them and yourself and will cause you to lose friends.

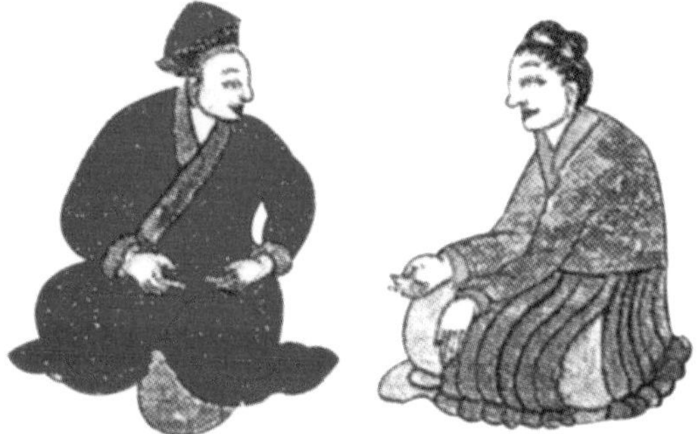

Do not cheat

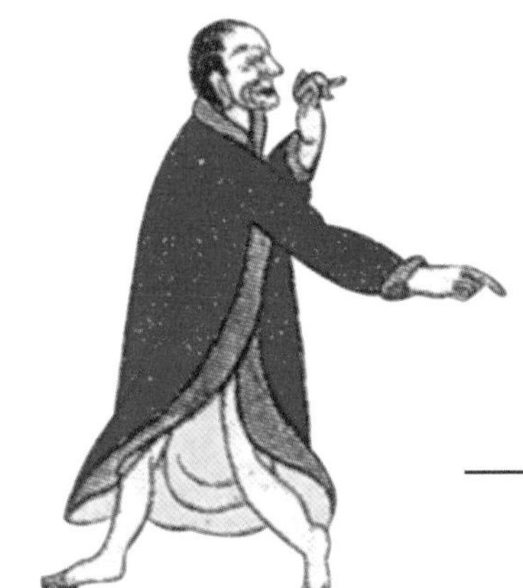

Do not hurt others with malicious language.

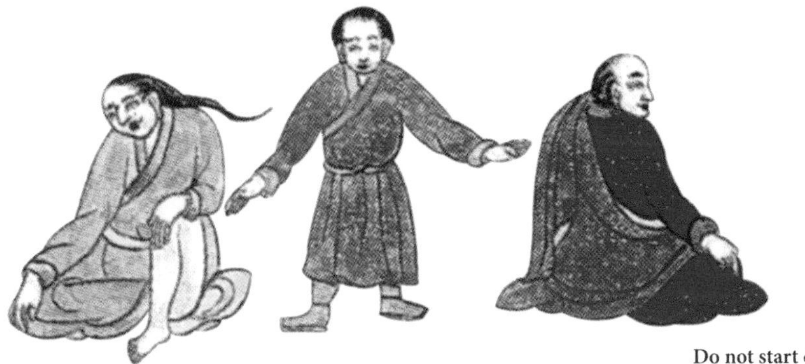

Do not start discord.

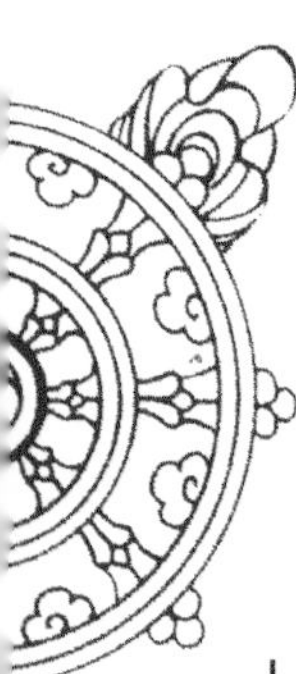

Taboo against wild fancies

This refers to immoral ideas to obtain wealth from other people. It is especially important not to have evil thoughts when other people have fame and wealth, as these will destroy a pure mind. Without a pure mind, how can anyone follow the teachings of Buddha?

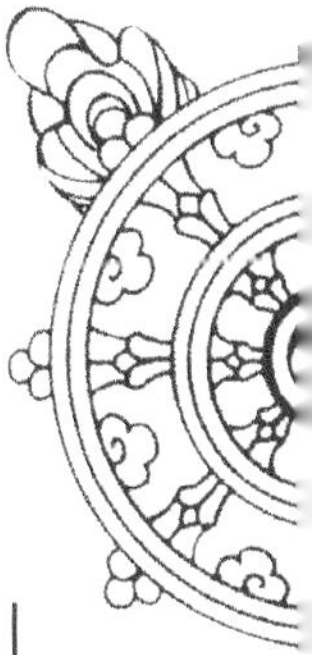

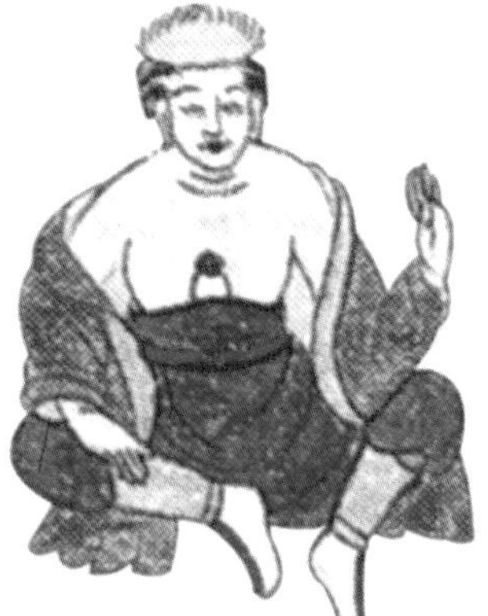

Do not envy other people's wealth.

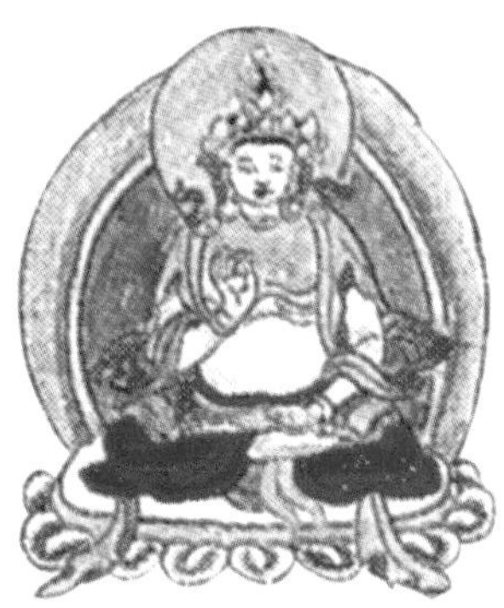

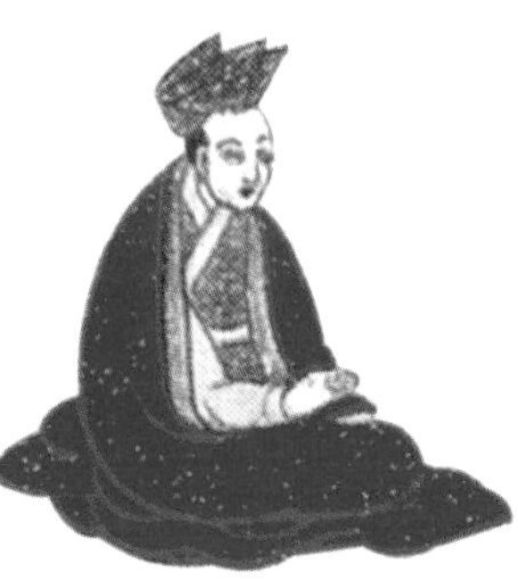

Do not harbor evil ideas.

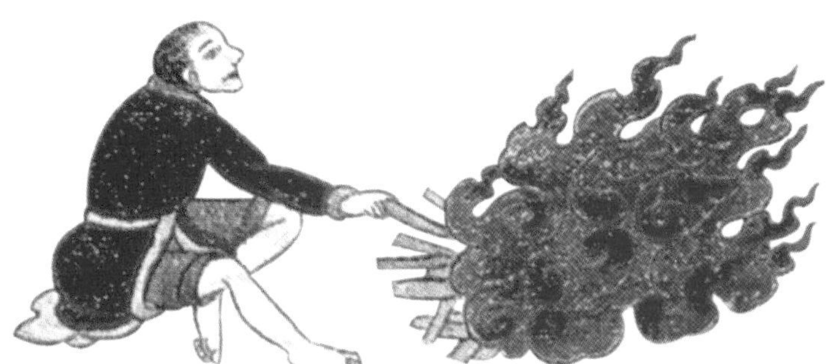

Do not generate ideas of hurting others.

In short, malicious behavior is outside the teachings of pure Buddhism. One must correct their behavior so it conforms to Buddhist teachings and live without performing malicious acts. Only then can the true essence emerge into your speech and acts.

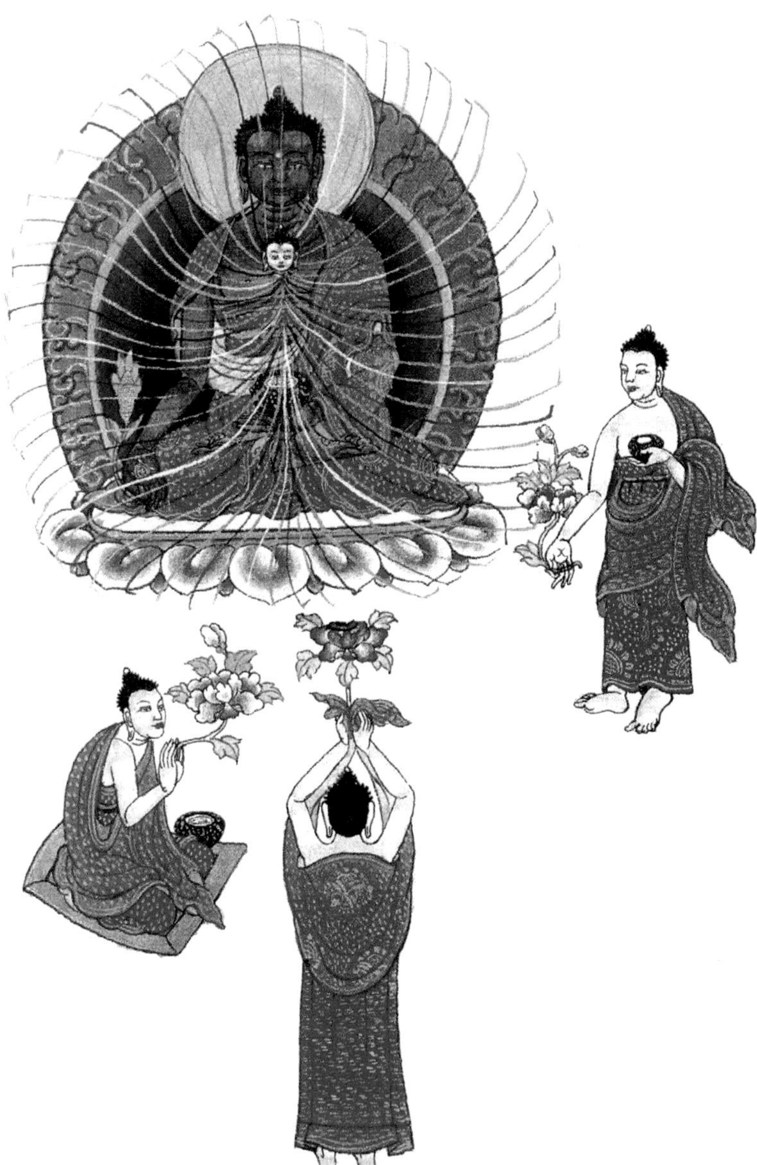

Correct you body, speech, and mind to fall in line with Buddhist teachings. This is the root of health cultivation (part of *Thangkha* two in the *Sman thang* series of *The Four Medical Tantras*).

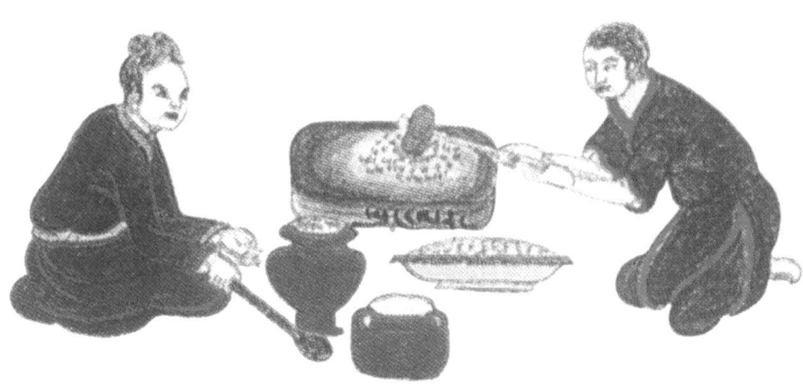

ཟས་སྐོམ་གྱི་ལུས་བྲུངས་གསོ་བ།

CHAPTER 5 HEALTH CULTIVATION THROUGH DIET

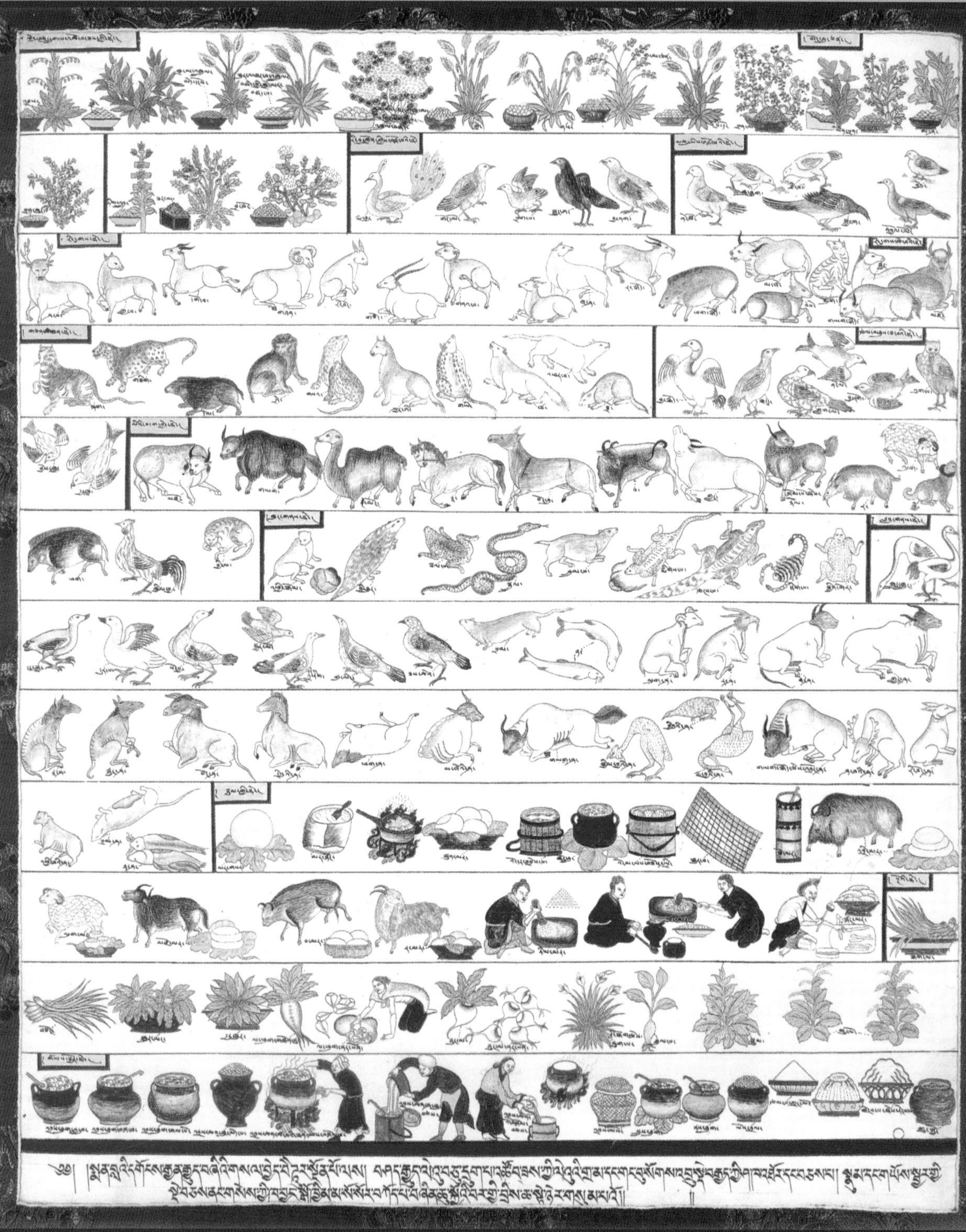

Diet, from *Thangkha* twenty-three in the *Sman thang* series of *The Four Medical Tantras*.

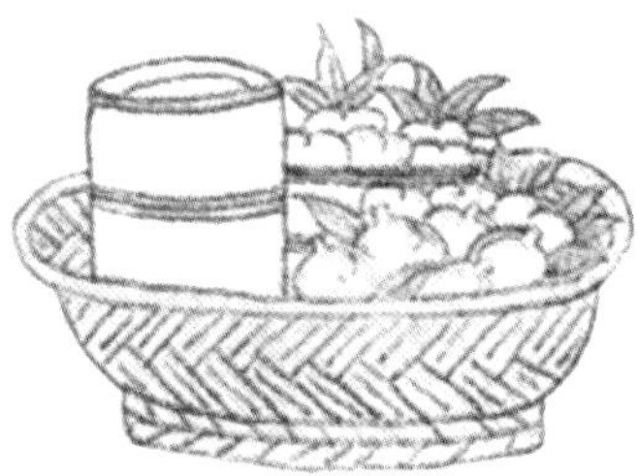

On the vast, snowy plateau of Tibet, the natural conditions have bestowed the living things there with the intelligence of the earth. All birds in the sky, fish in the water, and beasts on the earth follow the plants to absorb the essence of the universe.

People all over this snowy land communicate with the universe through religious practices on one end, and utilizing the food chain to establish the harmony between man and the universe on the other. Within the scope of Tibetan medicine, dietary theory is very comprehensive, and the functions of the different foods are extremely refined. It exemplifies the wonderful essence and the summation of experience of successive ages in Tibetan medicine. It is the basis for the reproduction and prosperity of the Tibetan people.

Drink

Tibetan medicine summarizes three categories of beverages: milk, water, and wine. Generally, these beverages have a light and loose nature and are beneficial to the body. However, drinking too much of any type is harmful. Milk treats *rlung* diseases, water treats *mkhris pa* diseases, and wine treats cold *badkan* diseases. Drinking too much milk may cause *badkan* diseases, drinking too much water may cause *rlung* diseases, and drinking too much wine may cause *mkhris pa* diseases.

Drinking milk

Most of the milk that is drunk in Tibet is cow or yak milk. Most kinds of milk are sweet, heavy, cool, moist, and have a suppressive nature. It strengthens the constitution, nourishes the spirit, makes the skin lustrous, moistens the muscles, and treats *mkhris pa* and *rlung* diseases. Tibetan medicine also categorizes other animal's milk, each with its own taste and nature.

Yellow cow's milk

This is the most nutritious kind of milk. It makes one intelligent and clever and is a tonic for strengthening the mind and body, moistens the muscles, and promotes lactation. It is indicated in stubborn lung diseases and chronic cases of frequent urination.

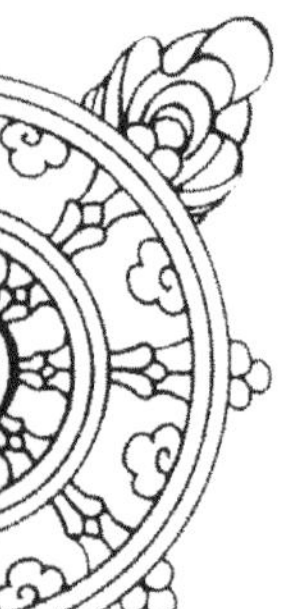

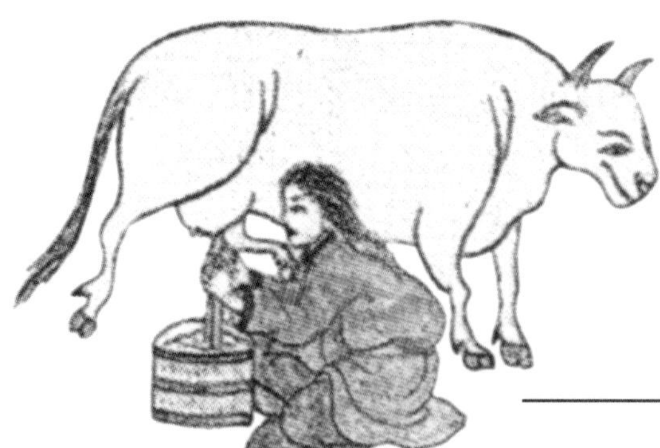

Yellow cow's milk.

Yak's milk

Yak milk is warm, heavy and nutritious, removes *rlung* diseases but is harmful to those with *mkhris pa* and *badkan* diseases. This is the main type of milk in Tibet.

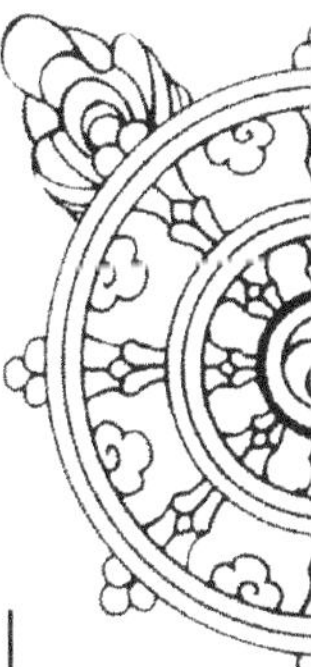

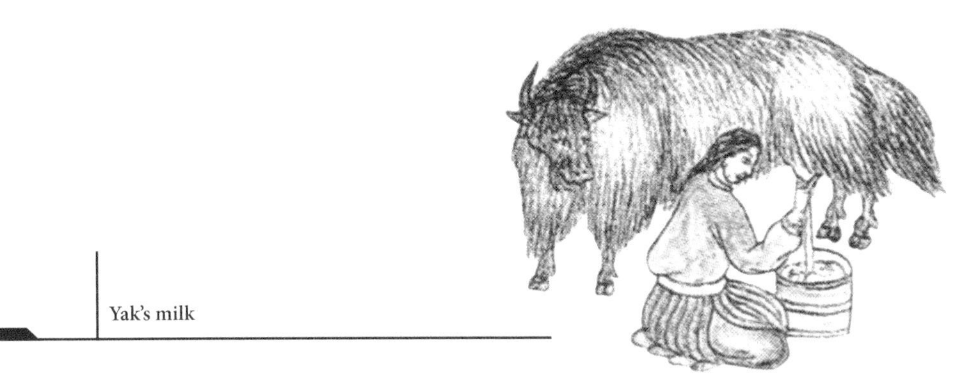

Yak's milk

Goat's milk

It is light, cool, calms wheezing, treats vexation and thirst, difficulty breathing, and epidemics.

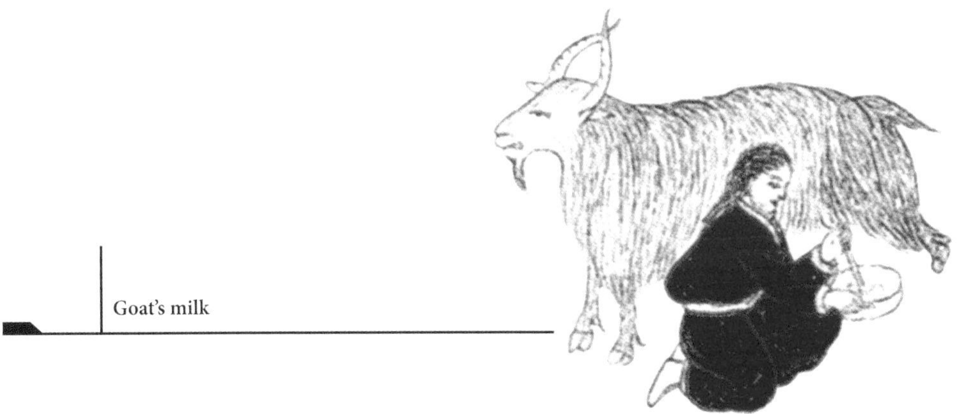

Goat's milk

Horse's milk, Donkey's milk

These kinds of milk are pungent, sour, and salty. They nourish the lung, eliminate wind, and treat lung abscesses. Drinking too much of these kinds of milk makes one dizzy. Donkey's milk is generally used as a medicine, not as a daily beverage.

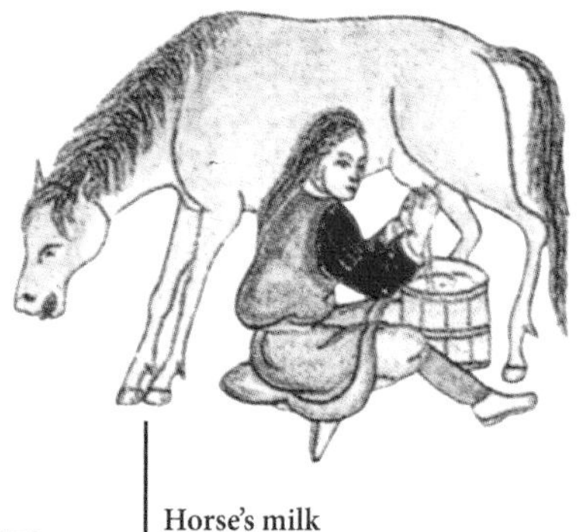

Horse's milk

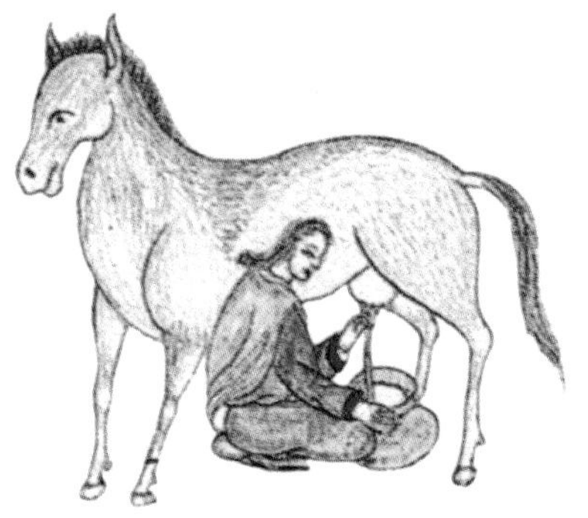

Donkey's milk

All kinds of milk are like nectar when just squeezed out. Fresh milk has a superior therapeutic action. When it cools down, its action becomes heavy and cool, and can result in *badkan* and worm diseases. Milk that is cooked for a long time becomes very heavy and can affect digestion. Milk should be carefully cooked for a proper amount of time.

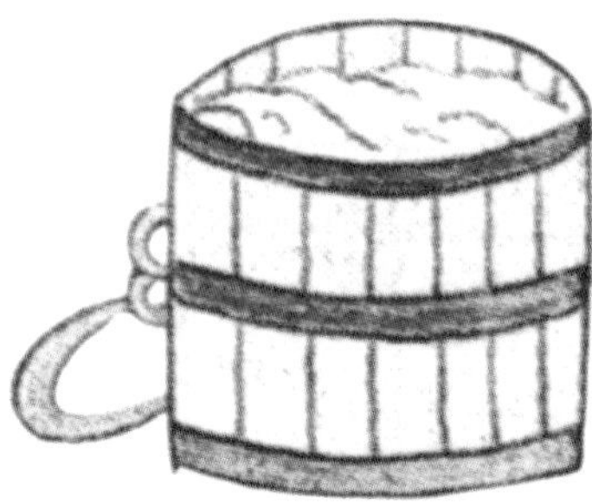

Fresh milk is like nectar and is a superior beverage.

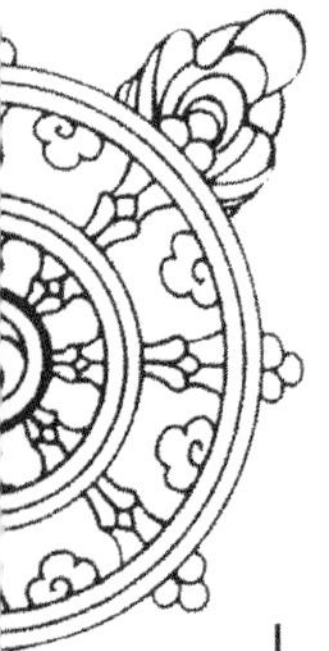

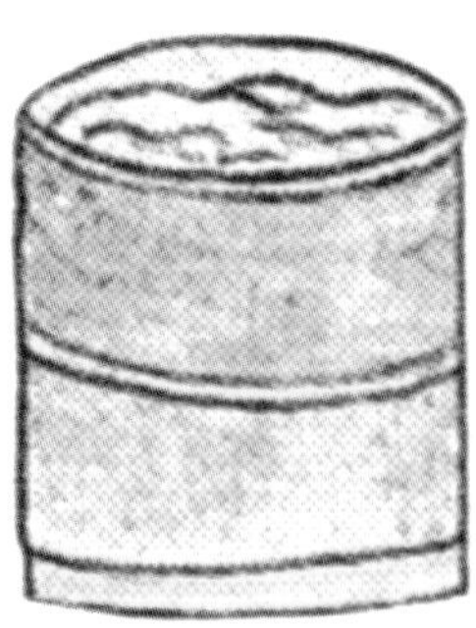

Raw milk is cool, heavy, and can cause worm and *badkan* diseases.
Cooking milk for too long makes it heavy and difficult to digest.

Dairy products eaten in Tibet include yogurt, dilute junkets, cheese, and the liquid residue from making milk and cheese. Yogurt is made from brewed milk, has a cool and moist nature, and is used to open the stomach, clear heat, and improve the appetite. It also treats constipation. Dilute junket is the cheese made by brewing the cream extracted from milk. The clear milk that separates from old milk treats epidemics, the common cold, and diarrhea. Fresh milk syrup is light, tastes astringent and sour, improves the stomach fire, and treats hemorrhoids, spleen diseases, tumors, and indigestion due to oily food. In Tibetan medicine, the watery residue from milk is called *Dala* Water, tastes sour, treats *badkan* disease, and prevents *badkan* and *mkhris pa* diseases. Cheese water is the liquid diffused from the process of making cheese. When it is fresh it treats diarrhea and watery stool. Cooked cheese is made of dehydrated cheese and liquid oil and treats constipation and heat diarrhea.

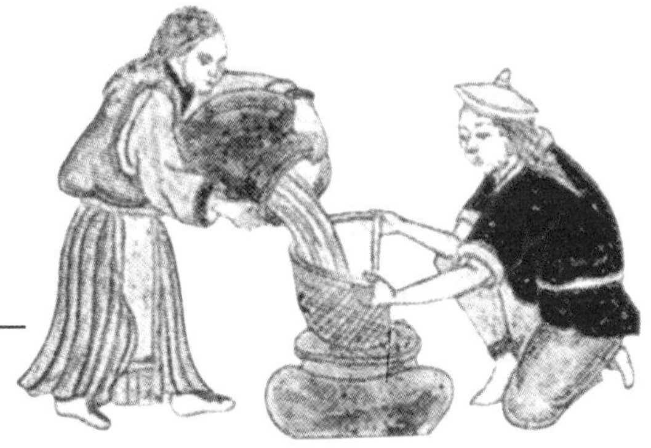

The watery residue from milk treats *badkan* disease.

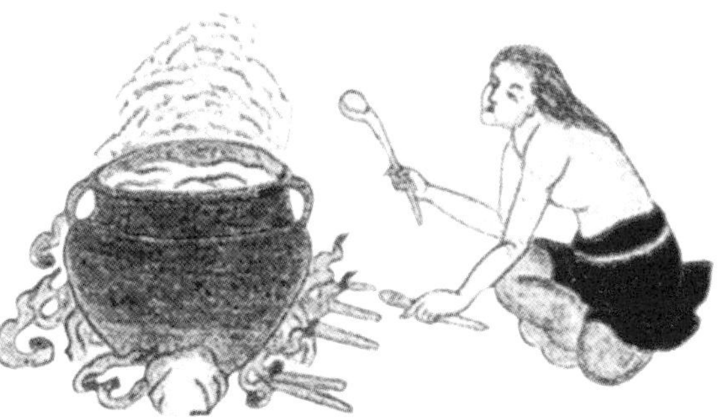

Milk cooked for too long is heavy and difficult to digest.

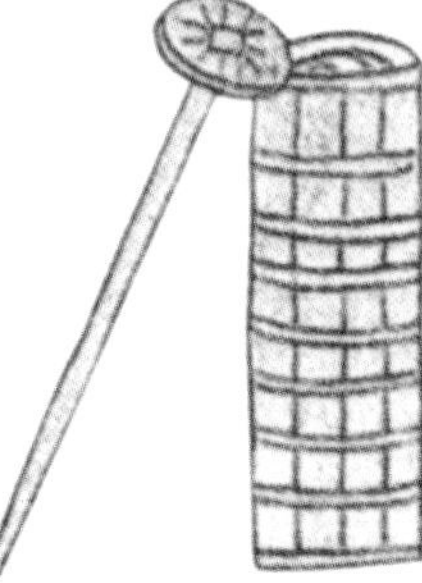

The clear liquid that separates from old milk treats common colds and diarrhea.

Milk is a fine beverage. Drunk in adequate amounts it treats disease. Conversely, it may damage health if too much is taken.

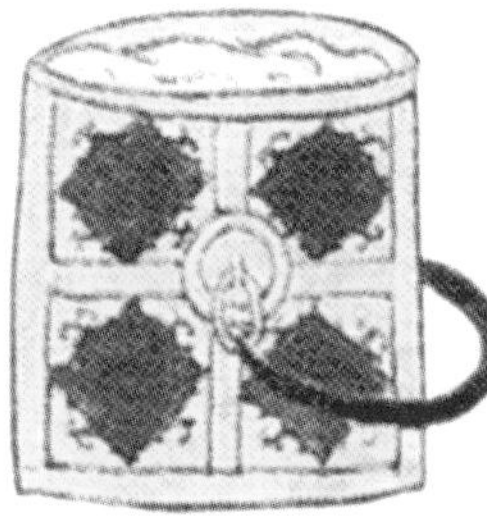

The water left from making cheese treats diarrhea and watery stool.

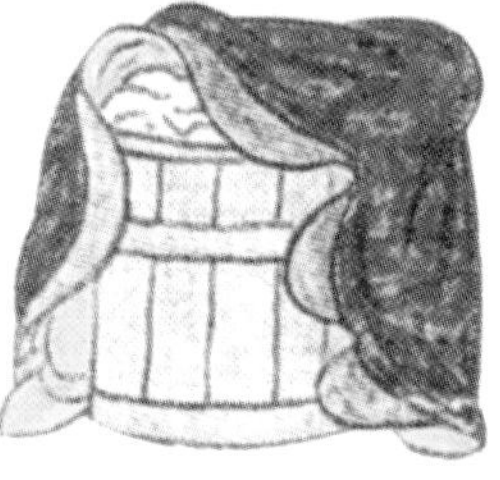

Yoghurt opens the stomach, clears heat and treats constipation.

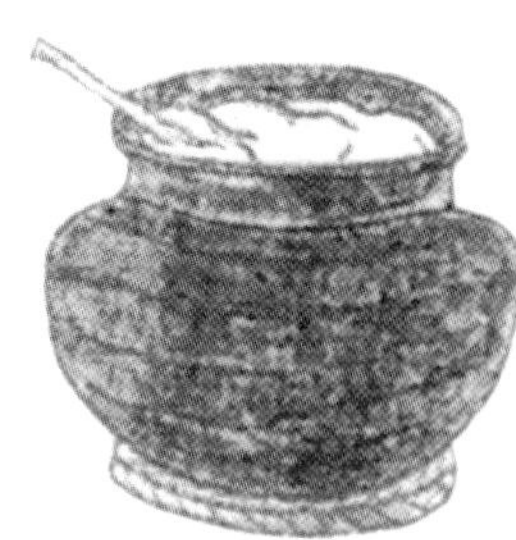

Fresh milk syrup treats hemorrhoids, abdominal masses, and poor digestion due to oily food.

Cooked cheese treats constipation and heat diarrhea.

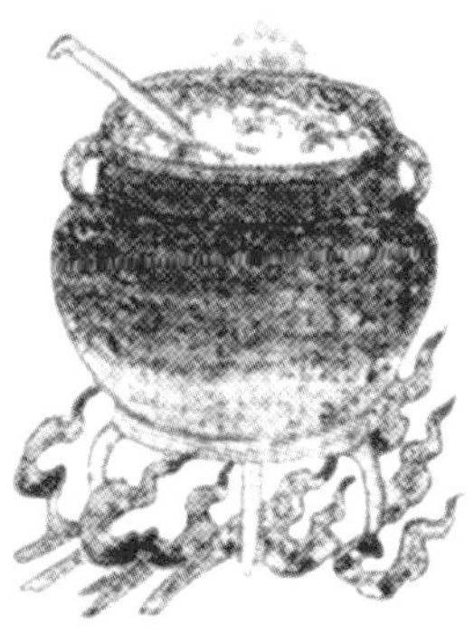

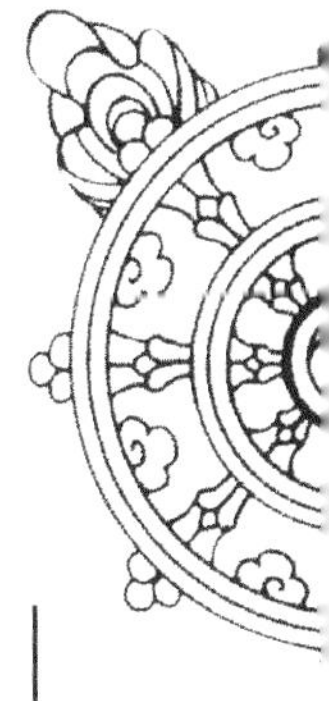

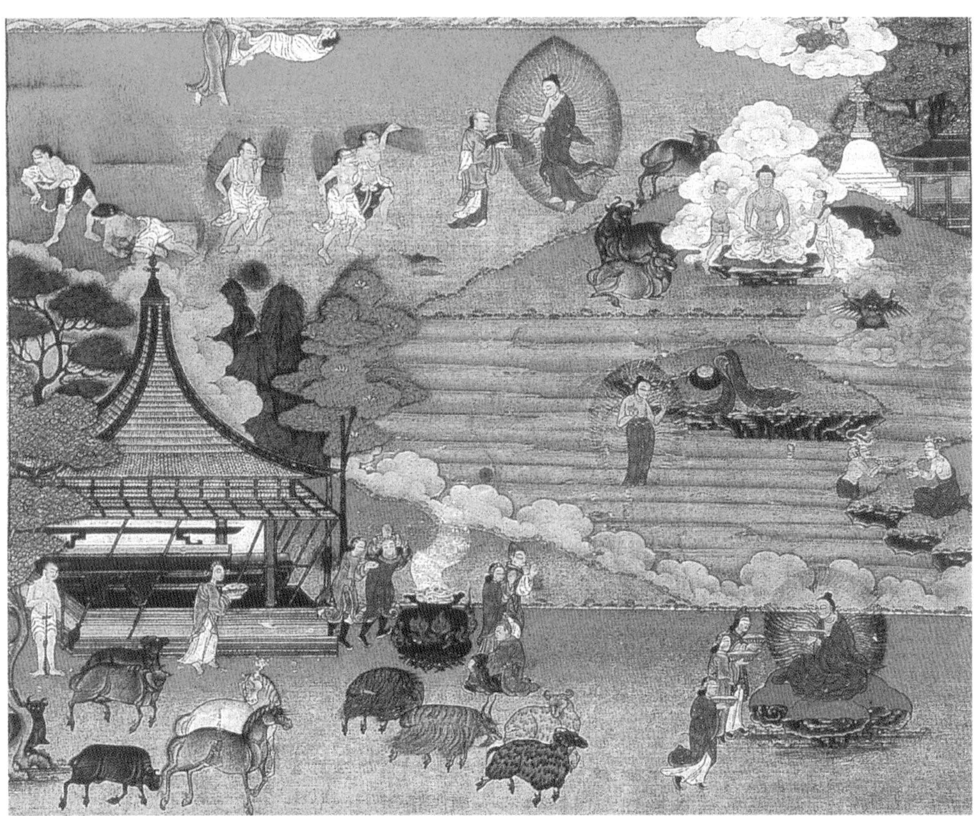

According to Buddhist history, after six years of painful asceticism, Sakyamuni accepted some mild junket from a herdswoman. He then started on his final practices that allowed him to become a Buddha (part of a *Thangkha*).

Water

Different types of water includes rain water, snow melt, river water, spring water, well water, salty water, and forest water. Rain water is considered the best, with the quality of the others descending in the order they are listed.

Rain water from the sky is like nectar, tasteless, light, and cool. It nurtures the body and spirit. It does not hurt the throat or stomach and because of this is the most excellent kind of water. Water running off a snowy mountain is even cooler than rain water and can decrease the stomach fire, so it is contraindicated for the elderly and those with weak stomach fire. Water from marshes, swamps, turbid and dirty water, spring water from where bryophytes (moss and lichen) grow, water found under trees without direct light from the sun or moon, water from deep wells and salty water are all inferior and not suitable for drinking. Continuous drinking of such kinds of water will lead to disease. Stagnant water or sluggishly running water may lead to worm diseases, elephantiasis of the lower limbs, beriberi, and heart disease.

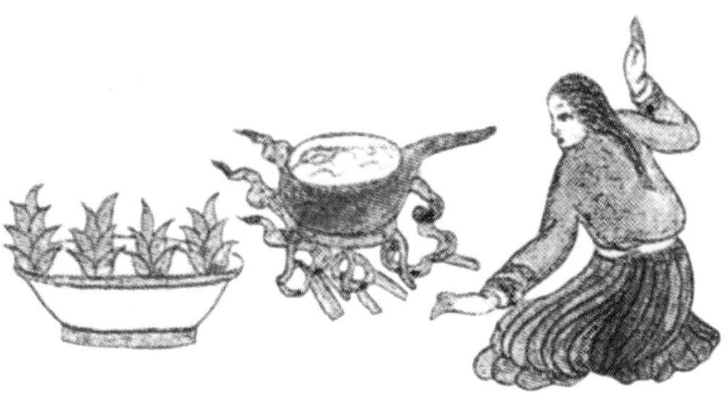

Rain water

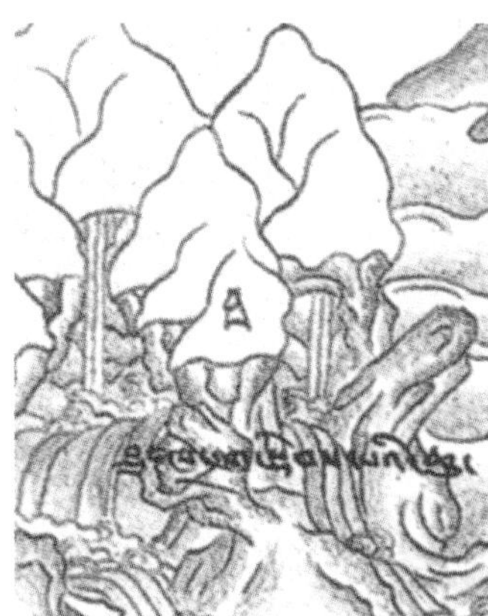

Snow water

In summary, all drinking water should be clean, always flowing, well ventilated and with direct sun, moon, and star light. After boiling, water becomes warm or hot, and is helpful in improving digestion, arresting hiccough, treating *badkan* disease, distended abdomen, difficulty breathing, and the initial stage of colds and epidemics. Boiled water treats *mkhris pa* disease after it has been cooled down. If left standing for an entire day, good water will become bad water, will lead to various diseases and should not be consumed.

The different kinds of water include rain water, snow melt, river water, spring water, well water, salty water and forest water. The quality of them descends in the above order.

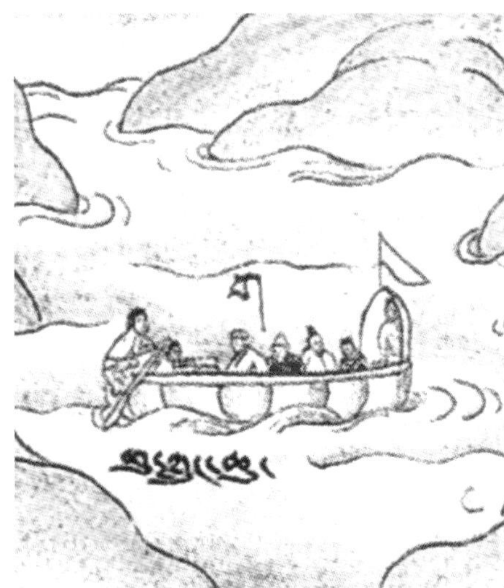

River water

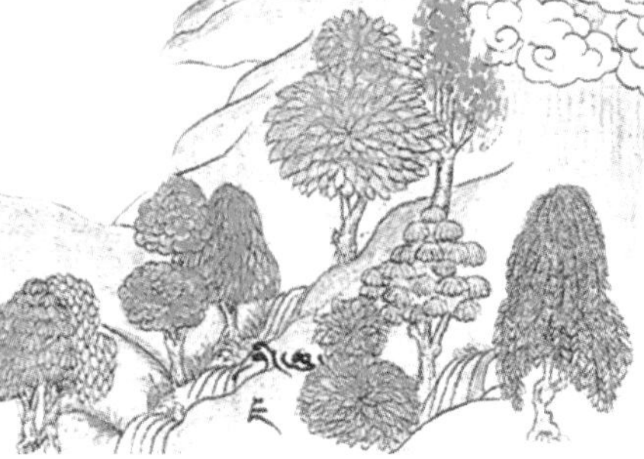

Water from forests

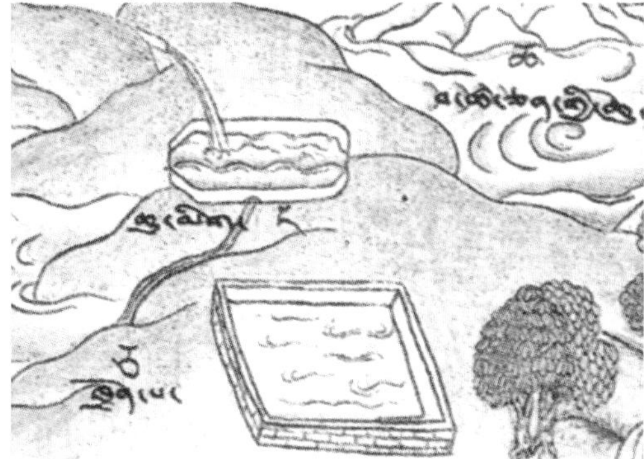

Spring water, well water.

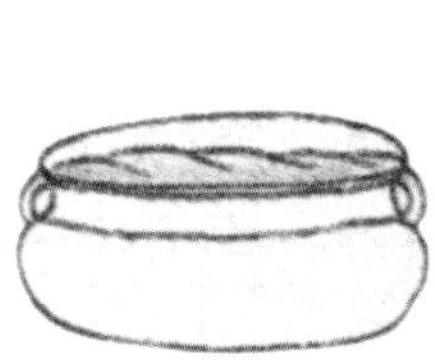

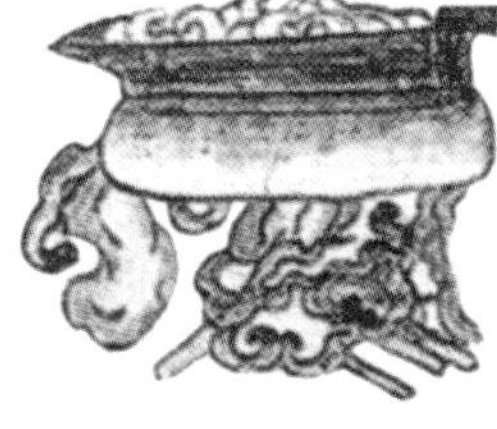

Rain water is tasteless, cold and light in nature, and is a superior kind of water.

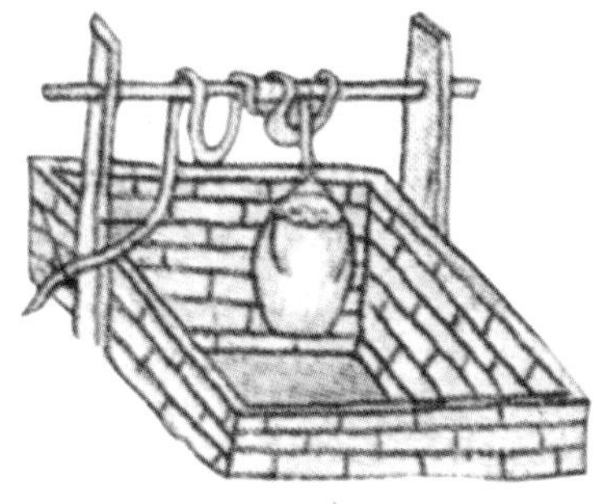

Water from deep wells is drinkable.

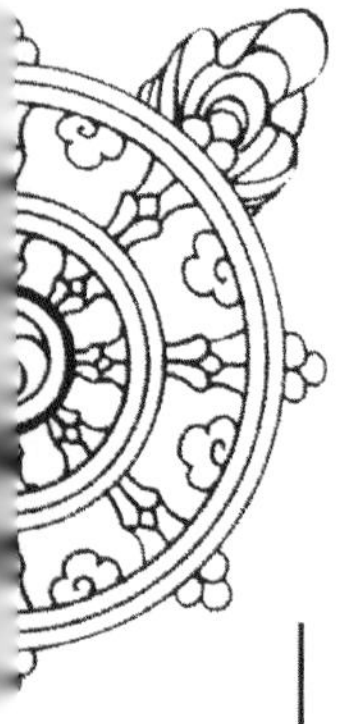

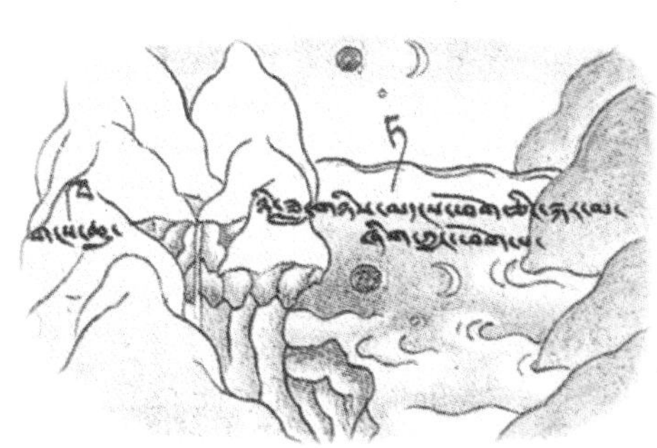

Snow water that is exposed to sun, moon and star light is excellent. It lowers stomach fire.

Cold water is not good for drinking.

Water becomes warm and hot after boiling. It helps digestion, arrests hiccough, treats *badkan* disease, abdominal distension, and the initial stage of common colds. Cooled boiled water treats *mkhris pa* disease.

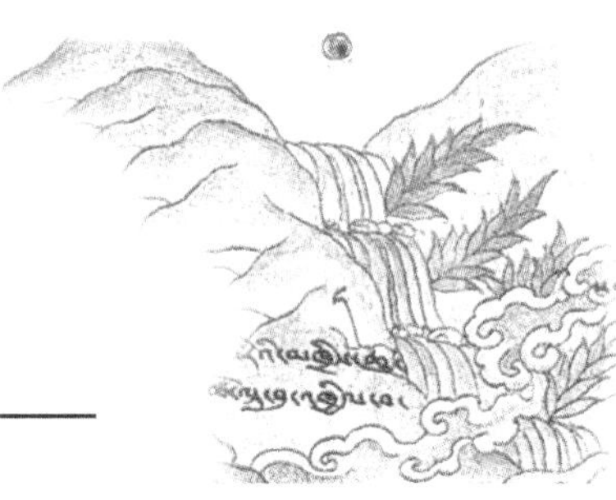

Water from snow capped mountains is drinkable.

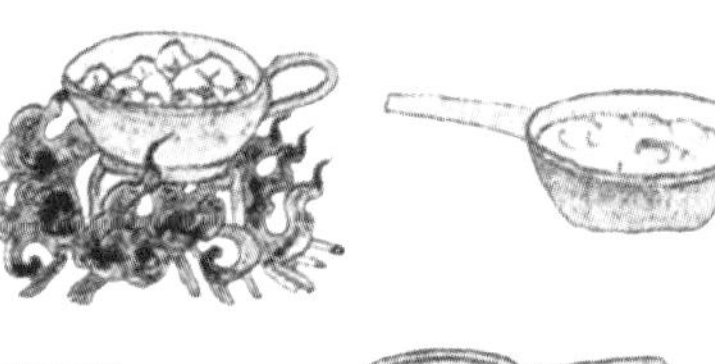

Boiled water left standing for a whole day can lead to disease.

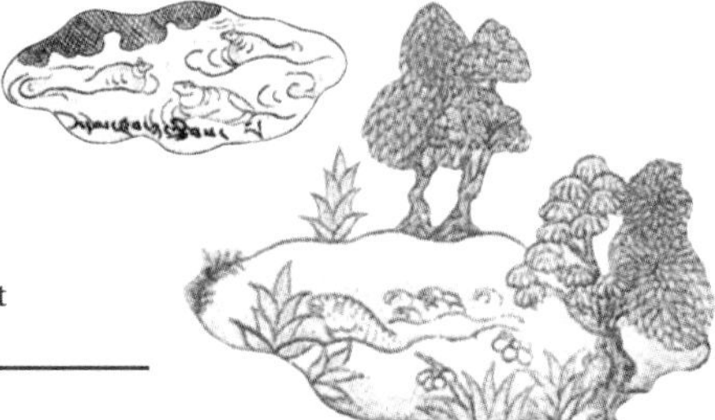

Stagnant water can cause worm diseases, heart diseases, and elephantiasis of the lower limbs.

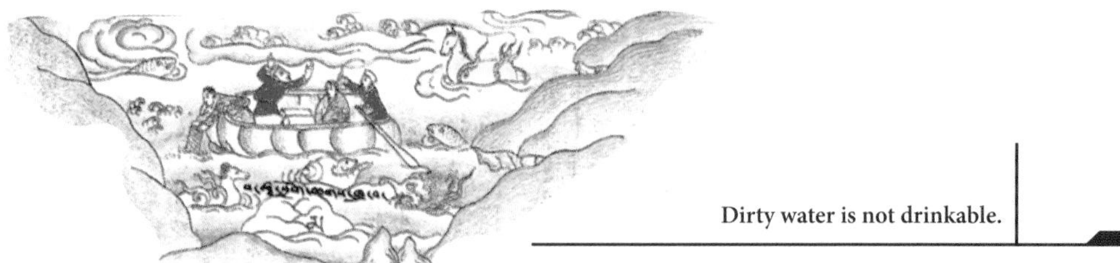

Dirty water is not drinkable.

Alcohol

The wines that are used in Tibetan medicine are mostly Tibetan wine, which is made by various traditional brewing methods. Through this kind of alcohol is not clear, it is fragrant, sweet and tastes mellow. Its alcohol content is relatively low, is rich in sugars, vitamins, amino acids, and other nutritious ingredients. The brewing process involves steaming, mixing with yeast, fermentation in a tightly covered container and the addition of pure water. During this process, the quality of the fire used, the temperature of the distiller's yeast, the duration it remains in the covered container, and the quantity of water added are strictly controlled. Many experienced householders can brew pure and excellent wine. The crude materials that are mostly used for brewing are highland barley, wheat, barley, oats, fried wheat, and rice.

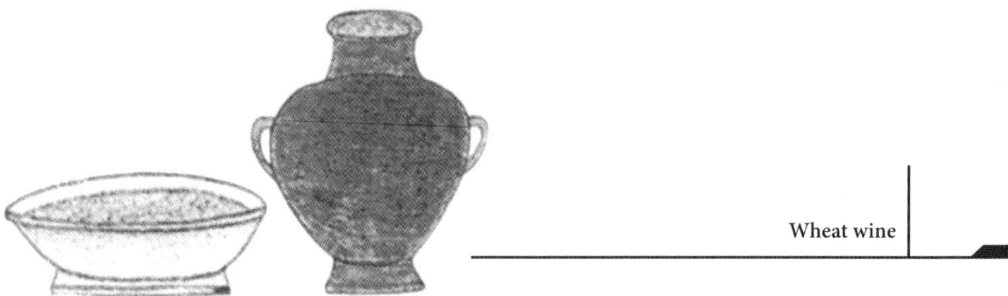

Wheat wine

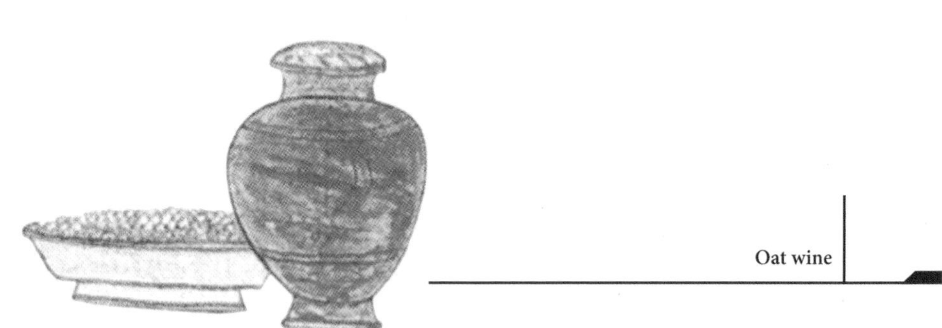

Oat wine

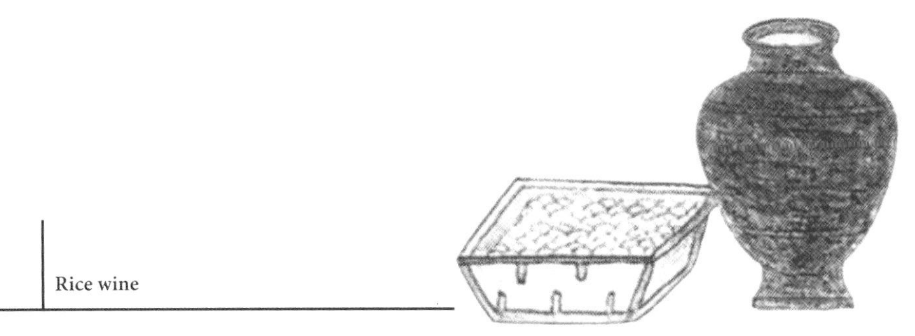
Rice wine

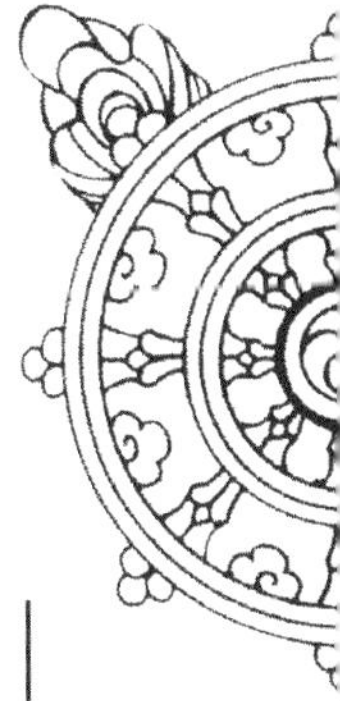

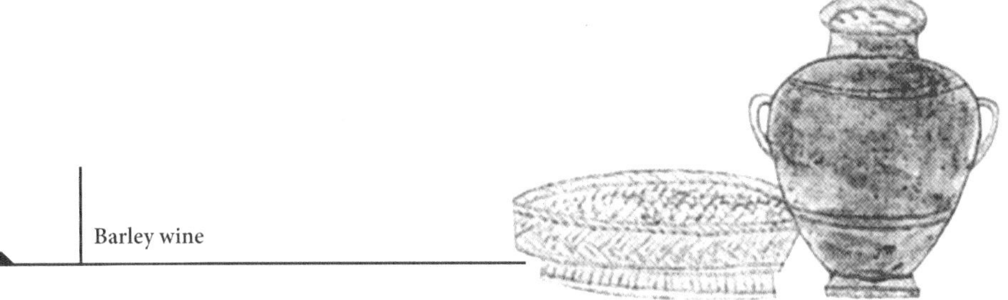
Barley wine

Wine can taste sweet, sour, or bitter. It tastes sour after being digested, has a sharp, hot, rough, fine nature, and can cause mild diarrhea.

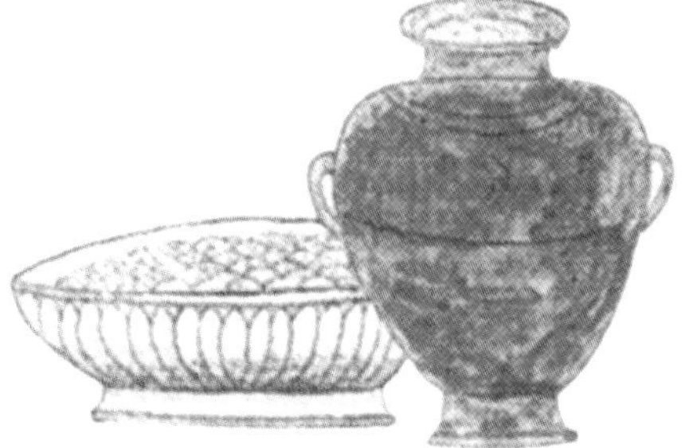
Highland barley wine

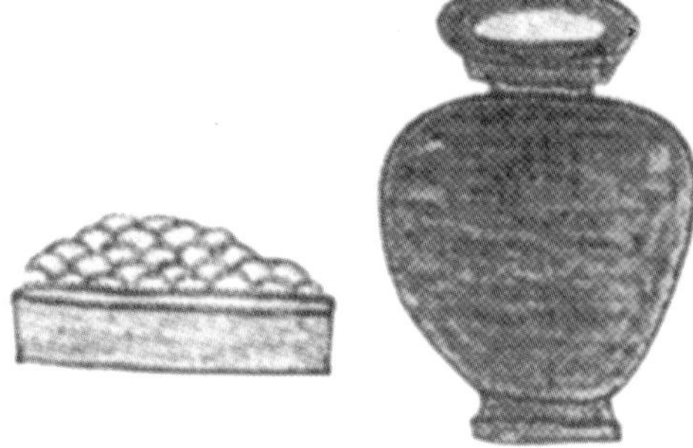

Fried wheat wine.

Tibetan wine tastes bitter, sweet, and sour. Its nature after digestion is sharp, hot, rough, oily, and has a mild purgative effect. Good quantity wine produces heat, strengthens the body, helps sleep, and treats *rlung* and *badkan* diseases. Excessive drinking results in uneasiness, unconventional and unrestrained behavior, ignorance, unconsciousness to bad acts, talking nonsense, or even illegal activities. Becoming drunk can cause coma, deep sleep, mania, or ignorance to the world. People who choose to drink wine should only drink a suitable amount and not take too much.

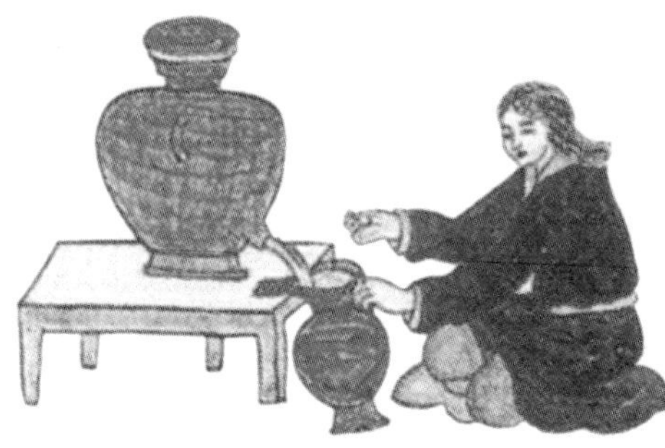

An adequate quantity of wine produces heat, aids sleep, and treats *rlung* and *badkan* diseases.

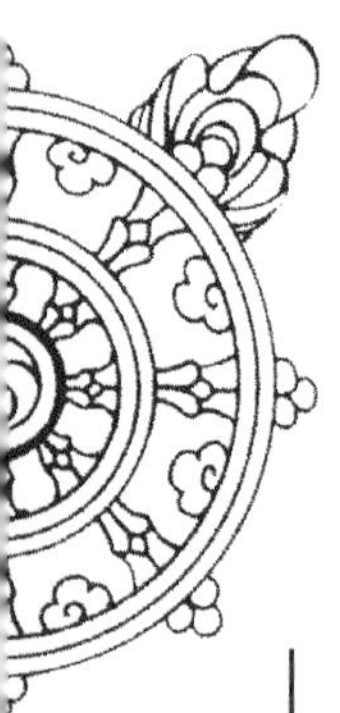

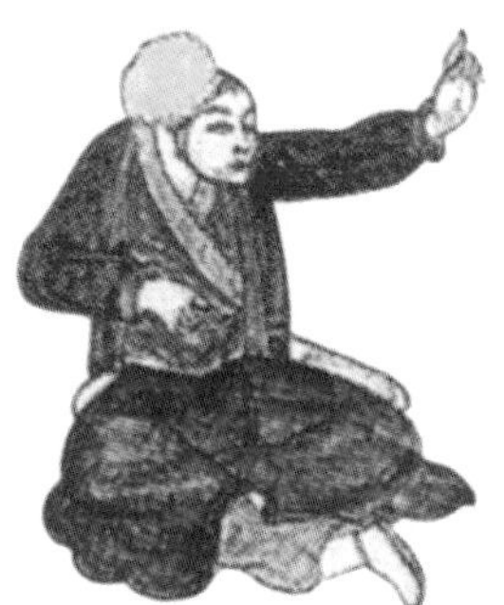

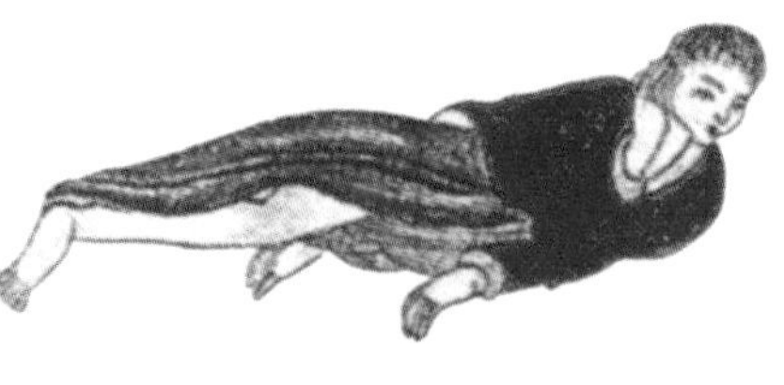

When drunk, people talk nonsense like a mad person and will lie anywhere.

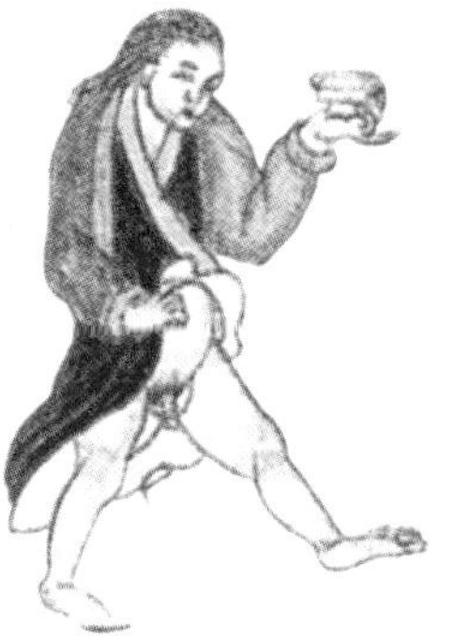
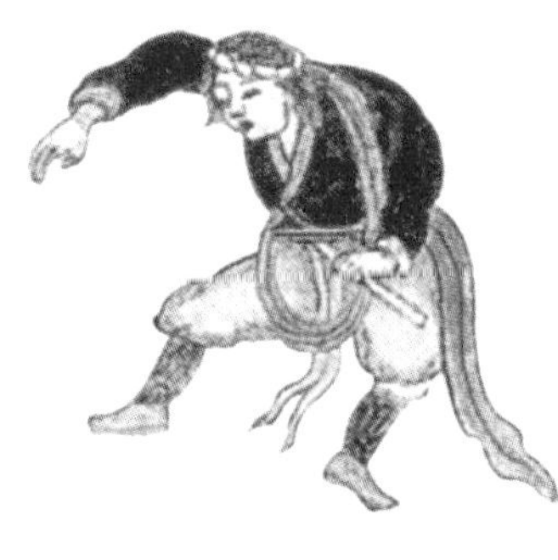

Excessive drinking makes one unconventional and unrestrained.

Freshly brewed wine is light, gentle, hot, and easily digested. All wine, when they become old and sour, treat blood diseases and *badkan* and *mkhris pa* diseases. Wines brewed with barley, oat, fried wheat and highland barley are gentle, while rice wine is strong, and wheat wine is even stronger.

All freshly brewed wines are gentle, hot, and readily digested.

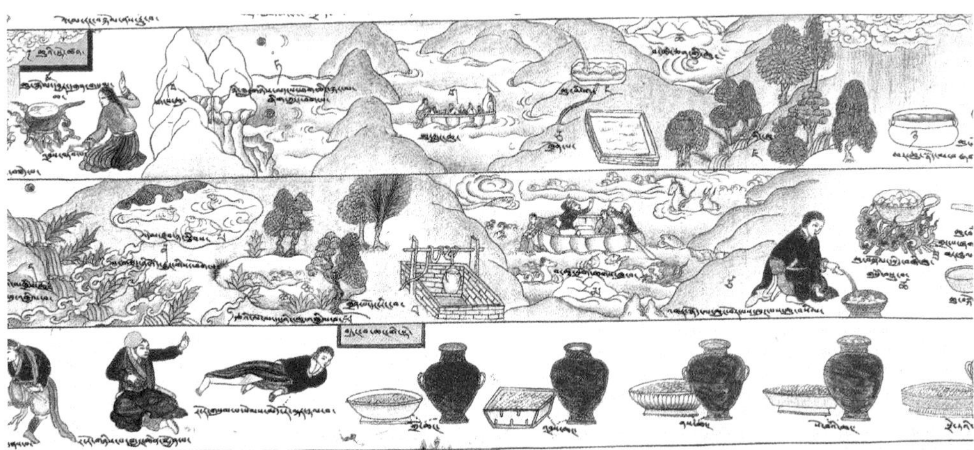

Seven kinds of drinkable water and wine (part of *Thangkha* twenty-four in the *Sman thang* series of *The Four Medical Tantras*).

Grains

Grains come in two categories, awns and pods. The former mainly consists of different varieties of rice; the latter of various beans. Generally, grains that are freshly harvested and have been stored less than one year are heavy, moist, difficult to digest, and likely to cause *badkan* diseases. Grains that are totally mature, completely dried, and have been stored over one year have a warm and light nature and are readily digested. Raw grains are heavy while cooked grains are light, and become even lighter after various ingredients are added. The lighter a grain is, the more readily digested it is, and the more beneficial to the body it is.

Awns

This category includes rice, millet, wheat, highland barley, barley and oats. They taste sweet, and the sweet taste stays after being digested. These grains strengthen the body's yang (warm, mobile aspect), improve strength and spirit, and eliminate wind. If misused they can lead to *badkan* diseases.

Rice

This is the main staple food in most parts of China. Its nature is soft, moist, cool and light, expels all *rlung*, *mkhris pa* and *badkan* evils, arrests diarrhea and vomiting, and strengthens the body's yang.

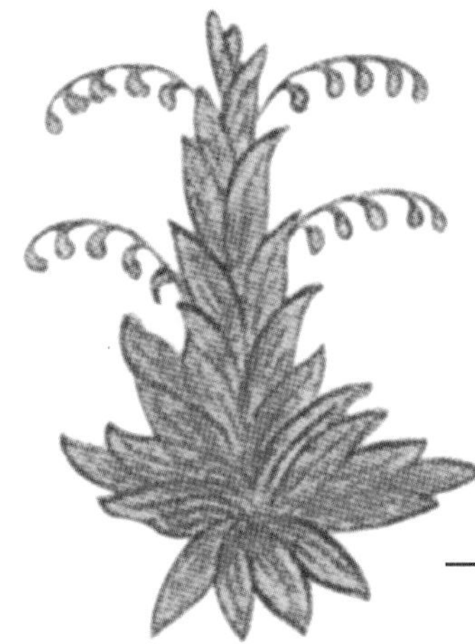

Rice removes the three evils, strengthens yang, and stops diarrhea and vomiting.

Grains are sweet and remain sweet after being digested. They strengthen the body's yang, increase strength, produce *badkan* diseases and eliminate *rlung* diseases.

Millet

Millet is heavy and cool, nurtures the body, and knits fractured bones. Immature millet is cool and rough, promotes digestion and improves the appetite.

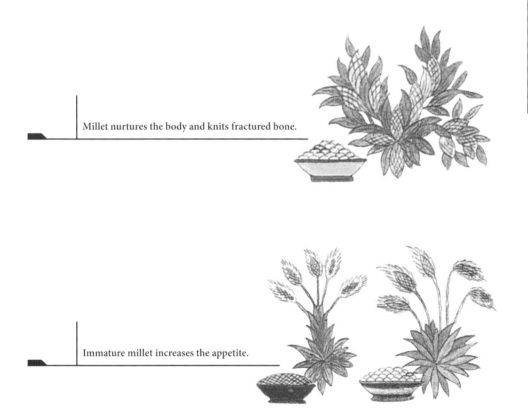

Millet nurtures the body and knits fractured bone.

Immature millet increases the appetite.

Wheat

This is also a main staple food in China. It is heavy and cool, nurtures the body, and treats *rlung* and *mkhris pa* diseases.

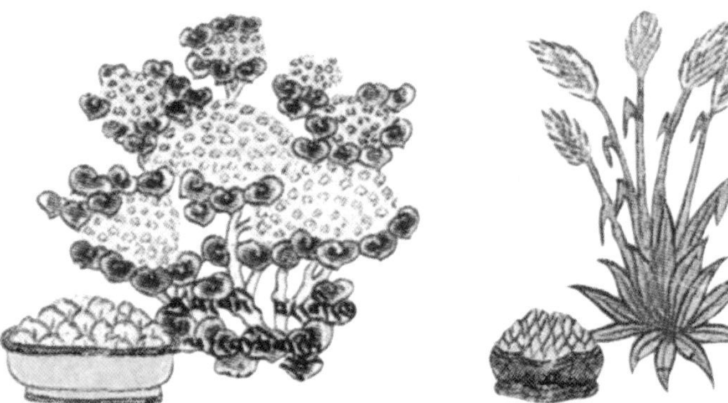

Buckwheat, wheat

Highland barley

This is the main grain produced in Tibet, and is the basic ingredient in *rtsam pa*, the main staple food of the Tibetan people. There are many species of highland barley, including white highland barley, blue highland barley, red highland barley, and immature highland barley. They are all heavy, cool, sweet, and able to strengthen the body and clean the digestive tract.

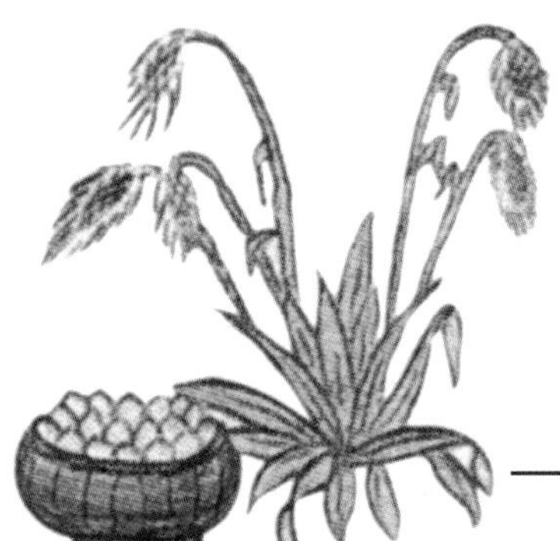

Highland barley

Barley and oats

These grains taste sweet, have a light and cool quality, eliminate *badkan* diseases and remove *mkhris pa*, accelerate delivery of a baby, and treat *rlung* diseases.

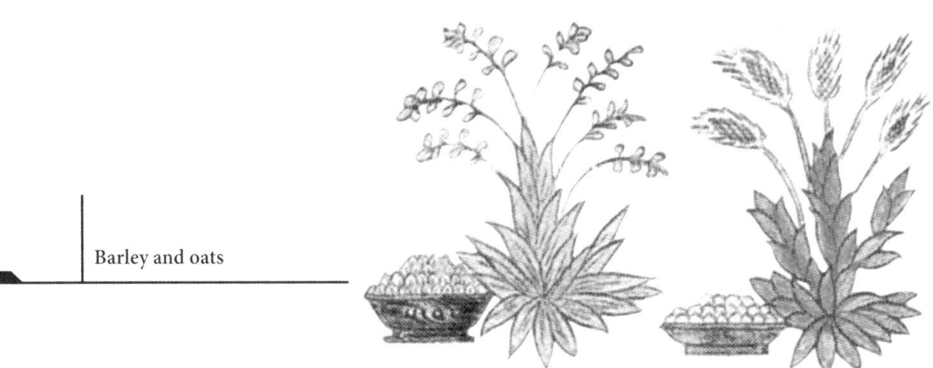

Barley and oats

Pods

This category consists mostly of beans, and includes peas, red beans, buckwheat, sesame, Indian white beans and flax. Most of them are sweet and astringent. After digestion they become sweet and slightly bitter, and their nature becomes light, cool, and rough. They can block the vessels, astringe the intestines, and dry the stool. Beans treat fever and diarrhea due to *badkan* and obesity of the *badkan* type. Over eating beans may cause *mkhris pa* diseases and blood disorders.

Peas

There are white and black peas and all are edible. Both are astringent and sweet, with a cool, light and dry nature. They can activate stagnant blood, remove stasis, treat fever due to *badkan*, poisoning that has spread to the internal organs, and diarrhea and discomfort due to too much oil.

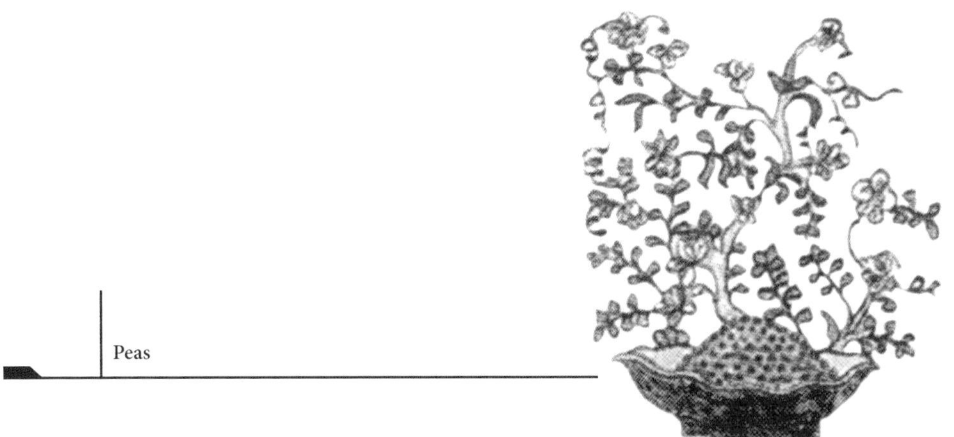

Peas

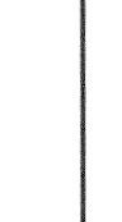

Indian white bean

Also called white broad beans, this type of bean is astringent and sweet, with a cool, light, and dry nature. It treats profuse sputum, difficulty breathing, hemorrhoids, and stones in the semen. It can also nourish blood, fluids, and bile.

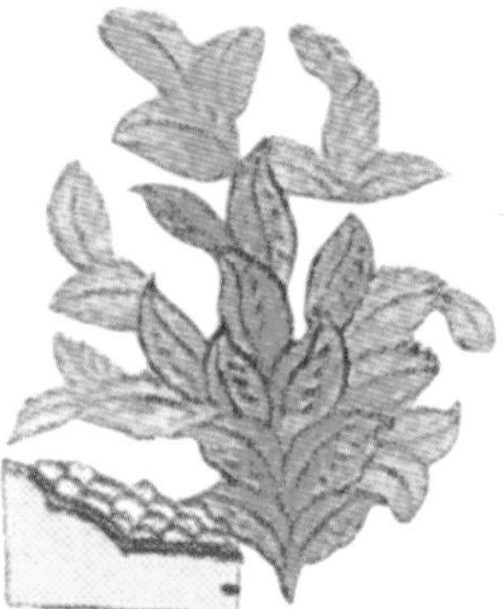

Indian white beans treat hemorrhoids, abnormal semen and difficult breathing.

Red bean

Red beans are used as food in most parts of China, but is only used as medicine in Tibet. The taste and nature are the same as Indian white beans, and are able to eliminate wind, benefit the spirit, and increase strength. It is used to treat *rlung* disease, increases *badkan* and *mkhris pa*, and elevate the spirit.

Red beans give rise to *badkan* and *mkhris pa* and elevate the spirit.

Buckwheat

Sweet and slightly astringent with a cool, light nature, buckwheat astringes sores and strongly activates blood. It is used to expedite the healing of wounds, but also can induce *rlung*, *mkhris pa* and *badkan* disorders.

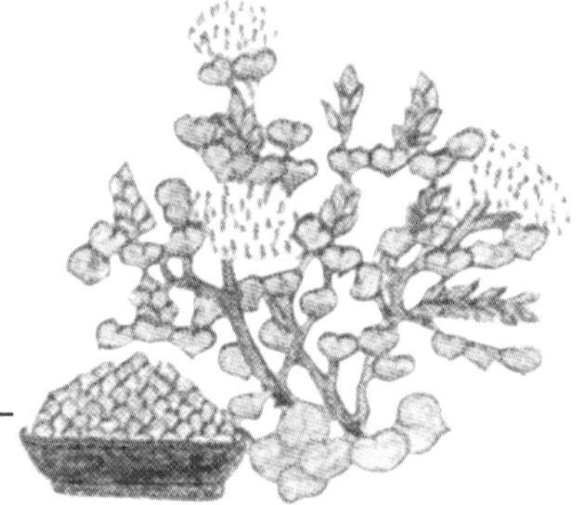

Buckwheat heals wounds.

Sesame

Sesame is heavy and warm, strengthens yang, and removes *rlung* evils.

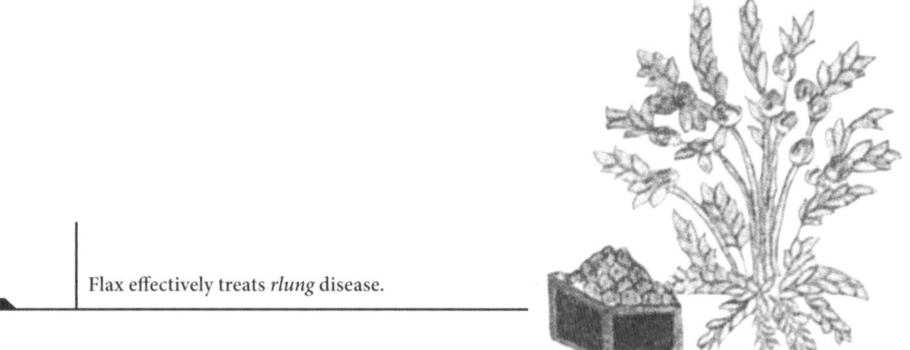

Flax effectively treats *rlung* disease.

Flax

Sweet and bitter, moist, and soft, flax treats *rlung* disease.

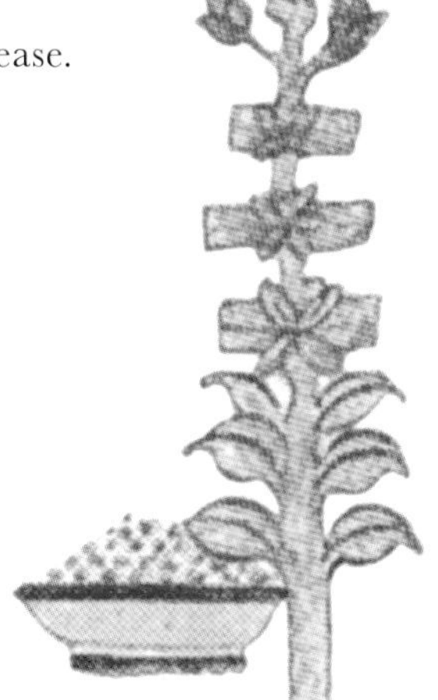

Sesame strengthens yang and treats *rlung* disease.

All raw and cooked grains including those that have been flavored are light, readily digested and good for the body.

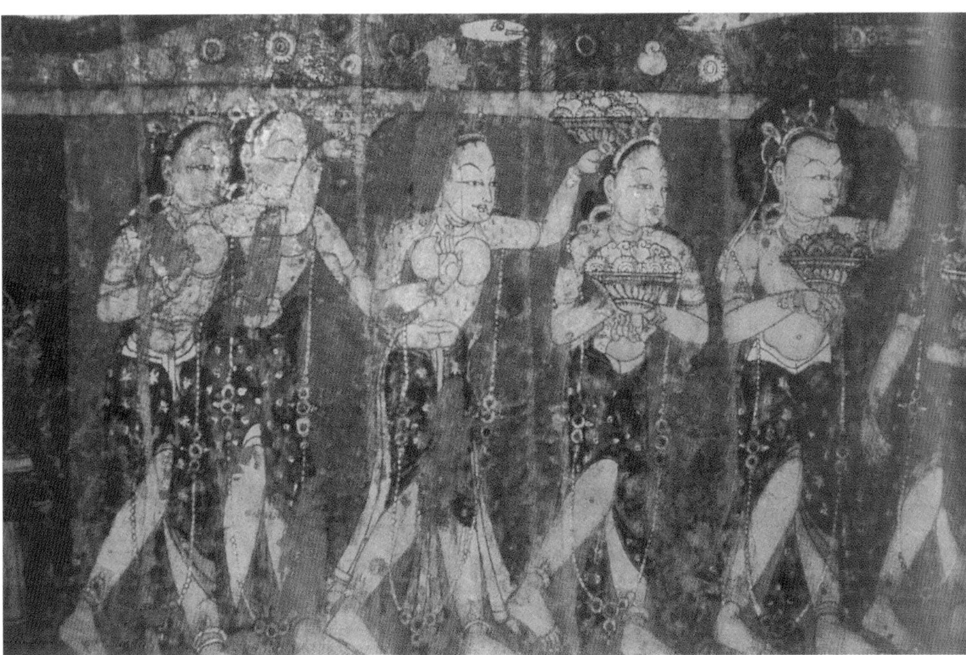

Grains are an important offering at alters (part of mural in a Tibetan monastery).

Meat

Living in a land locked region, the Tibetan people use mutton and beef as their main foods. Tibetan culture has a deep understanding of the natures and nutritional values of the various kinds of meat. People should select the meat they eat carefully and the choices should be based on their constitution and the conditions any diseases present.

Classes of meats

There are two basic kinds of classification. One separates the products based on the location the animal inhabits, such as dry land, wet land or moderate regions; another kind classifies the type of animal: birds, beasts, large beasts, fierce beasts, fierce birds, domestic birds and domestic animals, cave-inhabiting animals, and wet area-inhabiting animals.

Meat of animals from dry areas

This includes birds, beasts, large beasts, and fierce beasts. Meat from such animals is light, cool, and rough, and can cure illnesses due to heat and mixed *badkan* and *rlung*.

Birds

This includes mainly peacocks, snow chuckar, turtledove, crow, and other mountain birds that pick up food by digging with their claws. This category also includes parrots, cuckoos, magpies, pigeons, sparrows, thrush and other birds that pick up food by pecking.

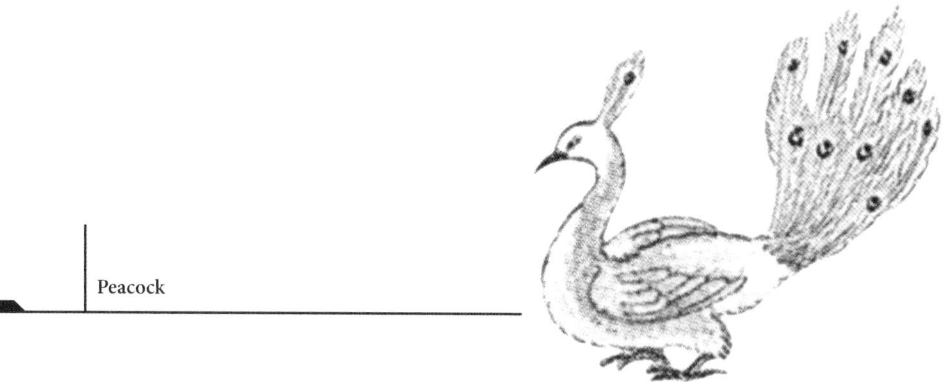

Peacock

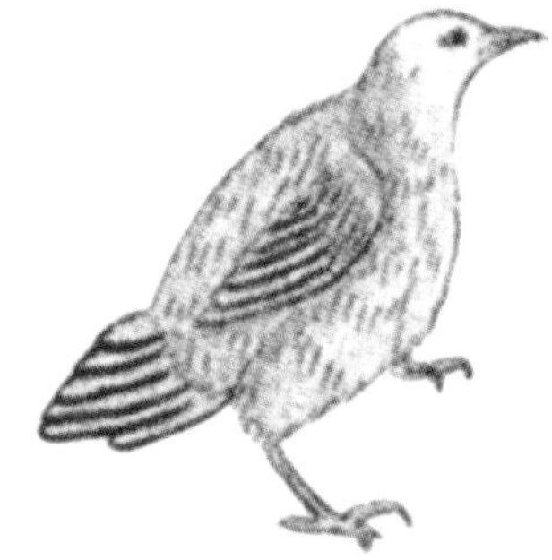

Snow chuckar

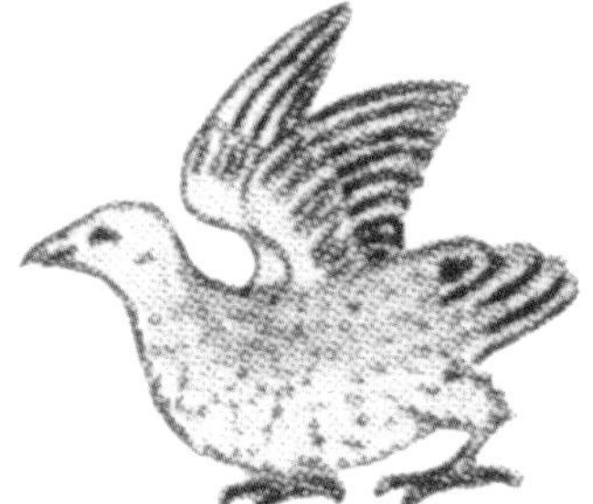

Turtledove

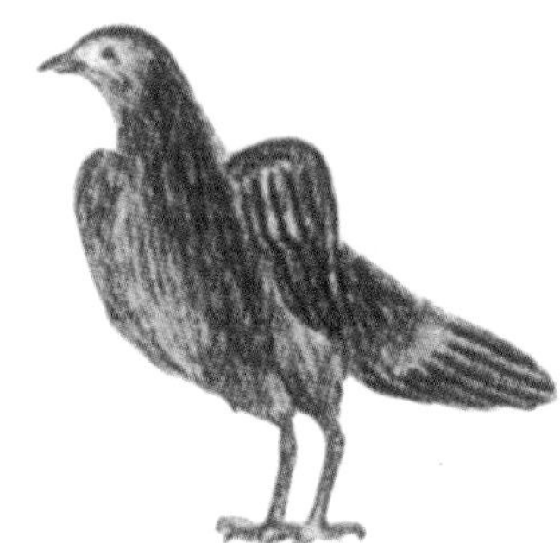

Crow

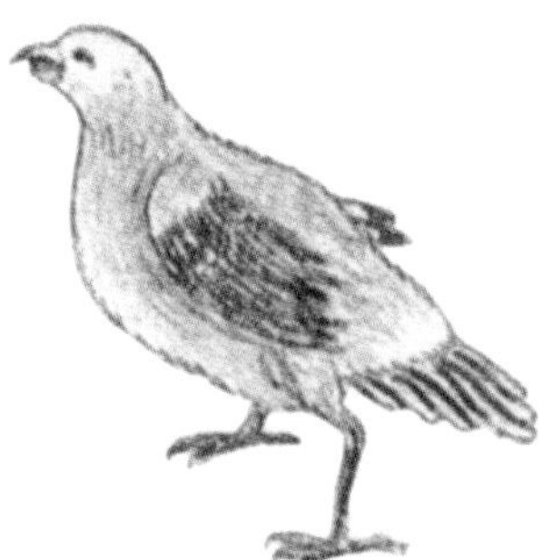

Mountain bird

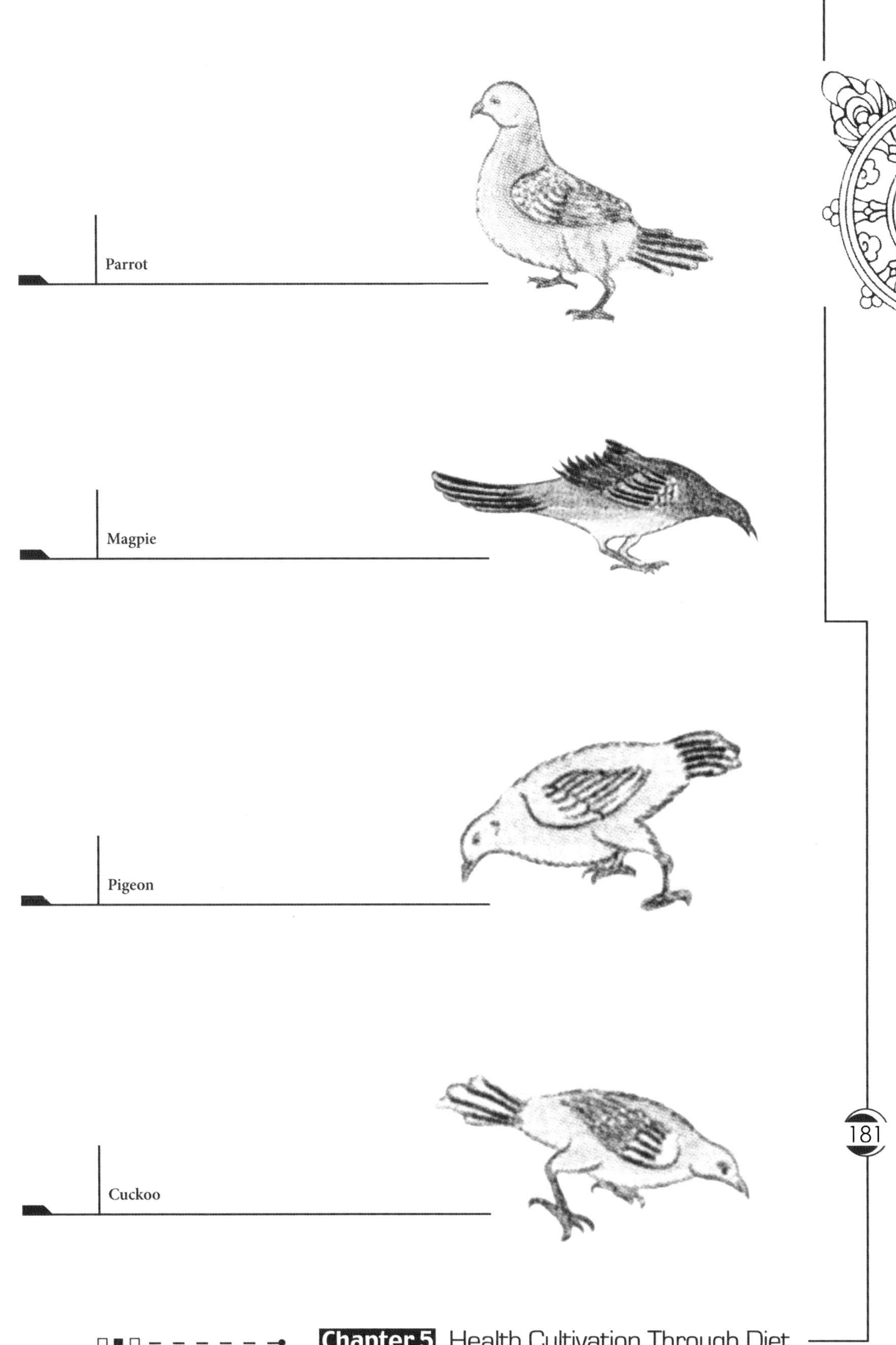
Parrot
Magpie
Pigeon
Cuckoo

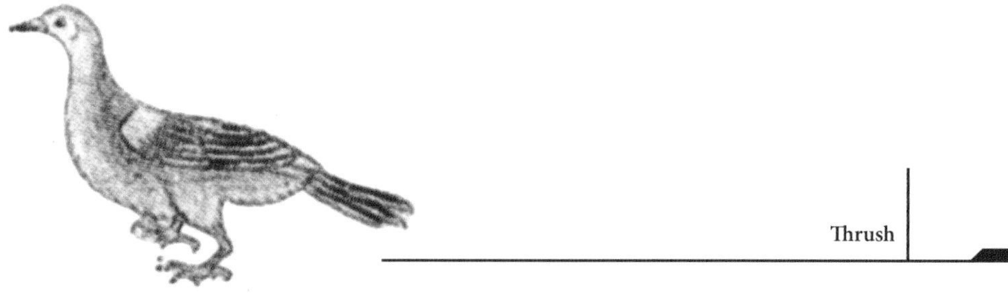
Thrush

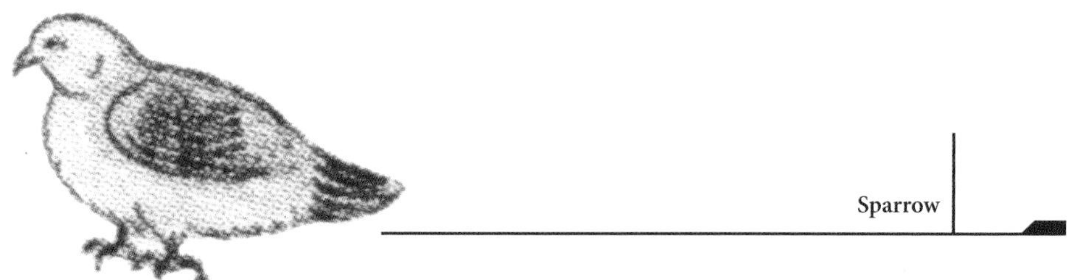
Sparrow

There are eight sorts of meat: bird, beast, large beast, fierce beast, fierce bird, domestic animal and bird, cave-inhabiting, and those that live on and in water. All are further classified as living in dry land, wet land, or moderate regions.

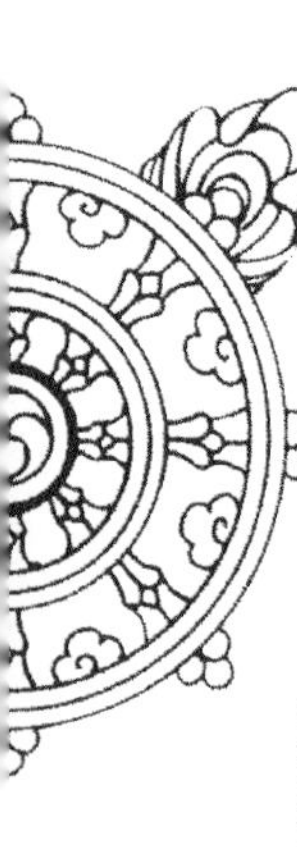

Beasts

This includes deer, musk deer, Mongolian gazelle, argali, wild rabbit, Tibetan antelope, and the yellow weasel.

Large beasts

Wild ox, wild donkey, water buffalo, rhinoceros, zupiko (a yak and cow mix), muntjac, polecat, wild goat, and wild boar.

Fierce beasts (predatory beasts)

Tiger, leopard, bear, brown bear, snow leopard, wolf, lynx, fox, and sandy fox.

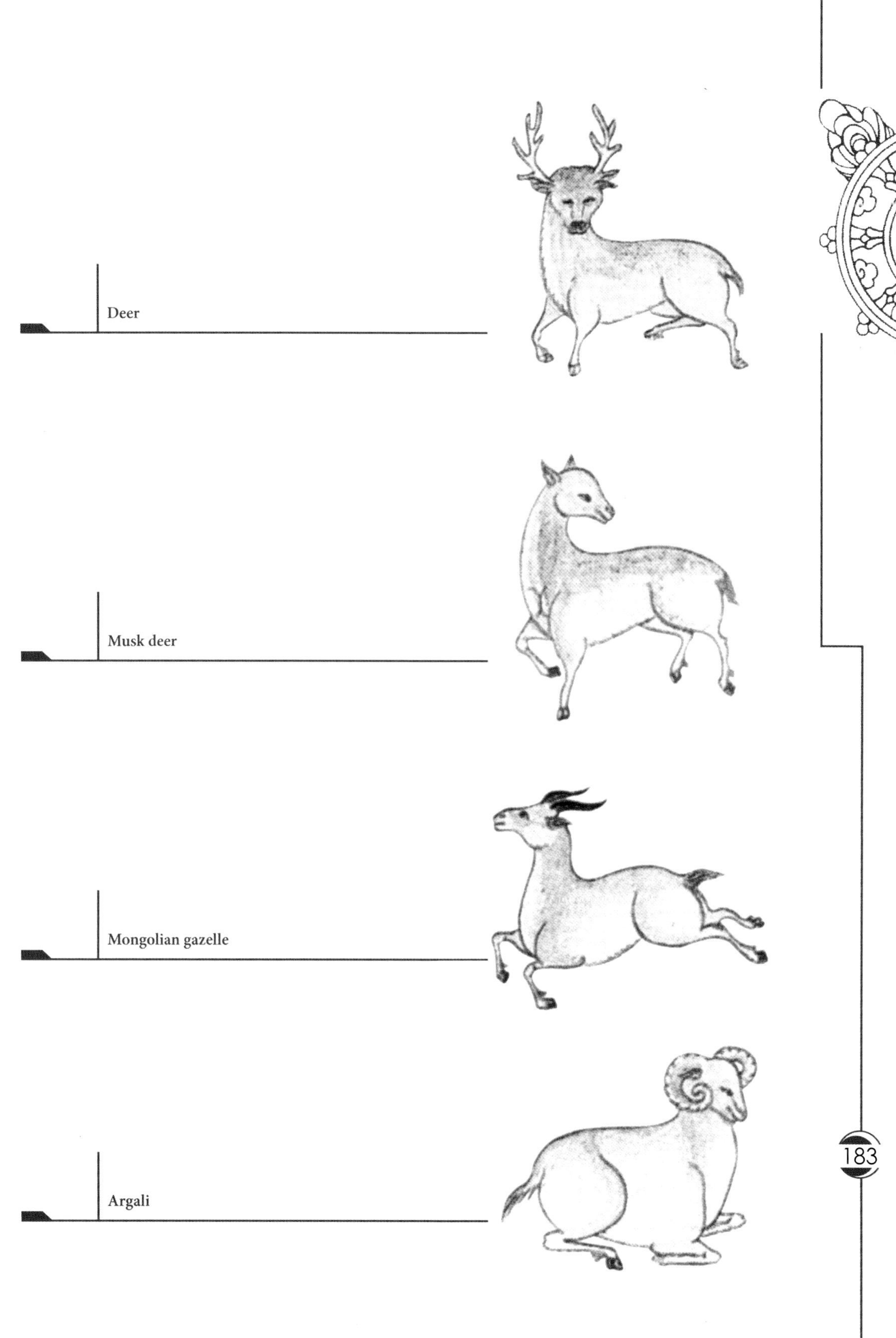
Deer
Musk deer
Mongolian gazelle
Argali

Wild rabbit

Tibetan antelope

Antelope

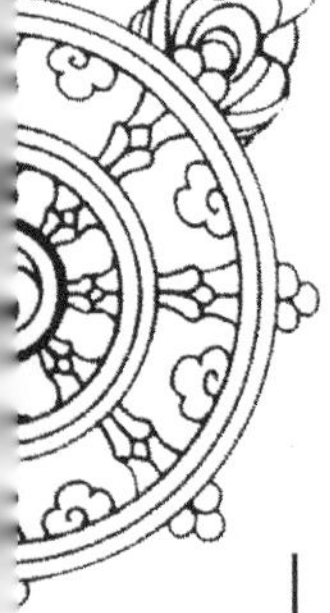

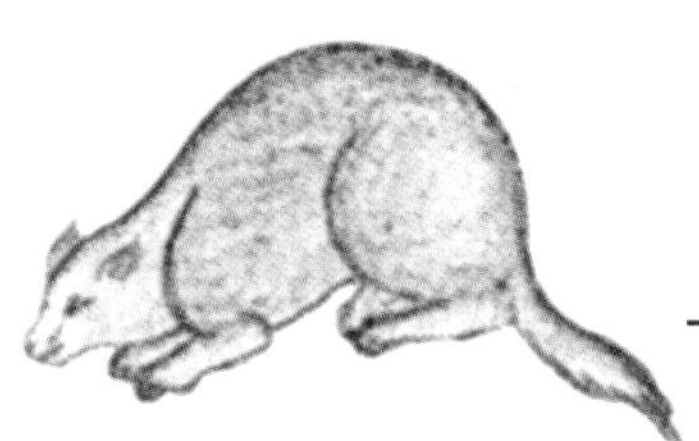

Yellow weasel

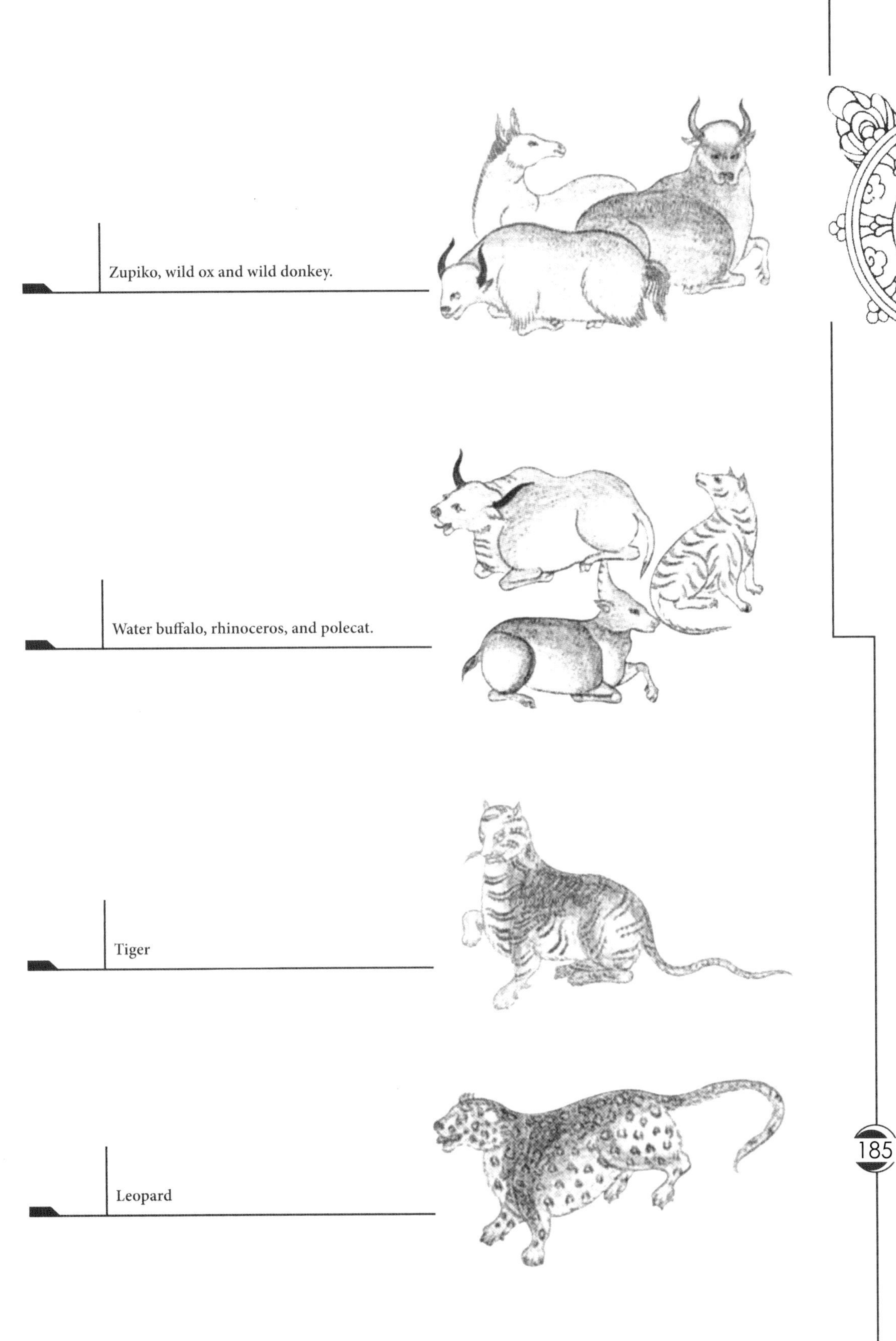
Zupiko, wild ox and wild donkey.

Water buffalo, rhinoceros, and polecat.

Tiger

Leopard

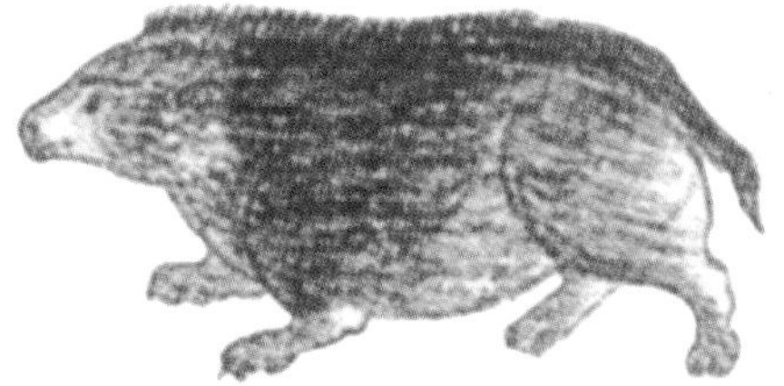

Bear

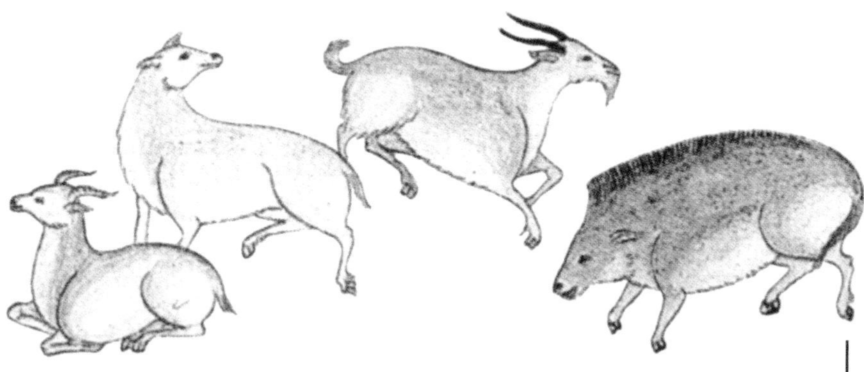

Muntjac, wild goat and wild boar.

The meat of animals from dry regions is cool, light, rough, and removes fever due to mixed *rlung* and *badkan* disorders.

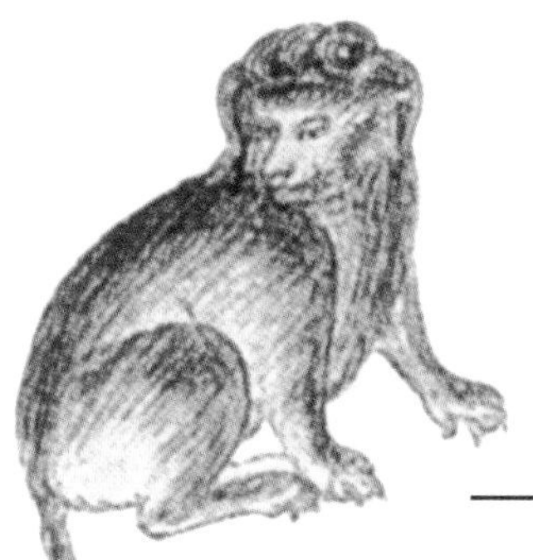

Brown bear

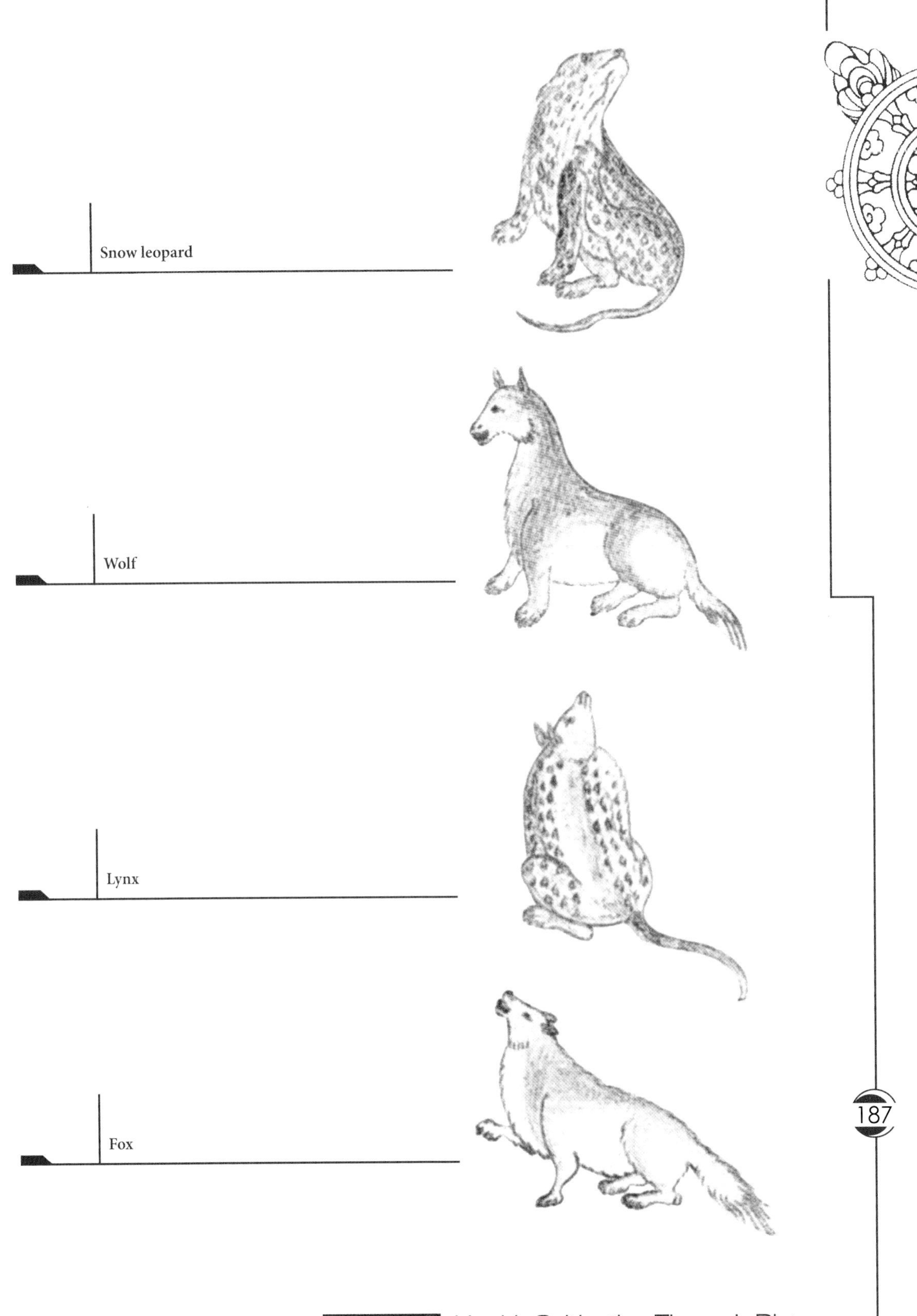
Snow leopard
Wolf
Lynx
Fox

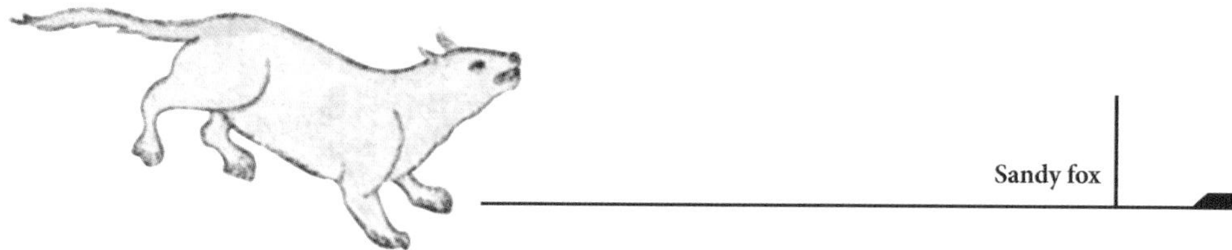

Meat of animals from wet areas

This includes wild goose, yellow duck, egret, yellow egret, aquatic birds, otter, and fish. The meat from these animals is greasy, heavy, and hot. It treats stomach cold, kidney cold, and cold *rlung*.

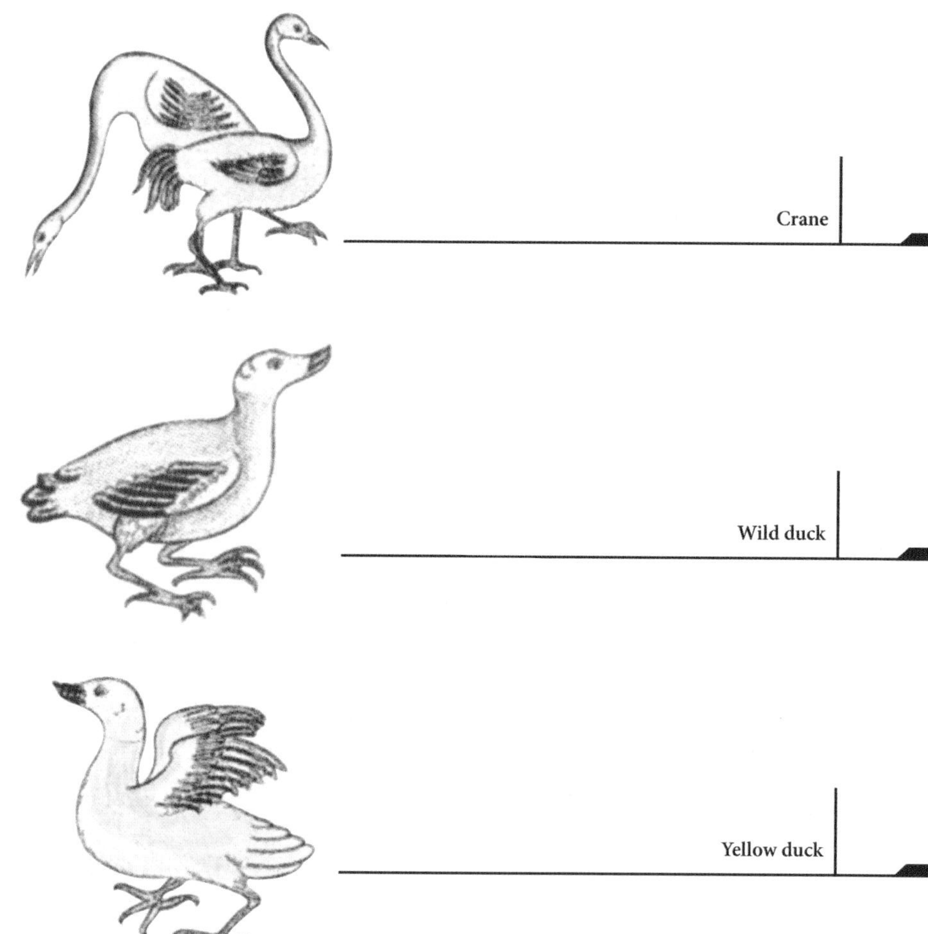

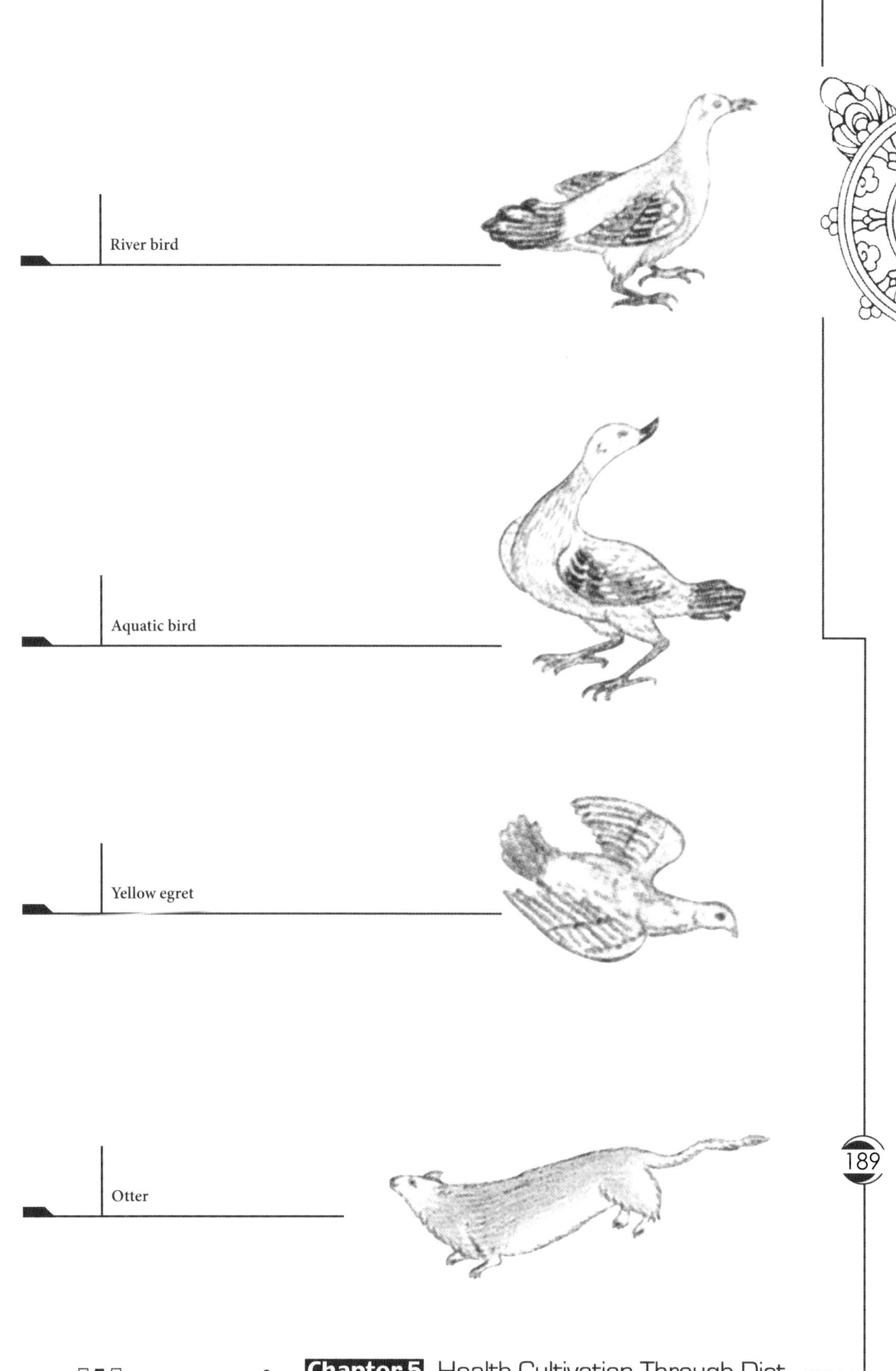
River bird
Aquatic bird
Yellow egret
Otter

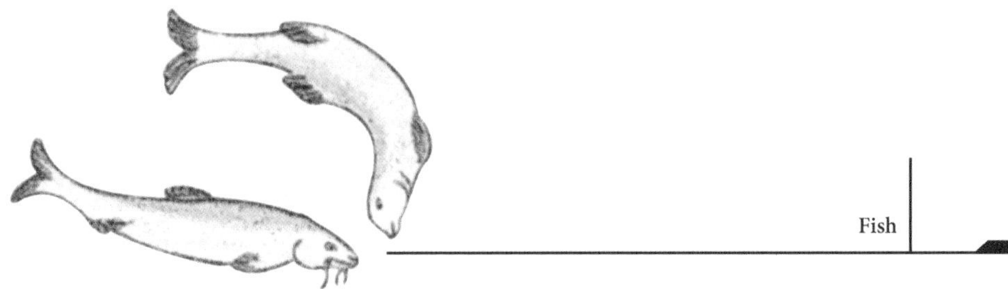

Fish

The meat of animals from wet regions is moist, heavy, and humid. It treats cold stomach, cold kidney, and cold *rlung* disorders.

Meats of animals from moderate areas

Animals that live in moderate areas include fierce birds, domestic birds and animals, and cave-inhabiting animals. Their meat includes characteristics from both the above two classes of animals. Fierce birds include crows, vultures, kites, and owls; cave-inhabiting animals include scorpions, marmots, snow toads, frogs, snakes, Tibetan badgers, sandy

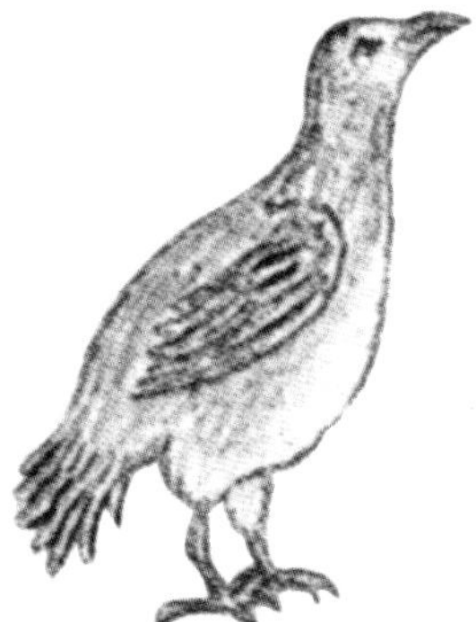

Small crow

lizards, and agama; domestic animals and birds include yaks, camels, horses, donkeys, dairy cows, yellow cows, goats, sheep, dogs, pigs, cats, and chickens.

Owl

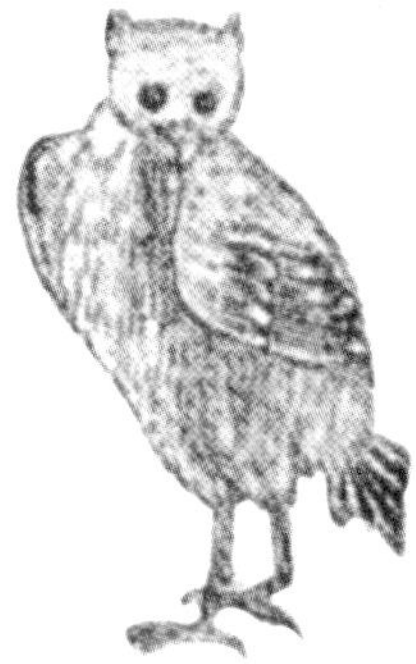

Turtledove

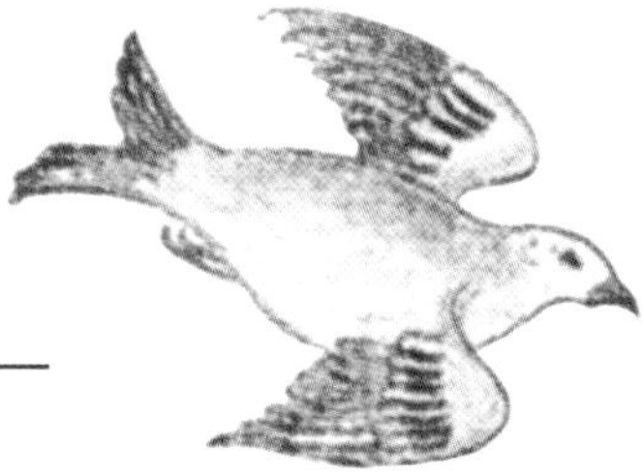

Vulture

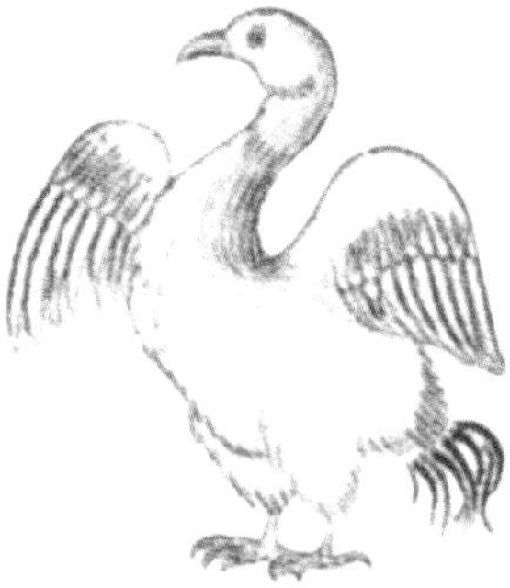

Eagle

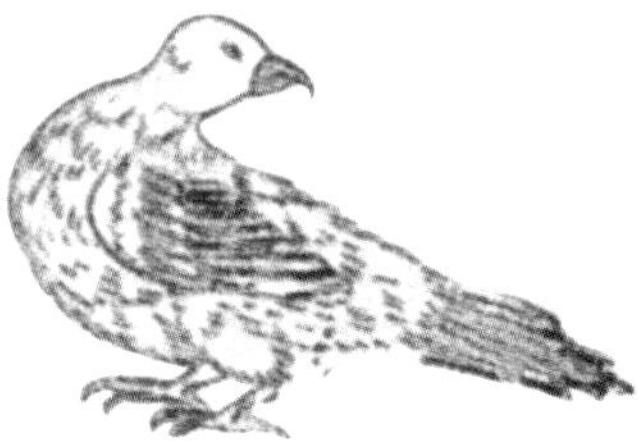

Sparrow hawk

Zupiko

Crow

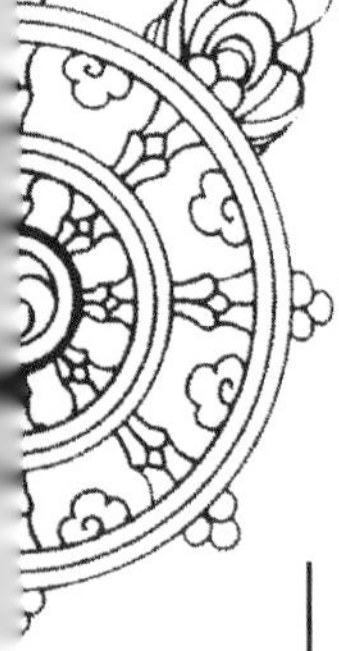

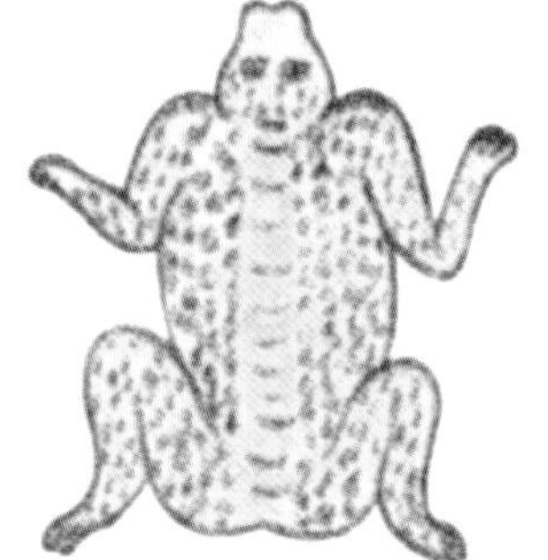

Snow toad

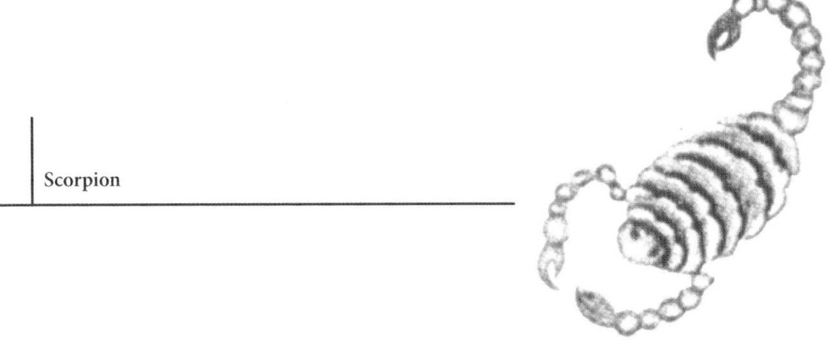

Scorpion

Meat from birds and beasts of prey and other carnivorous animals increases stomach fire, drastically eliminates masses, strengthens the muscles, and treats all cold diseases.

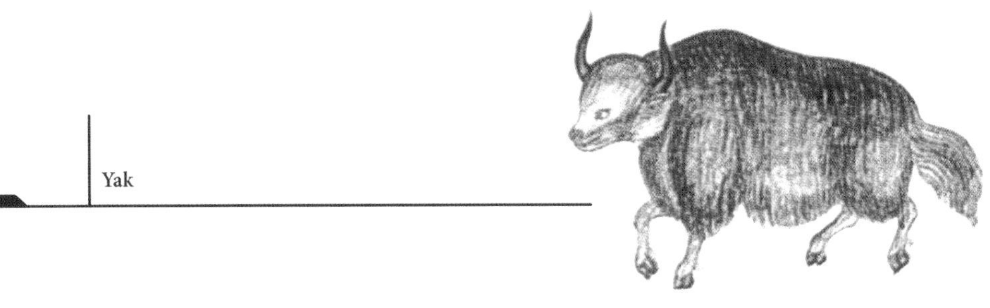

Yak

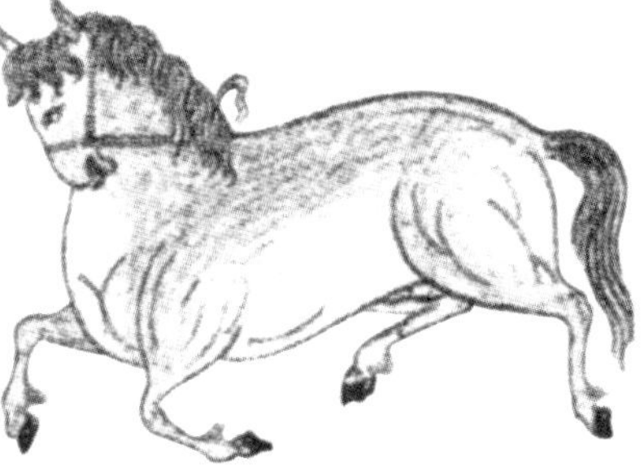

Horse

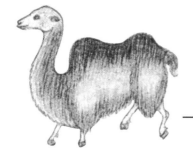

Camel

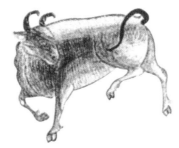

Milk cow

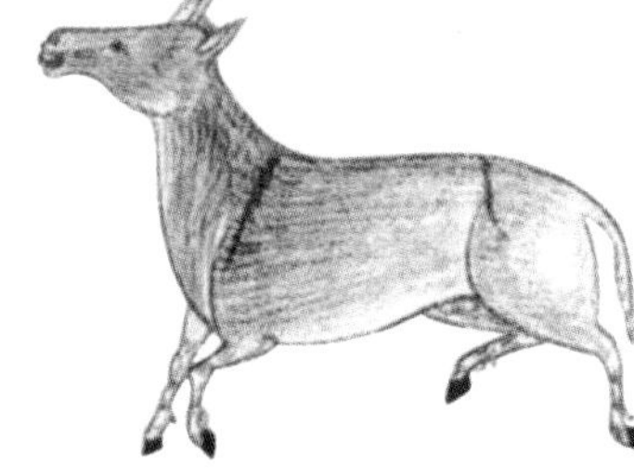

Donkey

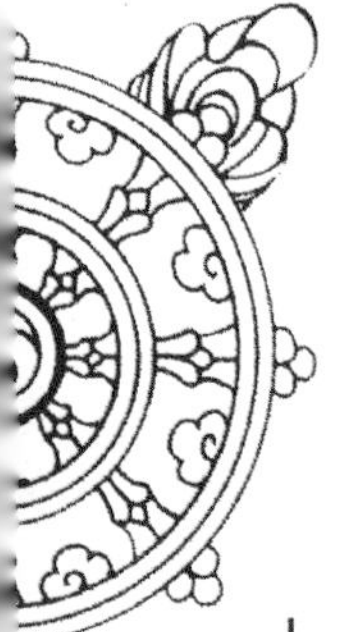

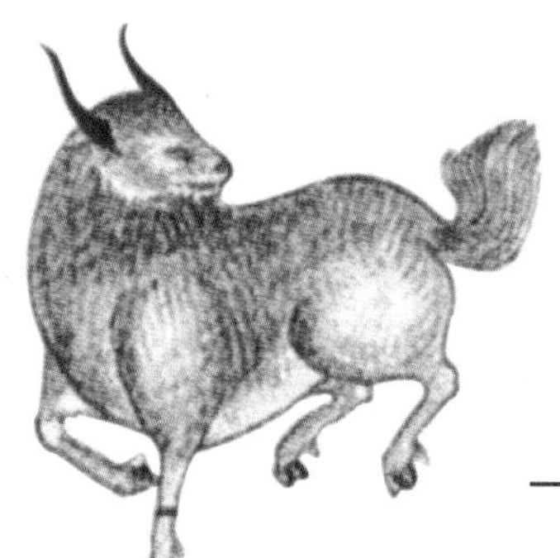

Female zupiko

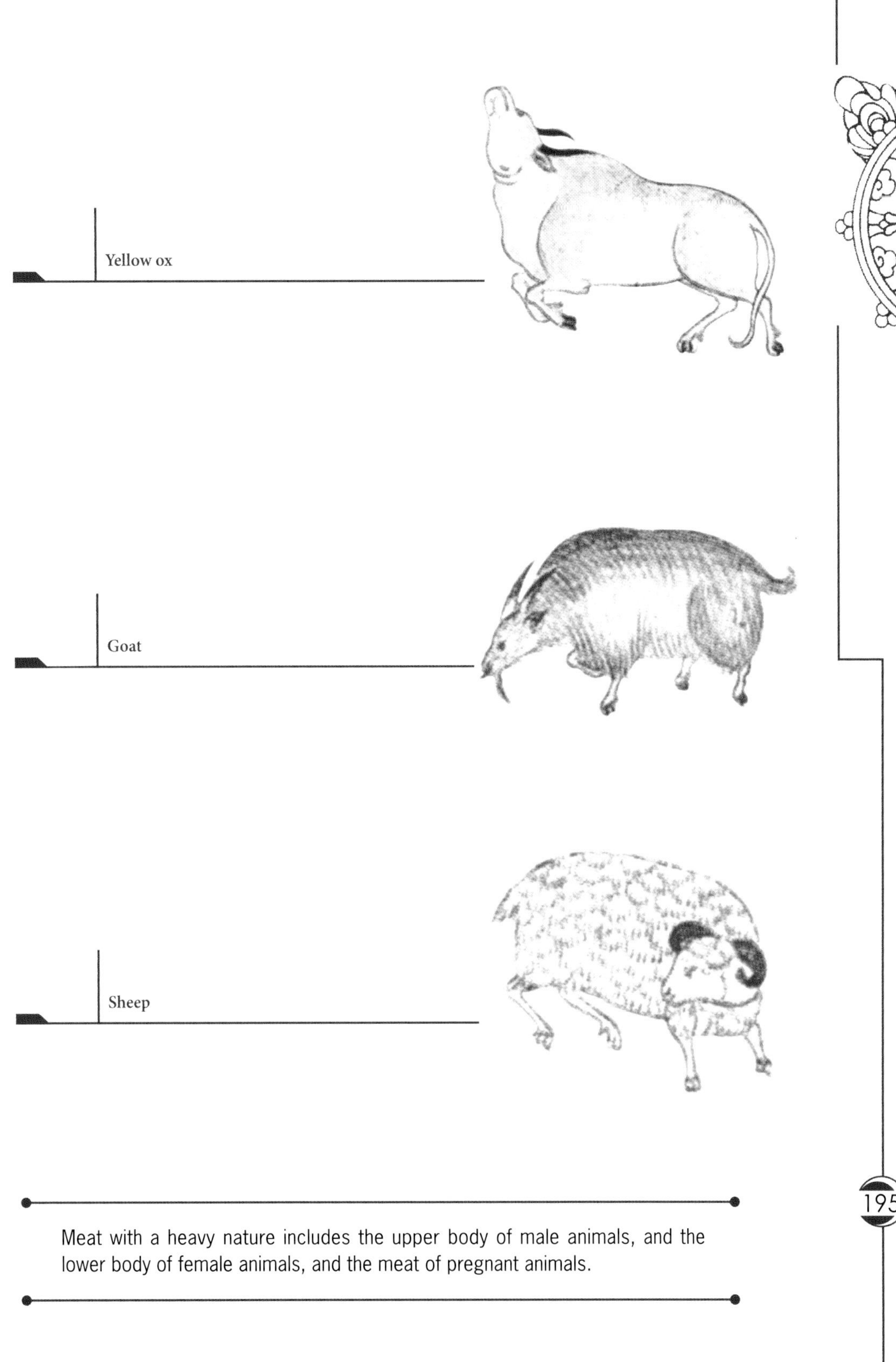

Meat with a heavy nature includes the upper body of male animals, and the lower body of female animals, and the meat of pregnant animals.

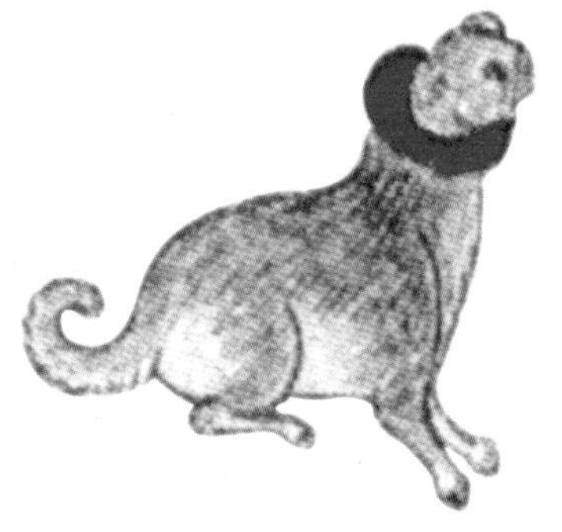

Dog

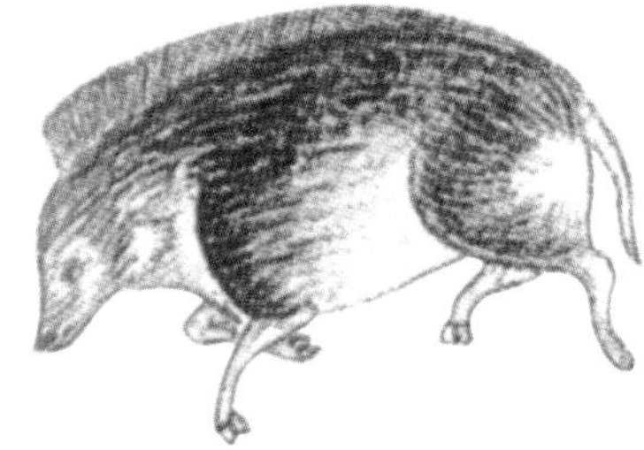

Pig

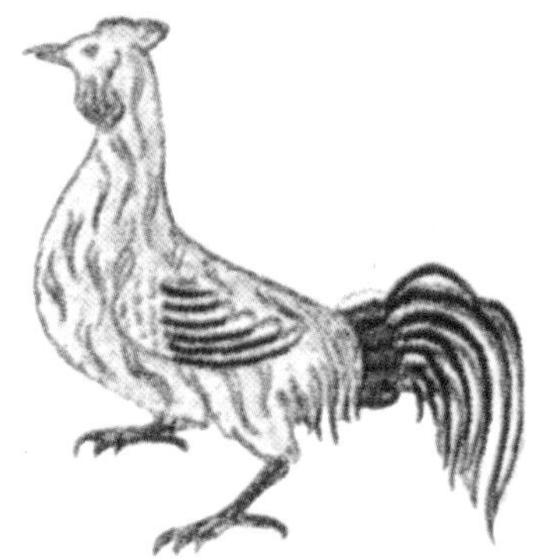

Chicken

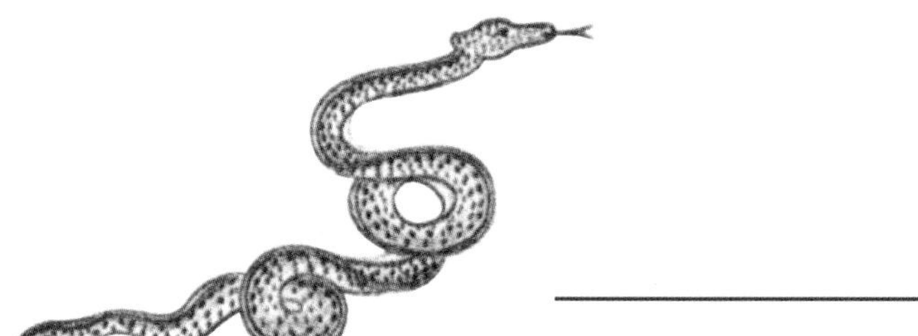

Snake

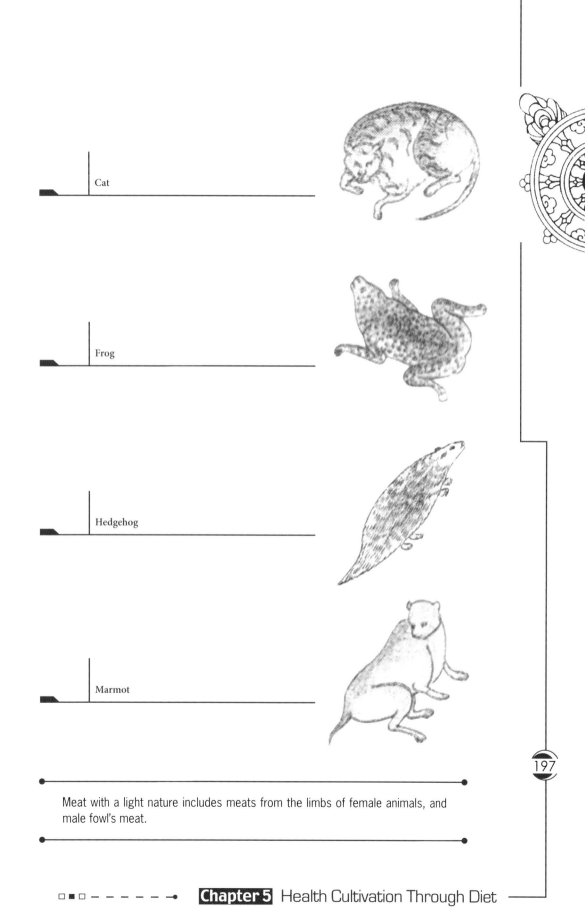

Meat with a light nature includes meats from the limbs of female animals, and male fowl's meat.

Tibetan badger

Sandy lizard

Agama

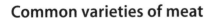

Meat from the head, upper body, chest, back, hip, and waist have a heavy nature, increasing in heaviness in the order listed.

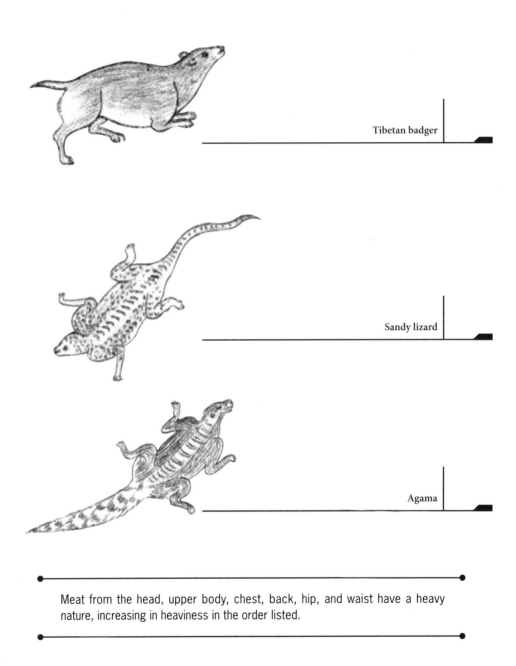

Common varieties of meat

Sheep meat (mutton)

This is the main kind of meat eaten in Tibet, and is well loved by the Tibetan people. It is warm, moist, nutritious, is helpful to the appetite and digestion, can strengthen the body, generate the original qi, and treat *rlung* and *badkan* diseases. It is good at resisting cold in winter.

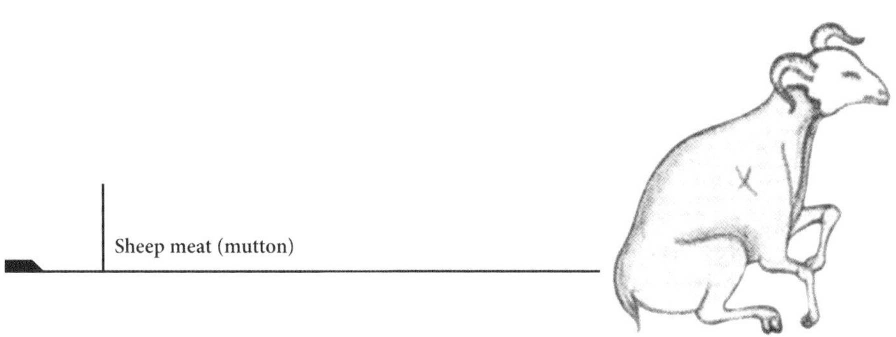

Sheep meat (mutton)

Goat meat

Goat meat is cool and heavy, difficult to digest, and treats syphilis, food poisoning, black smallpox, and burns. Since it is cool, it should be consumed in late spring and early summer when the weather becomes warm. During this time of year goats lose weight and the meat will be lighter. Since it is heavy and difficult to digest it will cause relapses of *rlung*, *mkhris pa* and *badkan* diseases. It should only be consumed with caution by the elderly, children, and those with chronic diseases.

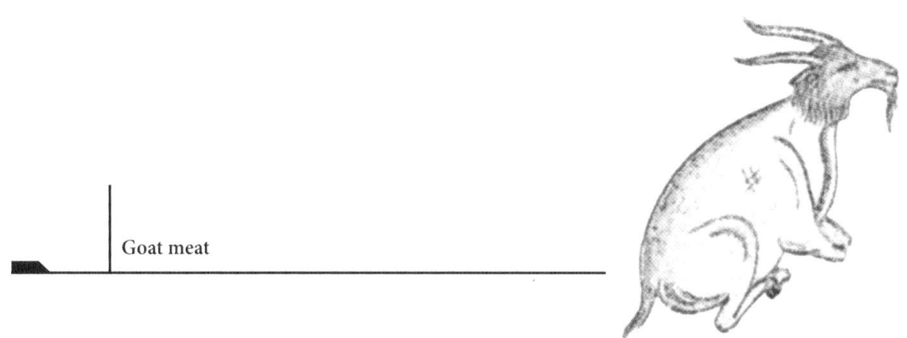

Goat meat

Yellow cow meat (beef)

It is cool and moist and it removes diseases of the fire-accompanying *rlung*. It can be consumed by patients with heat, phlegm fire, and damp-heat.

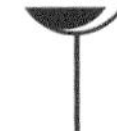

Water buffalo meat

It has a sedative action and helps sleep, strengthens muscles, and is indicated in insomnia, weakness, lassitude, sore and weak tendons. It can be sliced and boiled in porridge.

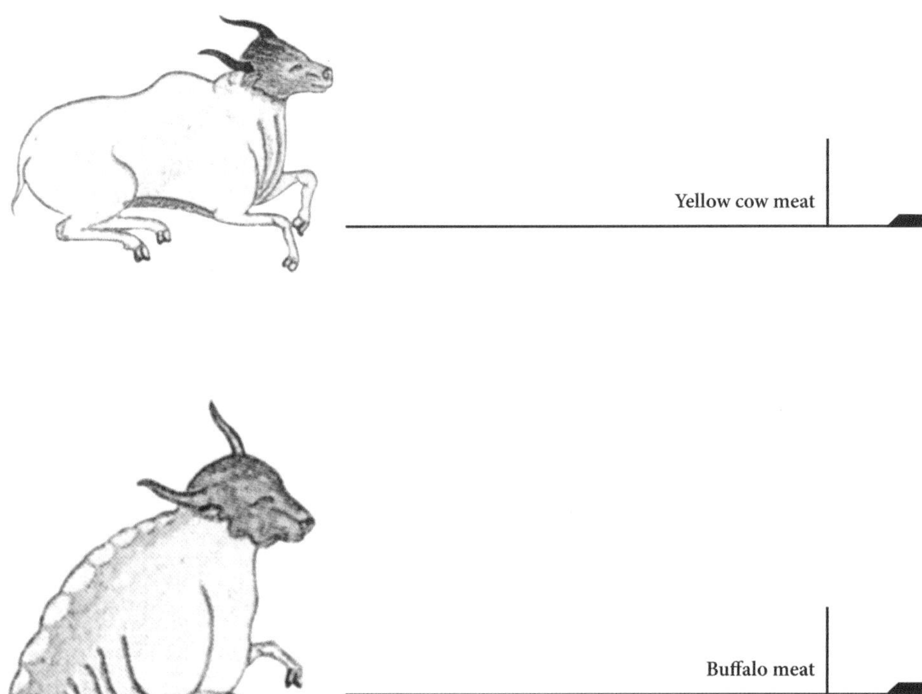

Pork

A very nutritious food, pork is cool, light, and moist. It clears heat, treats sores, and purple *badkan* disease. It is contraindicated in patients with the common cold.

Yak meat

This is a special product of the Tibetan plateau and is delicious, nutritious, has a low fat content and is an excellent tonic food. It is warm in nature, moist, and treats all cold syndromes, but it may cause blood and *mkhris pa* diseases. It is indicated in cases of deficient cold of the spleen and stomach, chronically weak patients with insufficient central qi, difficult breathing, pale complexion, diarrhea, and cold limbs.

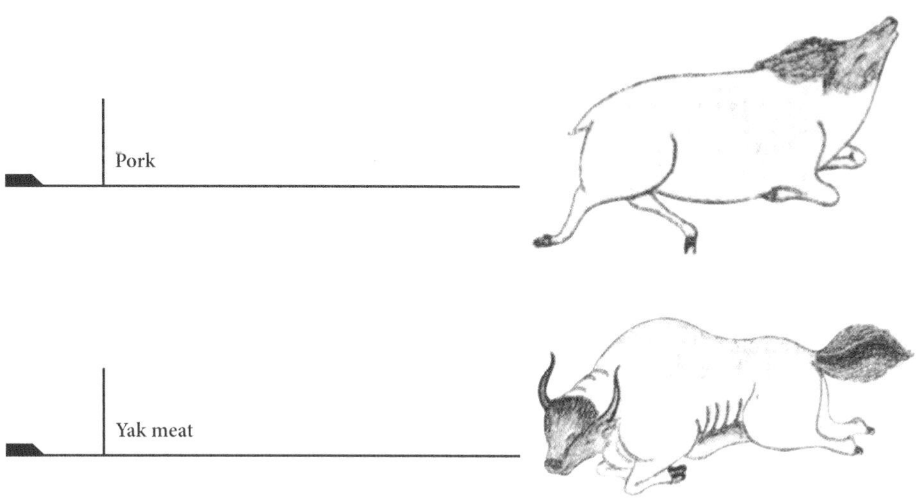

Meat of the wild ox

This kind of meat increases fire and heat, and treats cold diseases of the liver and stomach. Presently, wild ox is rarely seen.

Horse and donkey meat

The meat from around the spine eliminates wind, heat, and treats cold waist and yellow fluid diseases.

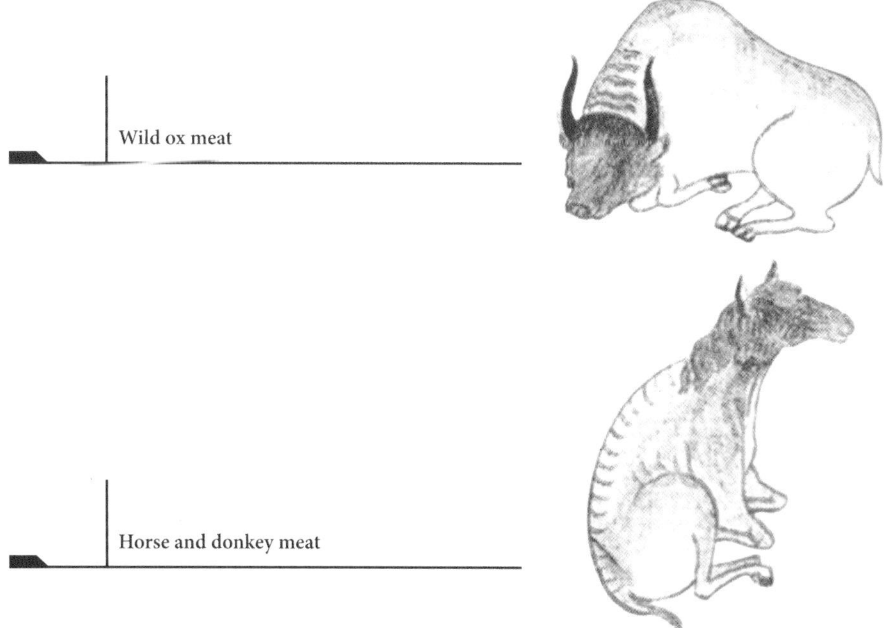

Chicken and sparrow meat

It is claimed that these kinds of meat increase semen and effectively treat sores. Black chicken meat is an antidote to many kinds of toxins. The *Crystal Materia Medica* says, "Black hen meat detoxifies."

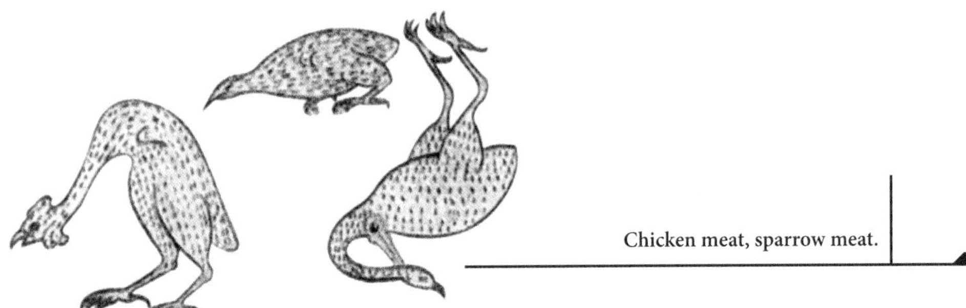

Chicken meat, sparrow meat.

Wild rabbit meat

It is warm and rough, increases heat, and stops diarrhea. Modern studies reveal that prolonged consumption of rabbit meat makes the skin soft, gives the body a smooth shape, and prevents and treats hypertension and coronary heart disease.

Marmot meat

This animal is frequently seen on the Qinghai-Tibet plateau and only used as medicine. It is warm, heavy, and moist and treats scrofula, sores, stomach disease, low back problems, kidney disease, head disorders, and cold *rlung* disease. It invigorates yang, and treats cold disorders of the low back and kidney.

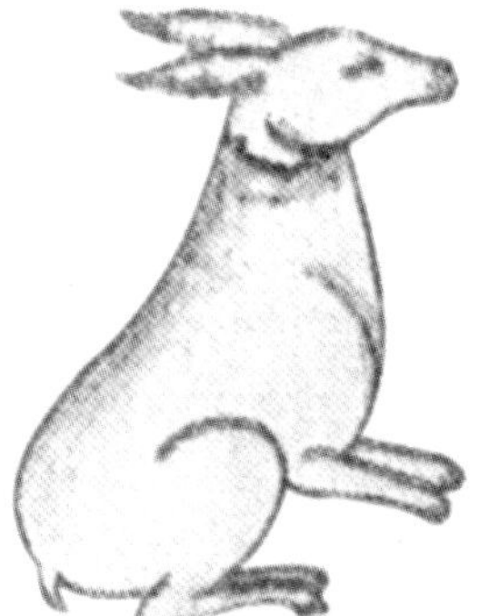

Wide rabbit meat

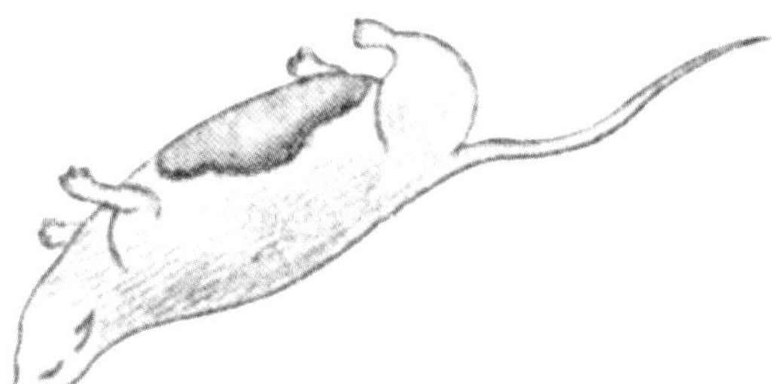

Marmot meat

Fish

Fish is sweet, warm, is good for the digestion and appetite, improves vision, and treats stomach disease, sores and ulcers, scrofula, and *badkan* disorders.

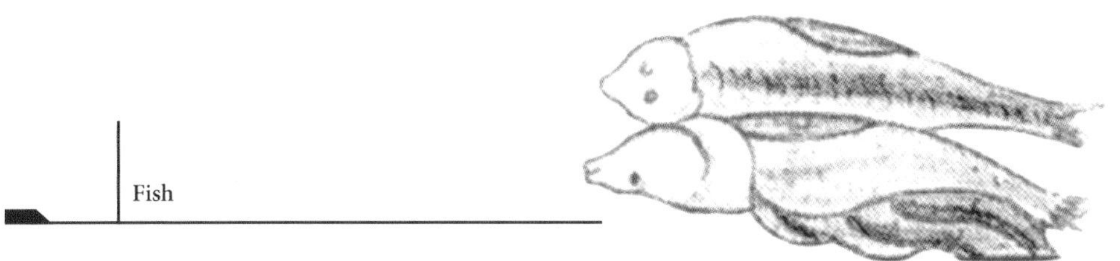

Fish

In summary, from the perspective of health cultivation, the sex of the animal, the freshness of the meat, and the body part all yield different functions therapeutically. Meat from a male animal's upper body is heavy, greasy, and that from the lower body is light. Meat from a female animal's upper and lower body is the reverse. Meat from pregnant animals is heavy. For animals walking on four legs, the meat from males is heavier than that from females. In terms of body parts, meat from female limbs, and from male birds is light; that from beasts' heads, upper body, chest, back, hip, or waist is heavy, with the degree of heaviness ascending in the order listed. Fresh meat is cool, cured meat is warm and more nutritious. Meat that is a number of years old can increase fire-heat, and boost stomach fire. Finally, meat from old, very young, weak, emaciated, diseased or animals that died due to toxins are inferior and should not be consumed.

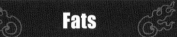

Fats

Fats are classified into butter, vegetable oil, marrow fat and animal fat. All fats are sweet in taste and heavy and cool in nature, becoming heavier in the order listed. Moreover, all fats are nurturing, blunt, fine, soft and moist. They are mild purgatives, can moisten the skin, and are excellent nurturing foods for the elderly, weak, those who are extremely emaciated with rough dry skin, people whose blood and spirit have been nearly consumed, and those who work with their minds. Fats are very helpful to these types of people if they are taken in an adequate amount.

Butter

Technically, butter includes fresh butter, aged butter, smelted butter, fresh cheese, edible latex, and barrel butter. Butter can come from many sources, such as yak, zupiko, sheep, or goat. The actions of each kind of butter are different depending on how they were prepared.

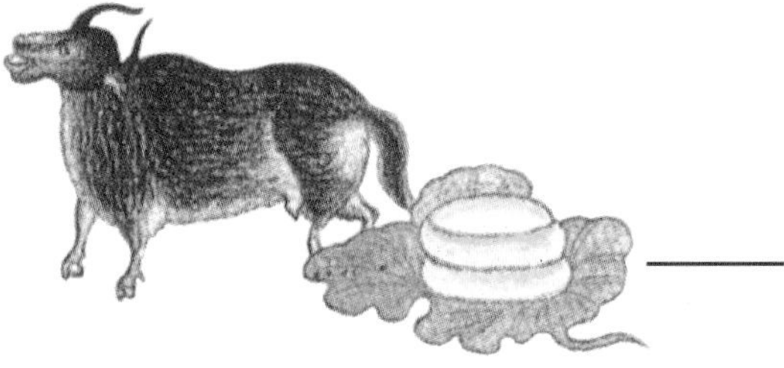

Butter prepared with zupiko milk.

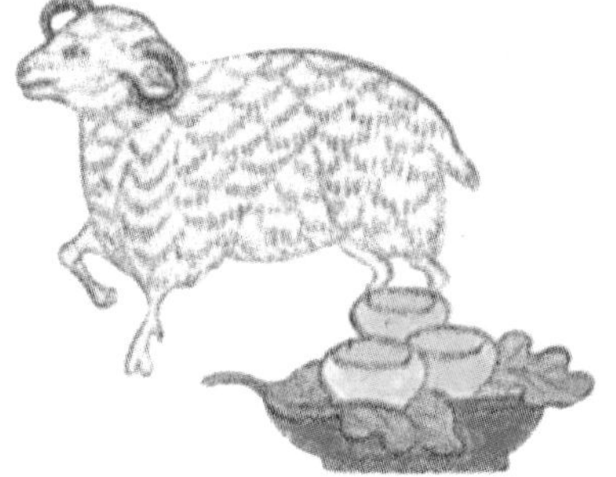

Butter prepared with sheep milk.

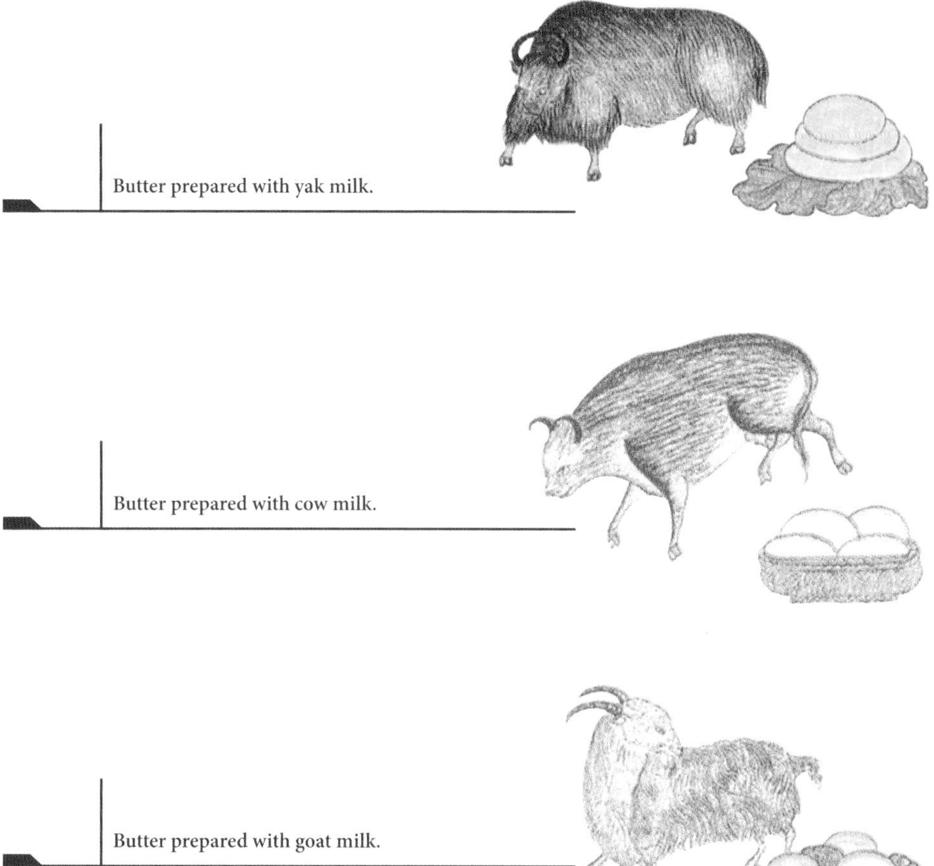

Butter prepared with yak milk.

Butter prepared with cow milk.

Butter prepared with goat milk.

Fresh butter

It is cool, strengthens yang, increases strength, improves the complexion, and clears *mkhris pa* fever, cures chronic lung disorders, *mkhris pa* disorders, blood disorders, cough and hemorrhoids.

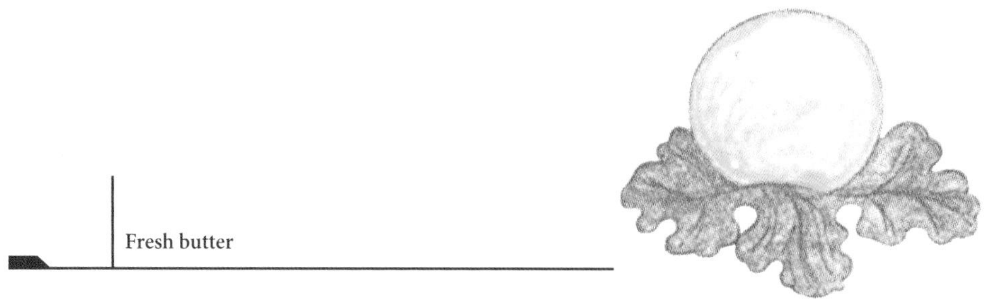

Fresh butter

Aged butter

This kind of butter dredges the heart orifice, removes *rlung* evils, mania, epilepsy, dizziness, forgetfulness, unconsciousness, and speeds the healing of ulcers and sores.

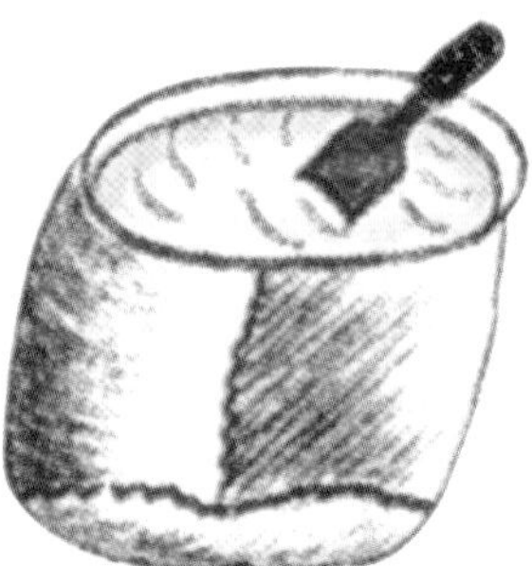

Aged butter

Smelted butter

Smelted butter energizes the spirit, improves the memory, increases strength, makes one keen and clear, moistens the skin, and solidifies the sense organs. This is the highest kind of butters and can be consumed frequently.

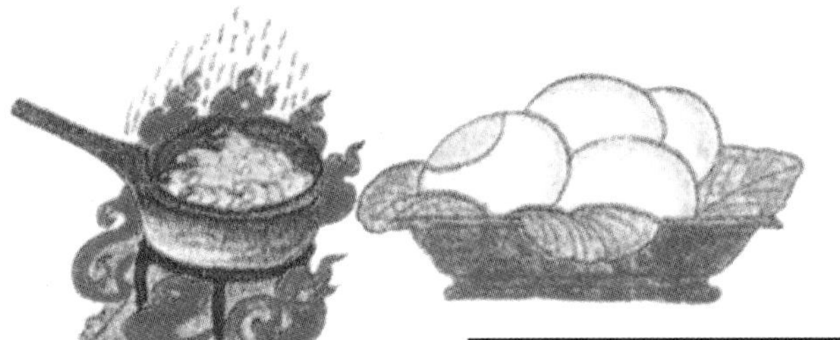

Smelted butter

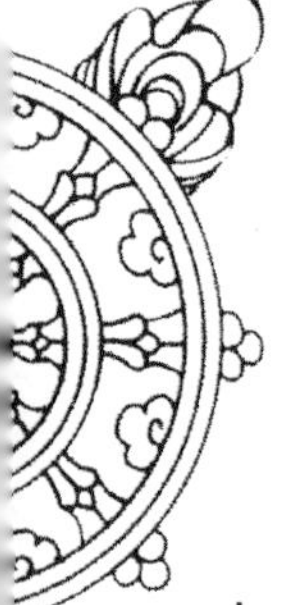

Fresh cheese, edible latex

Fresh cheese is similar to yoghurt, while edible latex refers to the milk secreted a few days after the delivery of baby animal, and has a fresh smell. They are both heavy, improve appetite and digestion, dry up stool, have sedative and strengthening actions, produce *badkan* and can induce *badkan* disorders.

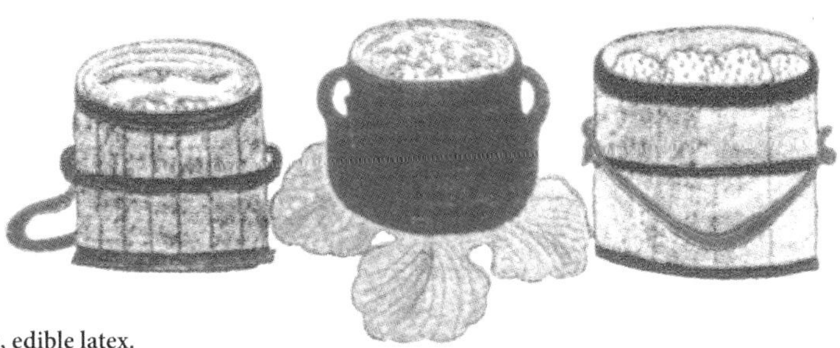

Fresh cheese, edible latex.

Fats are sweet and are mild purgatives. They are moist, blunt, fine, soft and wet, and are beneficial to the elderly, children, the weak, those with impaired blood and semen, cases of diarrhea, overstrain of mental work, and critical *rlung* disorders.

Barrel butter

This refers to the butter accumulated on the barrel wall. It is warm, increases heat and treats *badkan* and *rlung* disorders.

Butter from different sources has different actions, with quite different tastes and natures. Butters prepared from yak and sleep milk are warm, increase stomach qi, and treat cold *rlung*; those prepared with zupico milk are neither cool nor warm, eliminate wind and clears heat; those from goat and cow milk are cool, and treat fever due to *rlung*.

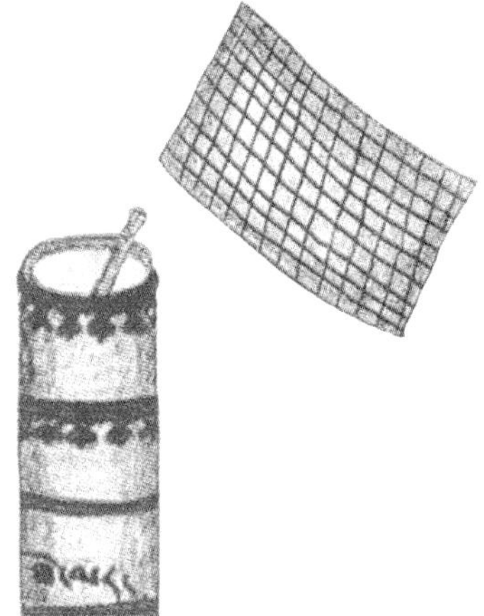

Barrel butter and milk residue.

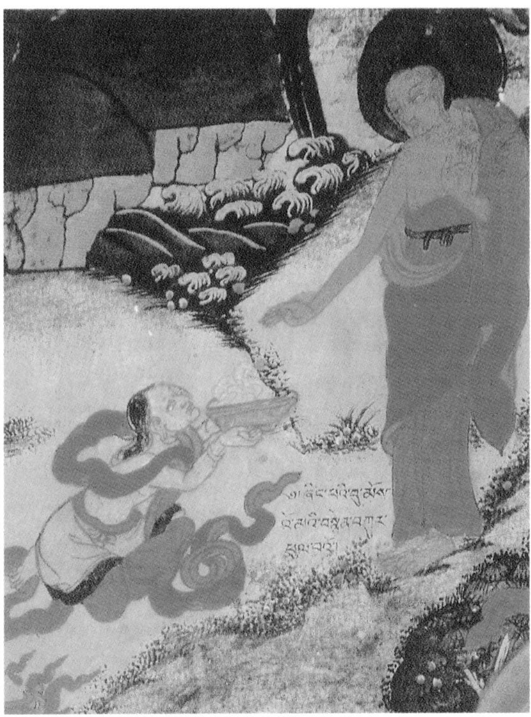

A rich variety of butter products are used as offerings at alters (part of a mural in a Tibetan monastery).

Plant oils

The most common plant oils in Tibet are vegetable oil, sesame oil, and mustard oil. Vegetable oil is the most common plant oil. It is sweet, warm, moist, is an antidote against toxins and a mild purgative. It is used topically for burns, sores of unknown causes, and itching. Sesame oil is mostly imported into Tibet. It is sweet, warm, and sharp. It increases muscles in slender people, but decreases weight in obese people. It treats *badkan* disease, *rlung* disease, stomach cold, dizziness, and constipation in weak patients. Mustard oil is astringent, heavy, treats *rlung* disease, but also induces *badkan* and *mkhris pa* disorders. It can't be used with mushrooms, or poisoning may occur.

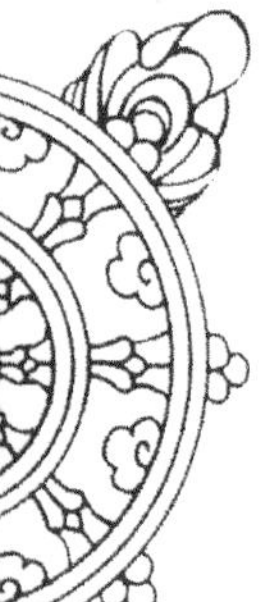

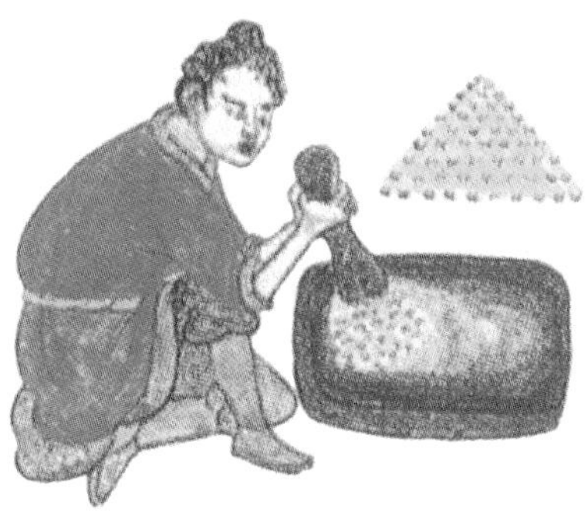

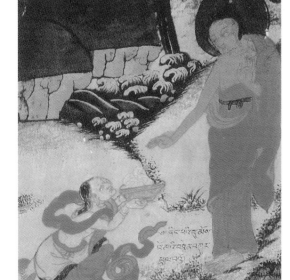

Sesame oil increases muscle in weak people, reduces weight in obese people, and treats *badkan* and *rlung* disorders.

Mustard oil eliminates *rlung* disorders, produces *badkan* and *mkhris pa*, but can't be fried with mushrooms.

Marrow oil

All animal marrow oils treat *rlung* disease, strengthen the spirit, but can induce *badkan* disease.

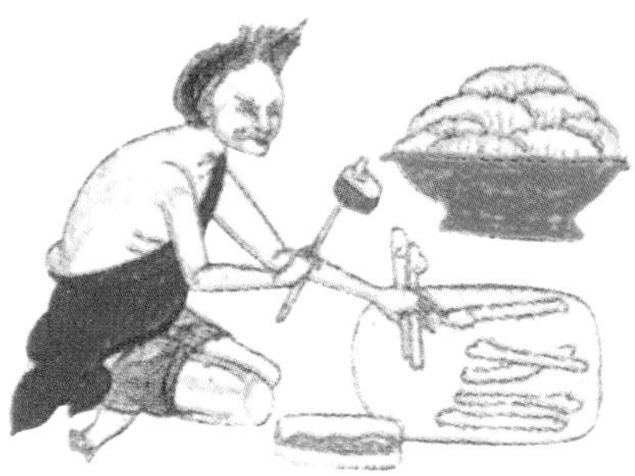

Marrow oil produces spirit and strength, and increases *badkan*.

Animal fats

All animal fats treat joint disorders, burns, *rlung* disorders, brain disease, ear disease, and uterine disorders. For ear problems and burns it is used topically. Fat from horses, donkeys and mules treat psoriasis; goat fat kills worms, and treats sores and syphilis.

Fats are nurturing, sharp, fine, soft, moist, are mild purgatives, moisten the skin, and are a superior tonic for the elderly, children, the weak, those that are extremely emaciated with rough skin, cases of extreme consumption of blood and semen, those who work with their minds and *rlung* patients.

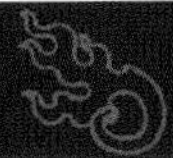

Vegetables and Seasonings

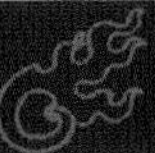

Due to geographical limitations, there are not many vegetables grown in Tibet. Because of this, vegetables only occupy a small portion of the diet of the Tibetan people. More seasonings are used to enhance the tastes of meat. Vegetables are not considered staple foods.

Vegetables

Tibetan medicine classifies vegetables into two different sub-categories. There are two kinds of climates, dry or wet, and four types of preparations, dried, fresh, cooked and uncooked, that vegetables are divided into. Dried vegetables, cooked vegetables, and those from a dry climate are warm and light, while fresh vegetables, uncooked vegetables, and those from a wet climate are cool and heavy. Warm and light vegetables treat *rlung* and *badkan* diseases, and cool and heavy vegetables treat *mkhris pa* disease. Vegetables also have individual tastes and natures which influence their selection. A patient with a fever, for instance, needs cold vegetables, and those with cold syndromes need warm vegetables. Furthermore, some vegetables may affect the action of certain medicine. Hence, one must carefully select vegetables during the treatment of disease.

In Tibetan region, common vegetables are radish, garlic, onion, wild garlic, Tibetan radish, carrot, potato, winter amaranth, pea and mustard.

Radish

There are two kinds of radish. The kind that is harvested before Venus appears is light and warm, pungent, slightly bitter, easy to digest, and slightly increases stomach fire. It drastically activates blood, removes stagnant blood, disperses nodules, arrests coughing and panting, expels sputum, treats insufficient stomach fire, hoarseness, disorders of the pharynx, constipation, and *rlung*, *mkhris pa* and *badkan* disorders. The kind is that obtained after Venus appears is an old radish and is astringent, cool, increases stomach fire, and induces *badkan* diseases. After being cooked, its taste becomes light, moist, and it nurtures the body, eliminates wind and opens the orifices.

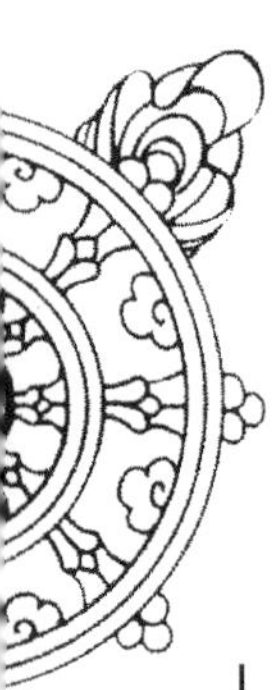

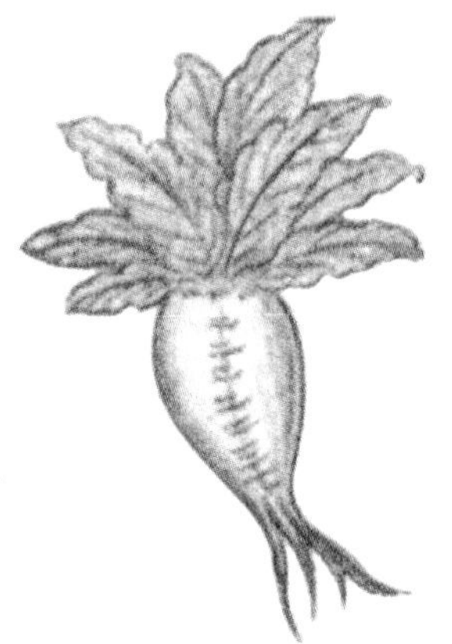

Fresh radish produces heat.

Tibetans consume radishes all year long, especially in the winter.

There is also a kind of Tibetan radish that is produced in the plateau. Its action is similar to that of the regular radish. Tender young Tibetan radishes are beneficial to the body, and old ones injure the body, but the old type help expel toxins from the body. Old Tibetan radishes are used as medicine.

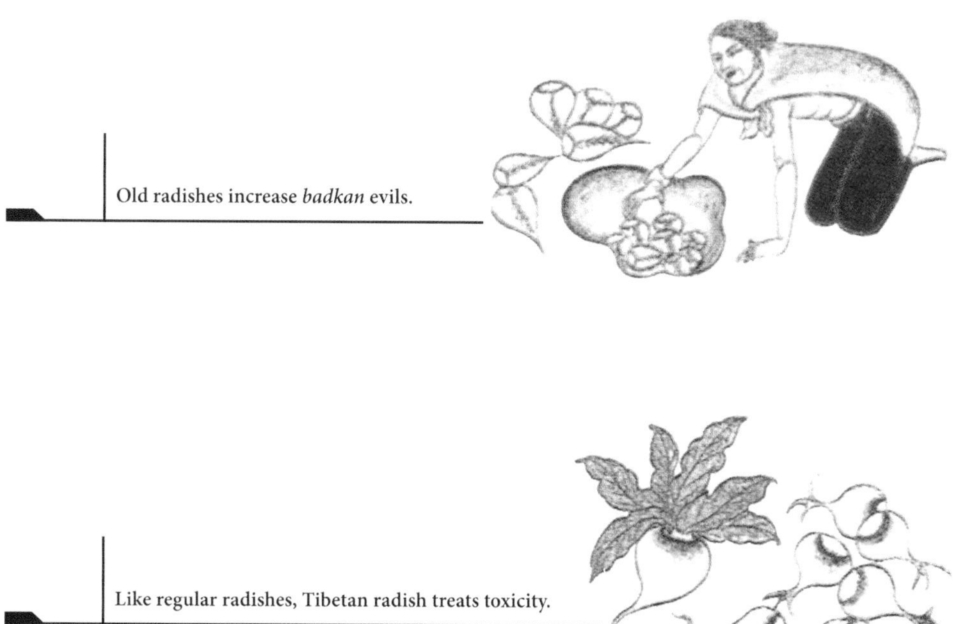

Old radishes increase *badkan* evils.

Like regular radishes, Tibetan radish treats toxicity.

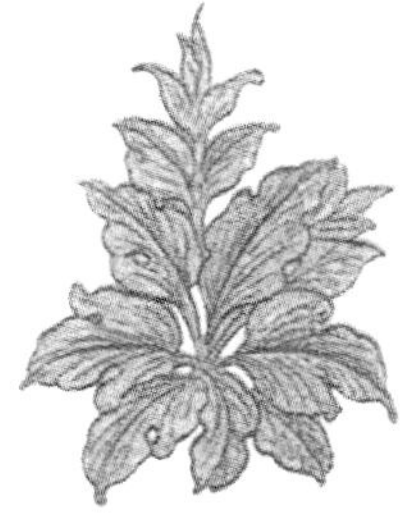
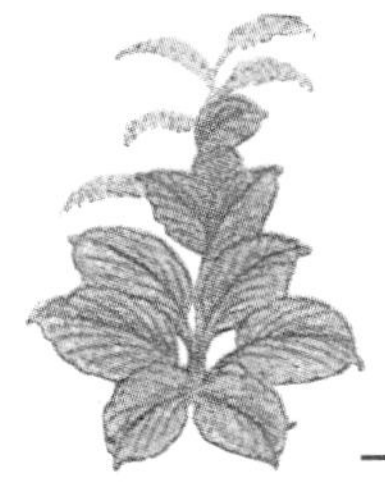

Leaves and seeds of rhubarb treat *badkan* disease and are good for digestion and the appetite.

Onion, garlic

Onions and garlic are good for digestion and the appetite, have a sedative action, and treat *badkan* and *rlung* disorders. Both are pungent, bitter and warm. Onion has a strong action of eliminating wind and cold, and is good for debilitated stomach fire, females that are averse to wind, and worm diseases. Garlic is good for resolving toxins, expelling worms, arresting diarrhea and eliminating indigestion, epidemics, sores and ulcers, and dysentery. Do not consume too much of either or the stomach will become distended.

There is a kind of wild garlic produced in Tibet, and is occasionally used as food. As is described in the *Crystal Materia Medica*, "All wild garlic is heavy, difficult to digest, but improves the appetite." Consume it only in an appropriate amount.

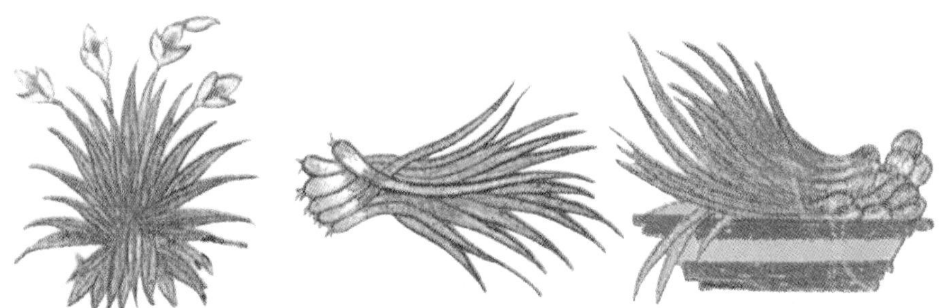

Wild garlic improves the appetite, but is difficult to digest.

Garlic and onion improves sleep and appetite.

Vegetables come from dry land or wet land, and there are fresh and dried vegetables, and cooked and uncooked vegetables. Those from dry regions, dried, and cooked vegetables are warm and light, while those from wet regions, fresh, and uncooked vegetables are cool and heavy. All green vegetables can be used as medicine and should be consumed in good quantity.

Seasonings

The common ones are:

Dried ginger

Warm, hot, generates fire, and treats *rlung* diseases.

Zanthoxylum

Can dilate the vessels and dredge the vessel gates, but can also induce *rlung* and *badkan* diseases.

Salt

Makes all food delicious, ascends stomach fire, improves digestion, and treats constipation.

Asafetida

Pungent, warm, disperses cold, kills worms, and treats *rlung* disease, stomach cold, abdominal distention and worms.

Tibetan fennel

Pungent, warm, improves the appetite, expels wind, regulates qi, and treats *rlung* disease, eye disease, and loss of appetite.

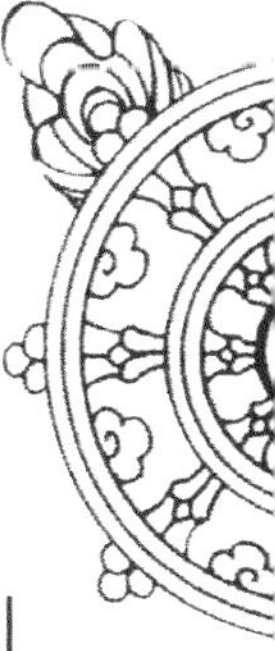

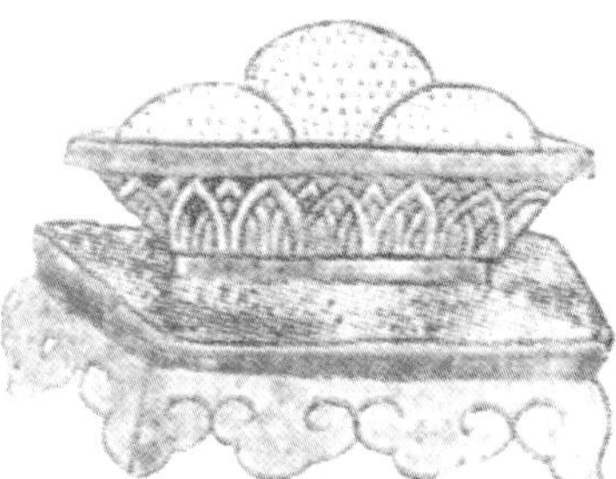

Asafetida eliminates *rlung* disease.

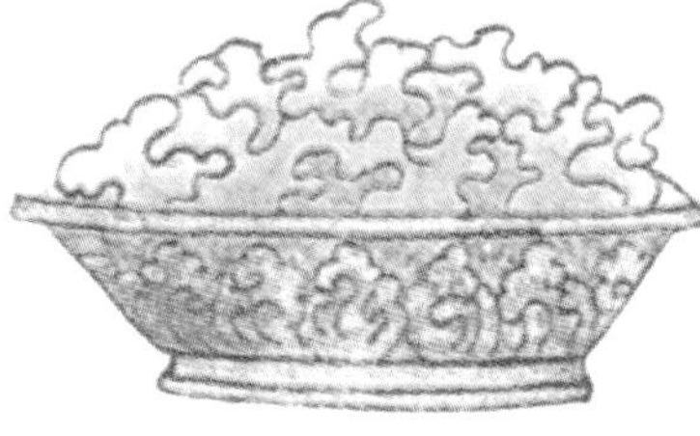

Dried ginger is warm and hot.

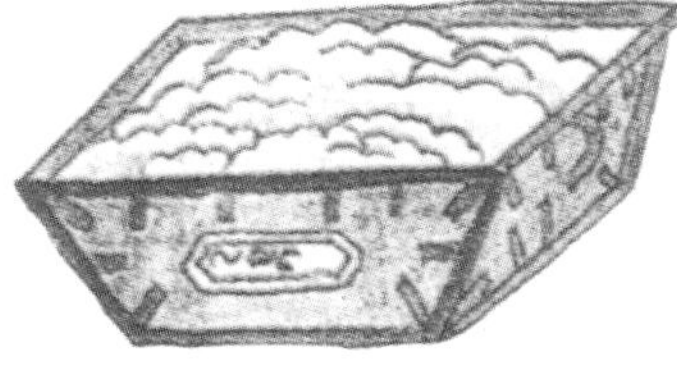

Salt is easily digested, gives a delicious taste to all food, and treats constipation.

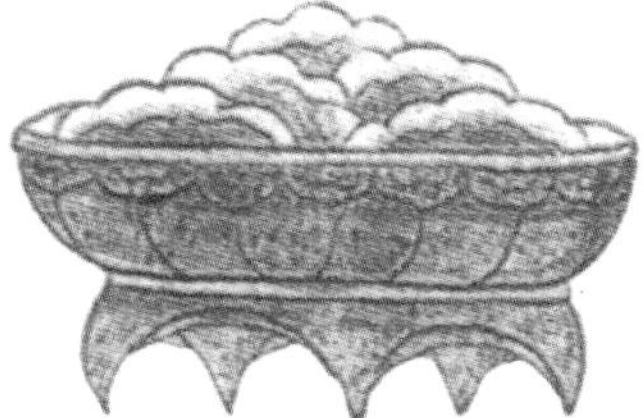

Tibetan fennel is warm and hot.

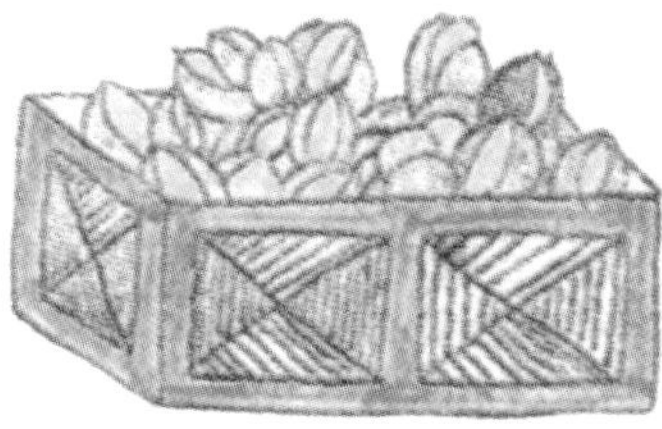

Zanthoxylum dredges the vessel gate, but also induces *rlung* and *badkan* disorders.

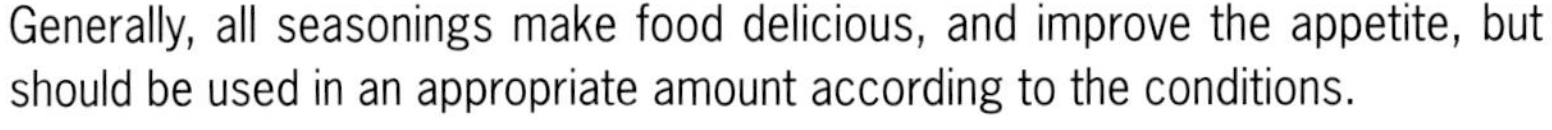

Generally, all seasonings make food delicious, and improve the appetite, but should be used in an appropriate amount according to the conditions.

Cooked Dishes

There are a wide variety of dishes prepared using the different kinds of food described above, using different cooking procedures such as boiling, stir-frying, or deep frying. Cooked dishes include staple foods and non-staple foods. Tibetan people have a unique view on the health cultivating functions of food. Generally, cooked foods are light and soft, readily digested, whereas raw food is cool, lowers stomach fire and is difficult to digest.

Staple foods

This mainly consists of rice porridge and *rtsam pa*, the latter being the most common staple food.

Rice porridge

This includes dilute porridge, dense porridge and sticky porridge, becoming lighter, more dilute, and easier to digest in the order listed. All are excellent for the elderly, debilitated, and patients with poor digestion. The more dense and sticky the porridge is, the better it is for weak people, while dilute porridge with warming medicinals added is best for nourishing patients with diarrhea. When milk and broth are added, it becomes even more heavy and difficult to digest.

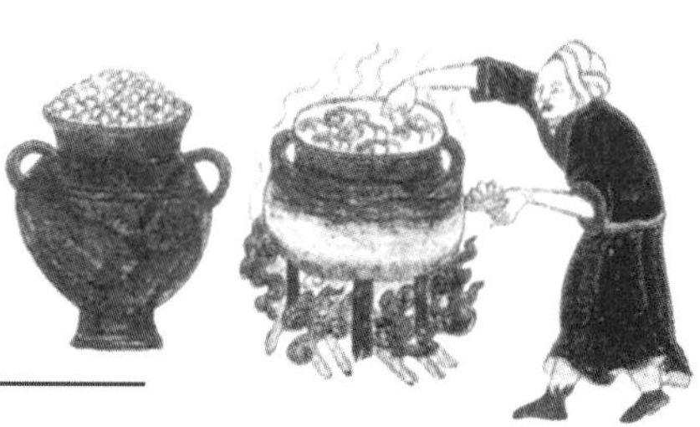

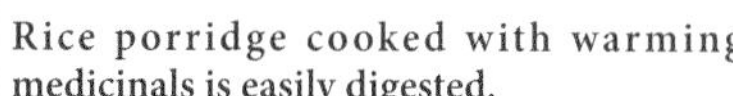

Rice porridge cooked with warming medicinals is easily digested.

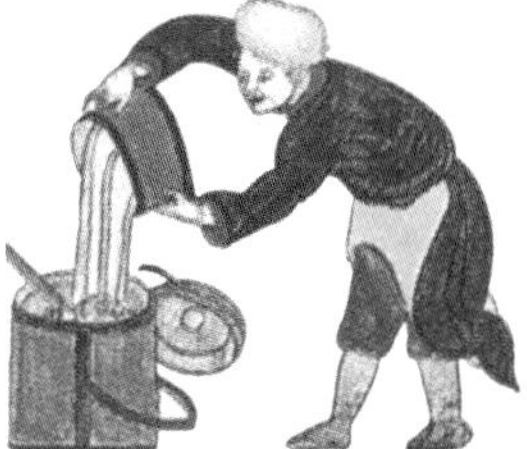

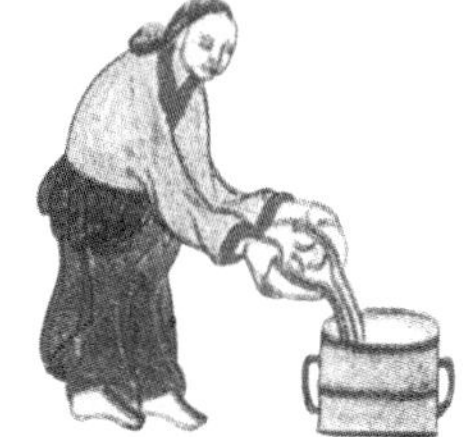

When milk and broth are cooked with porridge its nature becomes heavy.

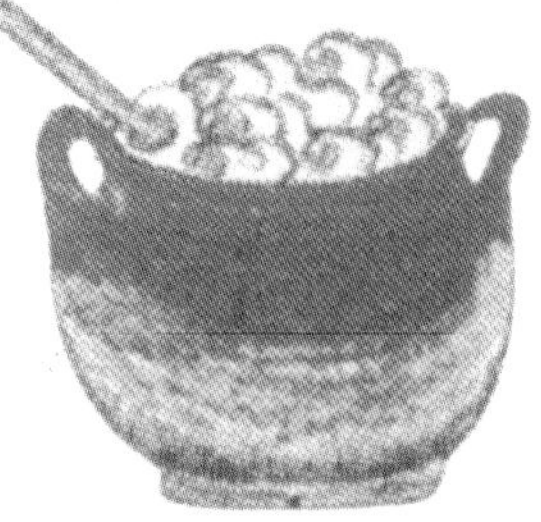

Dilute porridge helps digestion, increases body temperature, and prevents hardening of the arteries.

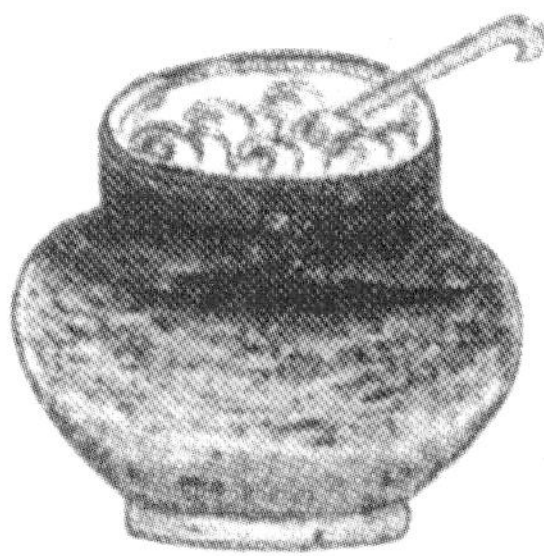

Dense porridge generates fire and heat, eliminates fatigue, and aids defecation.

Dilute porridge

This is a rice dish cooked with a large amount of water. Dilute porridge is easy to digest, helps to recover one's primordial qi, increase body fire, prevents hardening of the arteries, and eliminates evils that remain after diarrhea.

Dense porridge

A little bit denser than dilute porridge. It generates fire and heat, eliminates thirst and hunger, facilitates defecation and removes *badkan* disease.

Sticky porridge

Denser than the above, it stops diarrhea, eliminates hunger and thirst, and promotes digestion and the appetite.

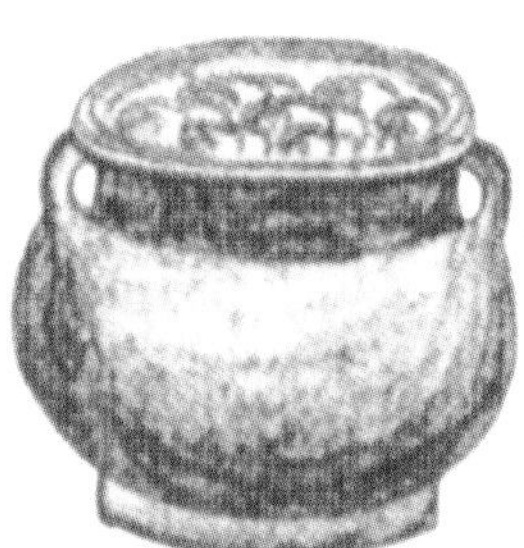

Sticky porridge stops diarrhea, strengthens the stomach and improves the appetite.

Stir-fried rice

When rice is stir-fried and then steamed, it can be eaten as food. It stops diarrhea and knits bone fractures.

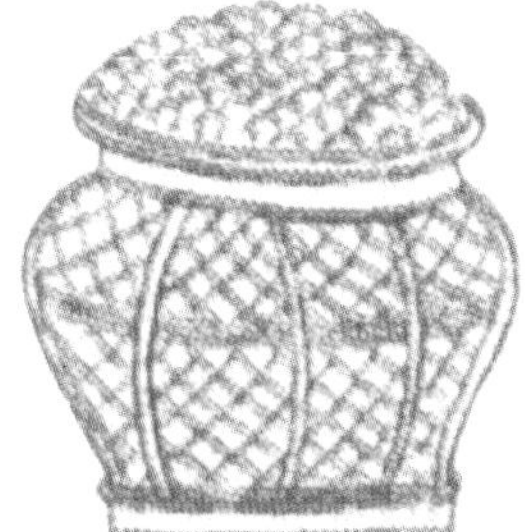

Stir-fried rice stops diarrhea and knits bone fractures.

Highland barley porridge

Cooking highland barley as a porridge hinders urination and defection. Adding vegetables to this kind of porridge makes it the best food to treat *rlung* disease. A modification is prepared by stir-frying the highland barley before boiling. Stir-fried highland barley is a tonic to the stomach, and the porridge prepared from it is light, warm, and readily digested.

The stir-frying of highland barley is somewhat difficult and the strength of the fire is very important. The barley grains should puff up like popcorn, with a pleasant fragrance, and a delicate, sweet taste.

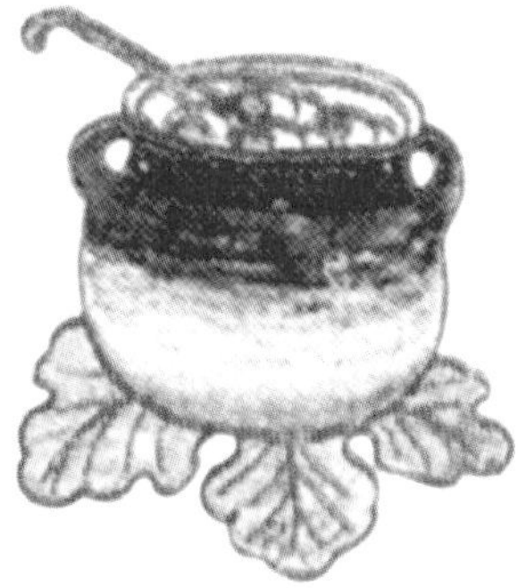

Highland barley porridge astringes the bowels.

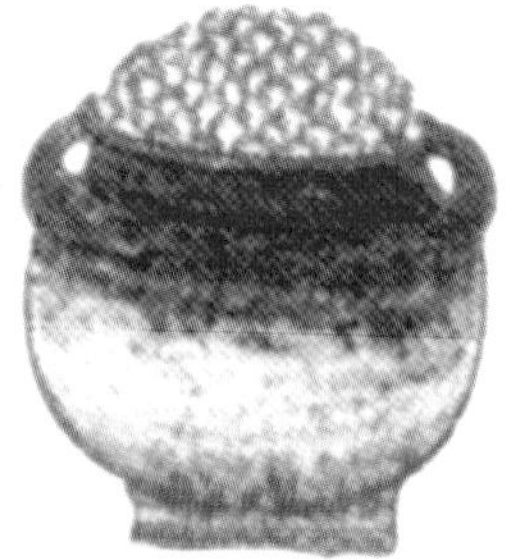

Stir-fried highland barley is nourishing to the stomach.

Rtsam pa

This is the main staple food of the Tibetan people. It is prepared with highland barley powder, and consumed in various ways. The most common method is prepared so that it can be eaten by hand. The powder is mixed with tea water and butter and prepared as a dough. It is heavy and strengthens the body.

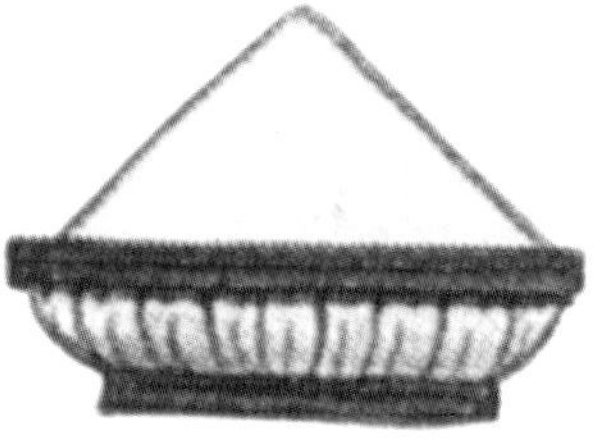

Cold *rtsam pa* increases one's strength.

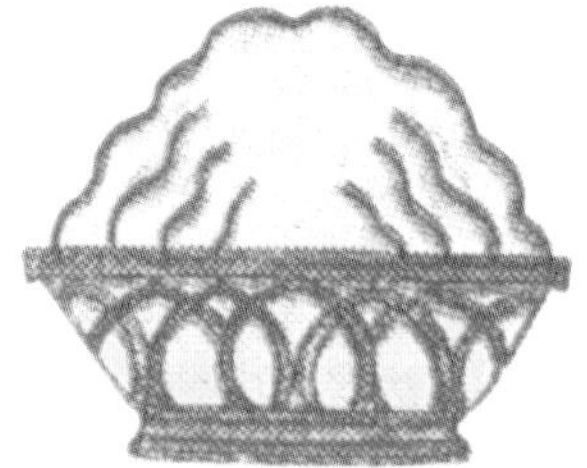

Boiled *rtsam pa* is easily digested.

Hot *rtsam pa* dumplings:

Small lumps of warm *rtsam pa* are made and then steamed. It is light and soft and digested rather easily.

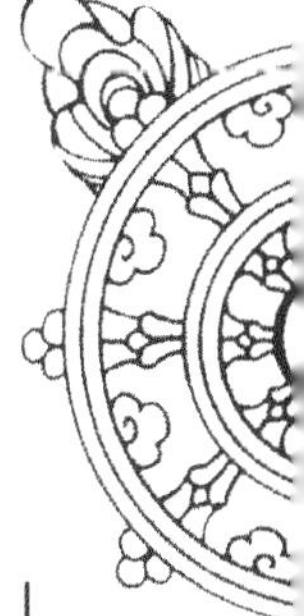

Yoghurt-*rtsam pa* dumplings:

Rtsam pa dough mixed with yoghurt can improve the appetite. It is easily spoiled, so should be eaten quickly. Another kind is made of dilute *rtsam pa* plus wine yeast. It treats *rlung* disease and improves the appetite. However, the residual fluid is harmful and induces diseases of the three evils so it should not be consumed.

Yoghurt plus *rtsam pa* improves the appetite.

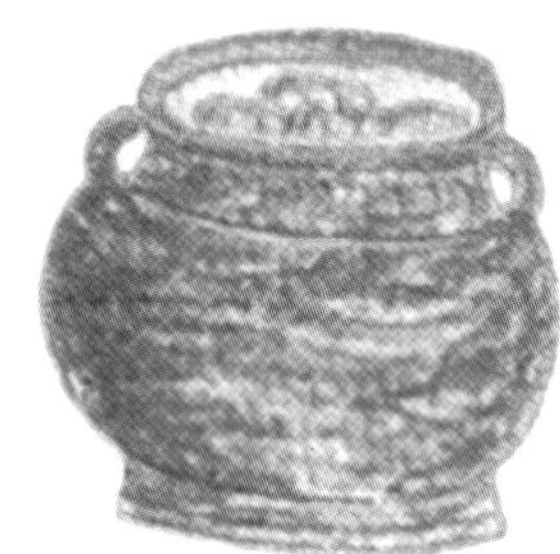

Rtsam pa plus seasoning is easily digested.

***Rtsam pa* paste:**

Add hot water or tea to *rtsam pa* to make a paste. It is easily digested and eliminates diseases of the three evils.

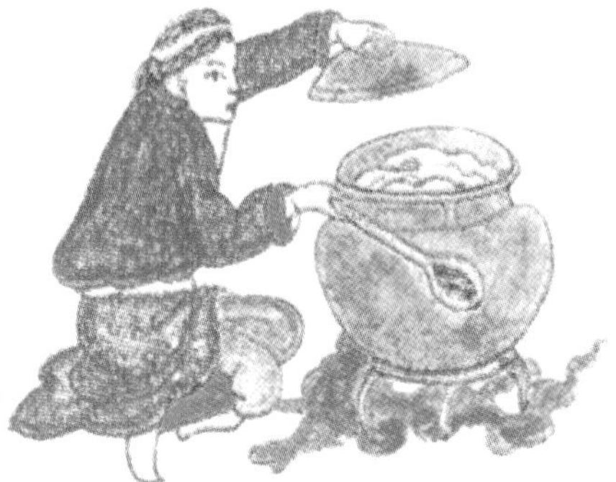

Rtsam pa paste with vegetables helps digestion.

Vegetable and meat dishes

Tibetan meat and vegetable dishes are very colorful and distinctive, and are mostly made from mutton, beef, radishes and winter amaranth. The cooking methods include steaming, boiling, stir-frying, deep frying.

Broth

Broth in Tibet is usually prepared by boiling the best mutton or beef. It is nurturing, increases body heat, and eliminates *rlung* disease.

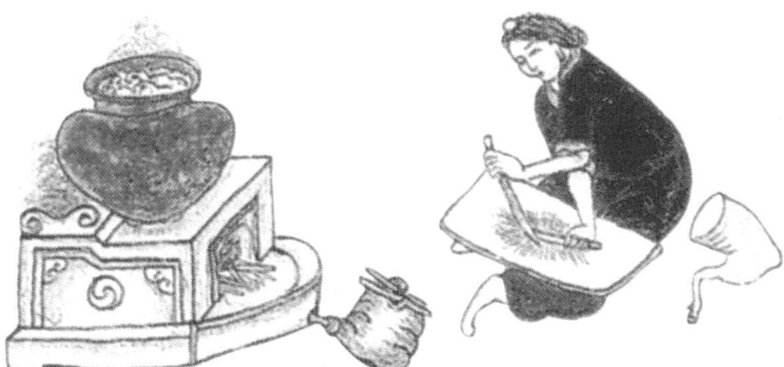

Broth generates heat and nurtures the body.

Nettles

These vegetables can be prepared by stir-frying, boiling in soup, or as stuffing in a bun. It eliminates *rlung* disease, and disperses *badkan* and *mkhris pa* diseases.

Winter amaranth

This plant is always stir-fried. It increases heat, and arrests diarrhea.

Peas

Peas are always stir-fried or boiled as soup. Fresh pea leaves are sweet, astringent, and have a neutral temperature. They resolve toxins and treat sores. Cooked pea leaves improve the appetite, remove excess grease, but are likely to induce *badkan* disease.

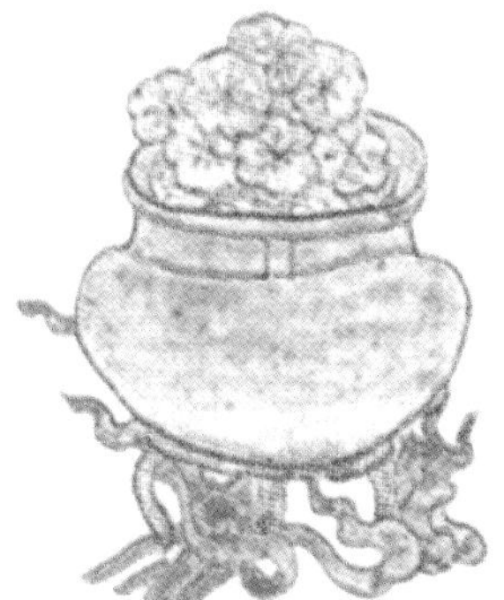

Winter amaranth generates heat and arrests diarrhea.

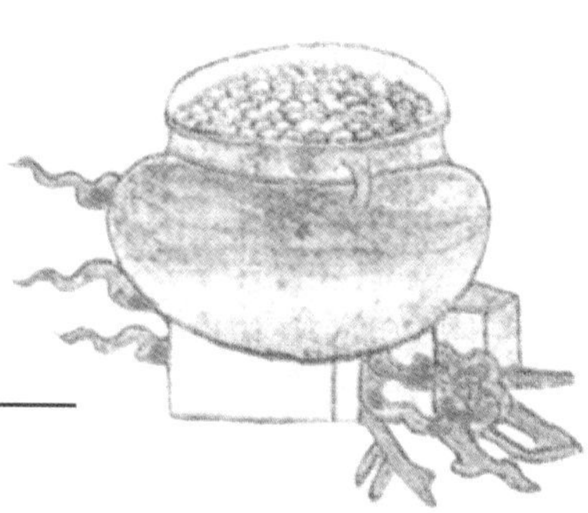

Peas improve the appetite and remove grease.

Gray striped vegetable

This type of vegetable is always prepared by stir-frying or boiled as soup. It moistens the stool, but can hurt the eyes. The type pioduced in the Menyu region treats diseases of the three evils

Radish

When cooked it stops diarrhea.

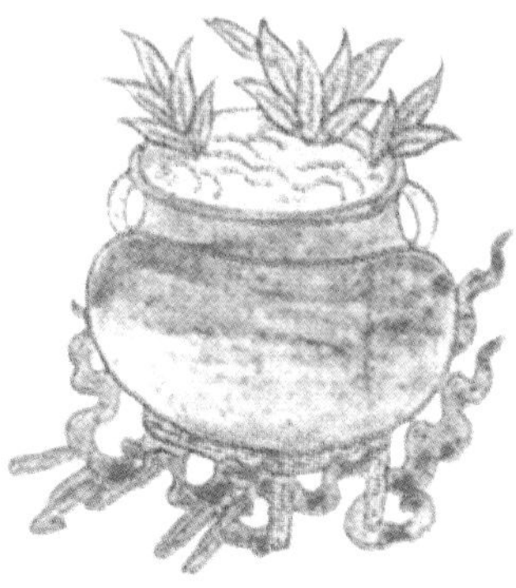

Gray striped vegetable harms the vision but treats constipation.

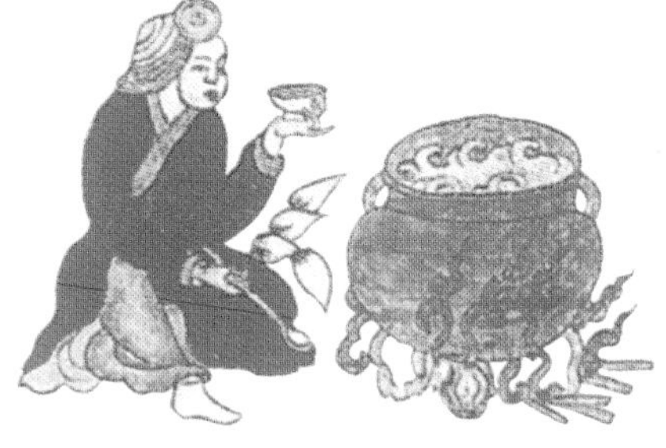

Radish stops diarrhea.

Dandelion

It is cool after being stir-fried, and treats heat diseases.

White garlic, green garlic

These become cool after being stir-fried, and treat heat diseases. Its soup is delicious and treats *rlung* disease.

Mustard

There are white and black kinds of mustard, they cause *badkan* and *mkhris pa* to be in disturbance.

Polygonatum and Rhizoma Ligustici Chuanxiong

These herbs can be stir-fried and treat *badkan* and *rlung* diseases.

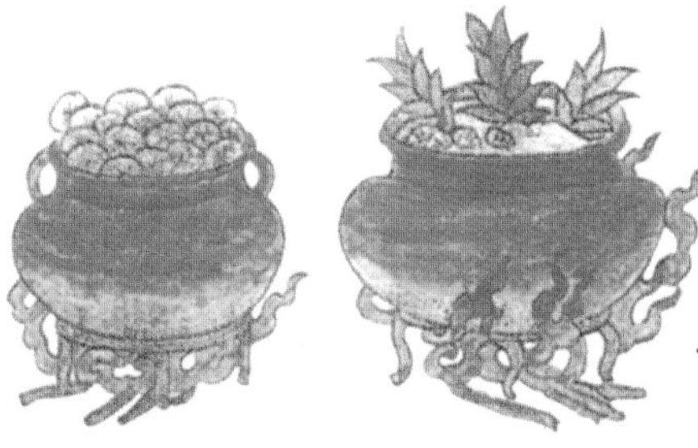

Polygonatum and Rhizoma Ligustici Chuanxiong treat *rlung* and *badkan* diseases.

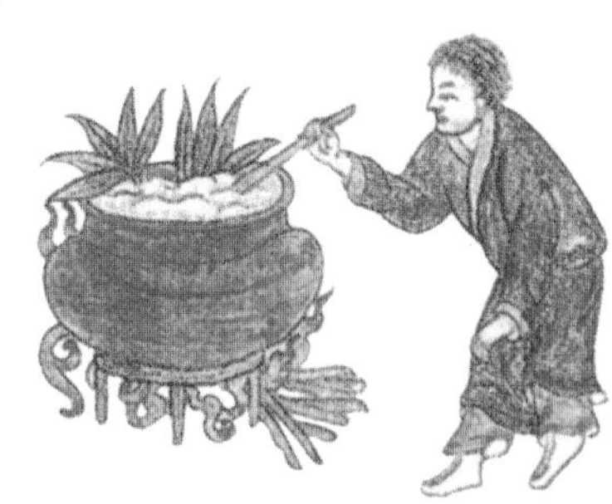

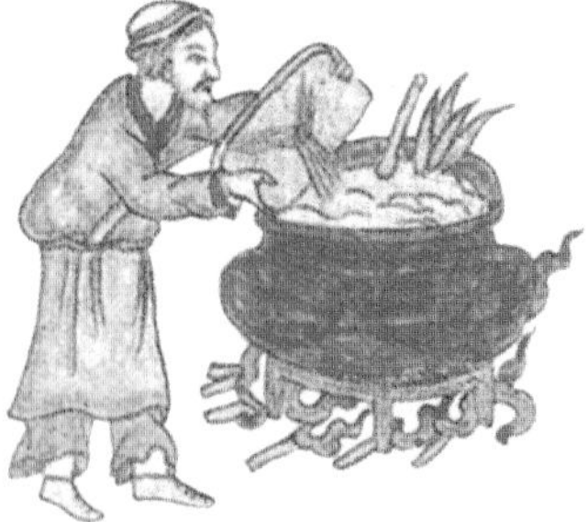

White garlic and garlic sprouts treats *rlung* disease.

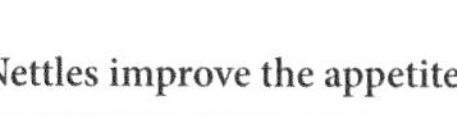

Nettles improve the appetite.

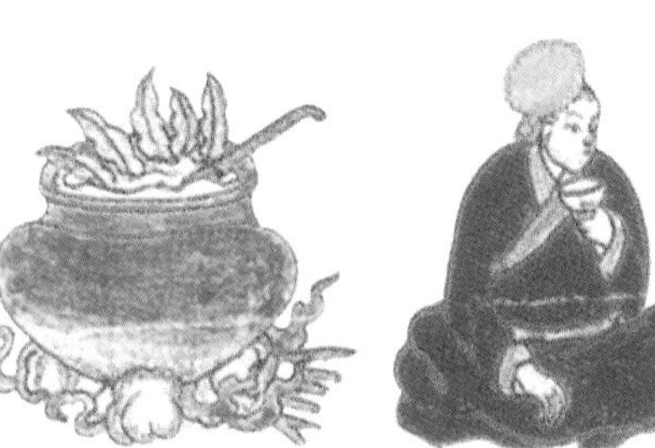

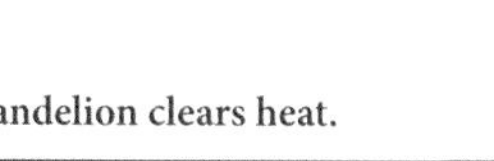

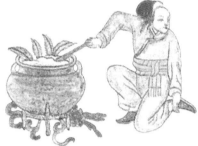

Dandelion clears heat.

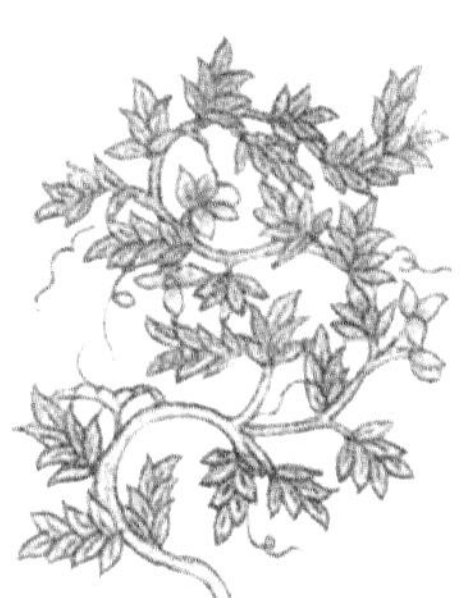

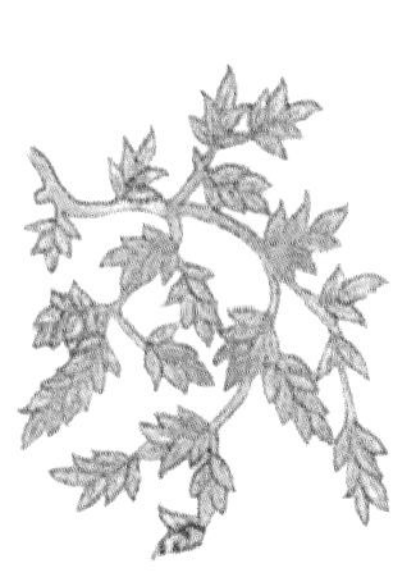

Fresh pea leaves have a neutral temperature.

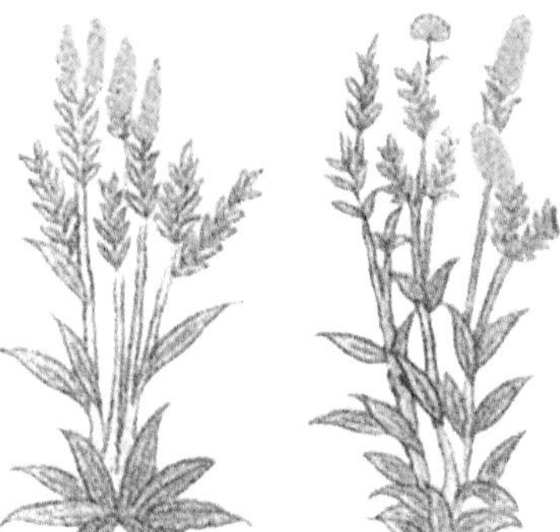

Mustard disturbs *badkan* and *mkhris pa*.

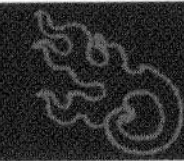

Food Amount and Dietary Taboos

Those who are conversant with the principles of health cultivation must not only know the nature and action of foods, but also understand the prohibitions and the appropriate quantity of food to be taken, and how to avoid poisonous foods.

Adequate amount of food and drink

Half of the stomach should be saved for food, one-quarter for drink, and the last quarter for the motion of *rlung*, *mkhris pa* and *badkan*. It is therefore essential to adjust the amount of food and drink according one's condition and the weight of the food. Some guidelines are:

When eating light food, one can eat until full. Heavy foods should be consumed until the stomach is only half full, so that digestion can proceed smoothly. This is the basis for adequate nutrition.

Those who wish to gain weight should drink some wine after meals. Those who wish to lose weight should drink honey mixed in water after meals. Drinking liquid before a meal will lead to a moderate body weight; drinking in the midst of a meal will lead to weight gain; and drinking after meals will help people lose weight.

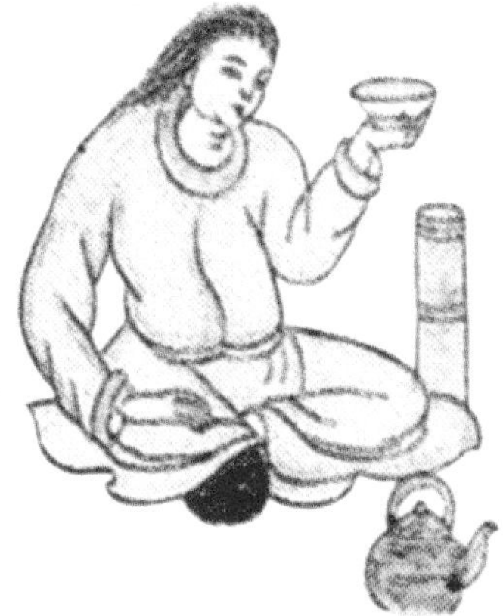

For obese people, honey water can be taken after meals.

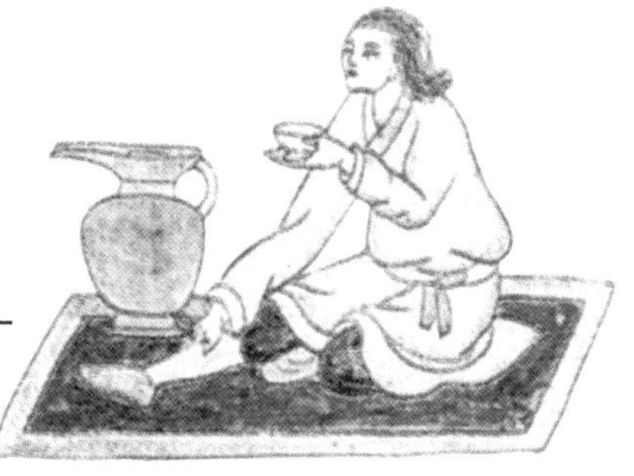

For slender people, wine can be taken after meals.

Water can be taken after meals, but its amount should not exceed one-quarter of the stomach. It can improve digestion.

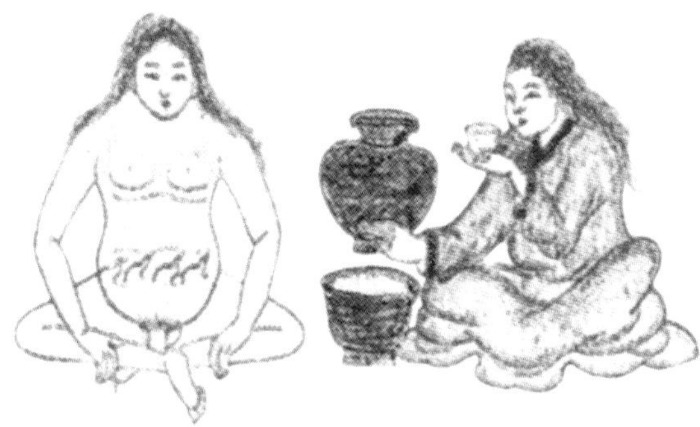

An appropriate amount of water after meals can improve digestion.

Those with weak stomach fire should drink wine after eating heavy meats to help digestion.

Drinking cold water after eating cheese, wine or contaminated food will help resolve toxins.

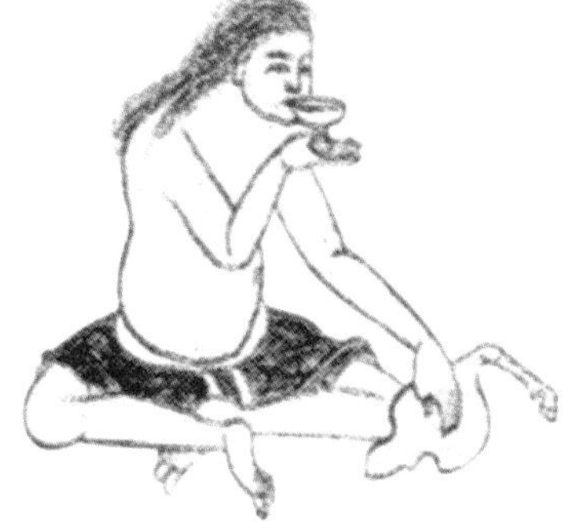

For those with weak stomach fire, an adequate amount of wine should be taken after eating meat.

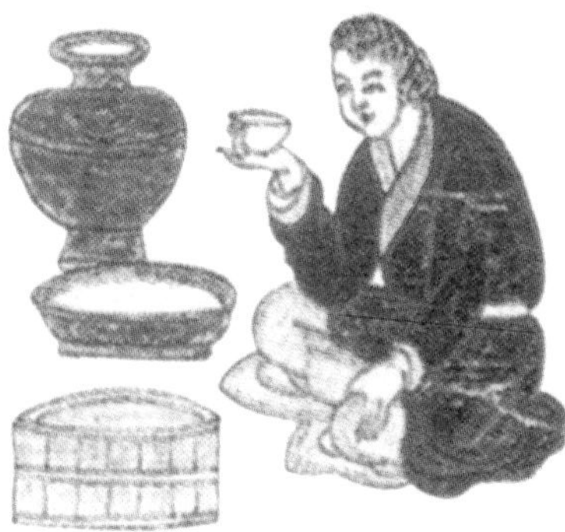

After taking cheese, wine or unclean food, drinking some cold water is helpful.

In short, only a proper amount of food and drink can make *rlung*, *mkhris pa* and *badkan* act normally. If the amount taken is insufficient, the body's needs won't be satisfied and will result in a bad complexion and *rlung* disorders. If one overeats, food won't be digested, *rlung* movement will be blocked, stomach fire debilitated, and many diseases will result.

Dietary taboos

The diet provides nutrition to the body, so if toxic substances are eaten or the food selection is poor, it will result in pain, discomfort, and disturbances of *rlung*, *mkhris pa* and *badkan* leading to disease. In serious cases, poisonous food might be fatal. Hence, dietary taboos are essential for everyone.

Avoid toxic food

One must pay attention to food that may be toxic or spoiled. Generally, people can't distinguish toxic food from non-toxic food. When a certain food is suspect, one should go to a specialist for inspection. Since toxic food is different from regular food, animals may react unusually to toxic food, so toxic food can be recognized through the reactions of these animals.

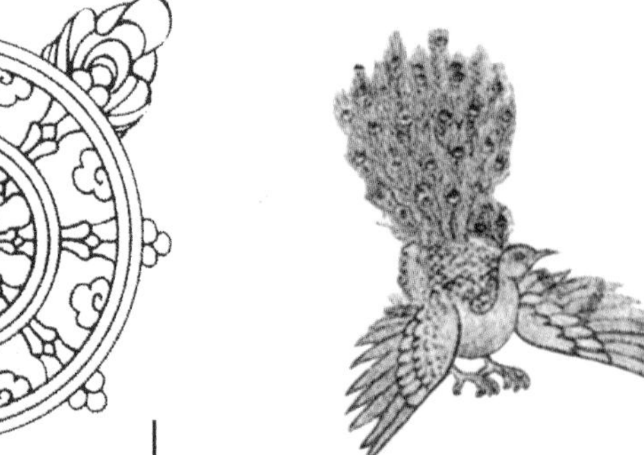

A peacock will spread its tail feathers in front of toxic food.

When the toxic food is cooked, the flame doesn't go upward but will burst outward, and will be a blue color.

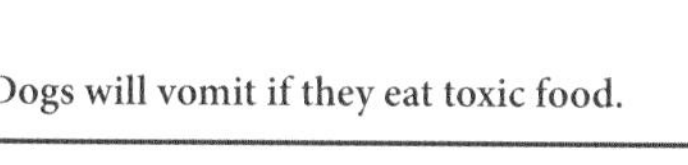

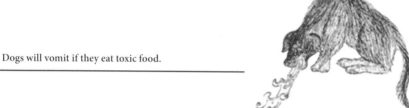

Dogs will vomit if they eat toxic food.

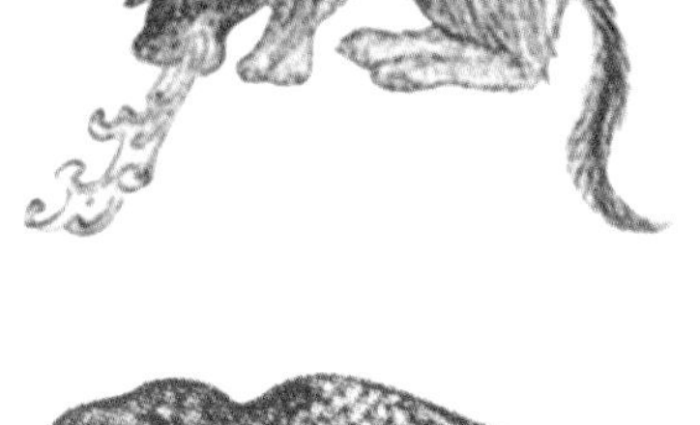

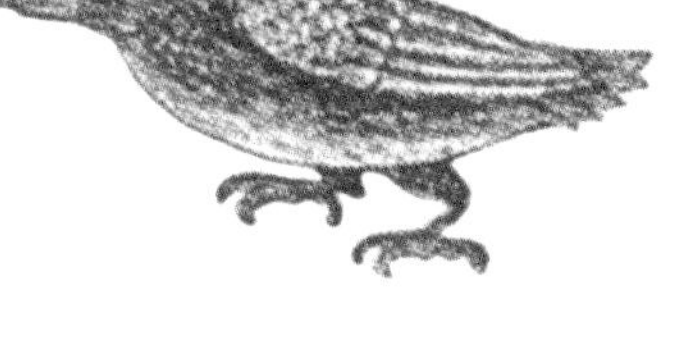

A crow will cry out in fear upon encountering toxic food.

Generally speaking, toxic meat is redder than healthy meat, is slightly swollen, and does not stick to a pan when cooked. When wine is poured on toxic meat, the steam is irritable to the eyes. When cooked over a fire, a multicolor flame like peacock's feathers will appear. Furthermore, the fire doesn't ascend upward but goes in other directions, and the flame may burst out. A crow when coming across toxic meat would cry in fear, while a peacock would spread its tail feathers in joy like it is going pick it up, and a dog will vomit immediately after eating it. If any of these things happen, the meat should be abandoned.

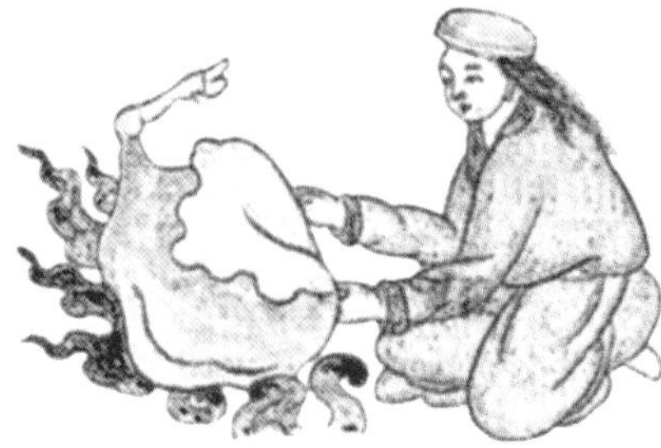

Toxic meat has a deep red color and doesn't stick to the pan when cooked.

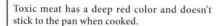

If someone intentionally poisons food, they will seem frightened, tremble, sweat profusely, look uneasy, dull, or spiritless, and will not dare to look directly at other people. If such a person is found, the food to be eaten should be carefully inspected.

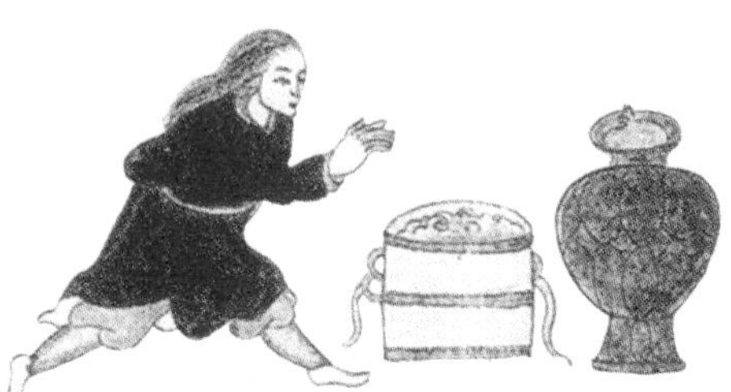

Someone intentionally poisoning food will be trembling, sweating, thirsty, and uneasy.

Toxic meat is a beautiful color, swollen, and doesn't stick to the pan; when roasted, the flame shoots outward rather than ascending upward.

Taboos of food combining

Most foods are non-toxic, but when combined with certain other food items can cause disease or poisoning. It is, therefore, essential to understand the interactions between some food items that should be avoided. The important ones are:

Pea leaves with brown sugar and cheese. Do not eat these together.

Do not stir-fry mushrooms with mustard oil.

Chicken meat with cheese.

Bee honey with an equal amount of clear oil.

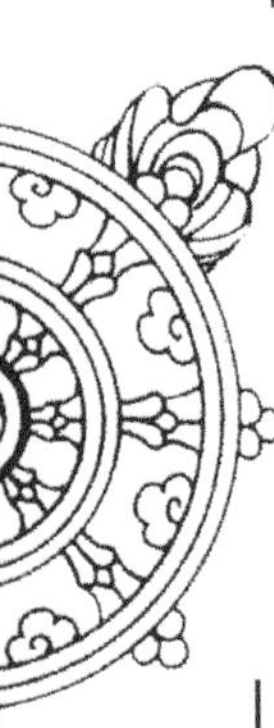

Do not put fresh butter in a copper container for over ten days, or poisoning will occur.

Do not roast wild rabbit meat with barberry wood.

Do not eat rabbit meat, chicken meat and lion meat together.

Fish, beef and milk have incompatible natures and tastes. Don't eat them together.

Do not eat sallow fruit and cow milk together.

Eggs and fish can't be eaten together.

Do not fry mushrooms with mustard oil.

Pea leaves, brown sugar, and cheese can't be eaten together.

Do not eat chicken and cheese together.

Bee honey and clear oil can't be eaten together.

Do not put fresh butter in a copper container for over ten days.

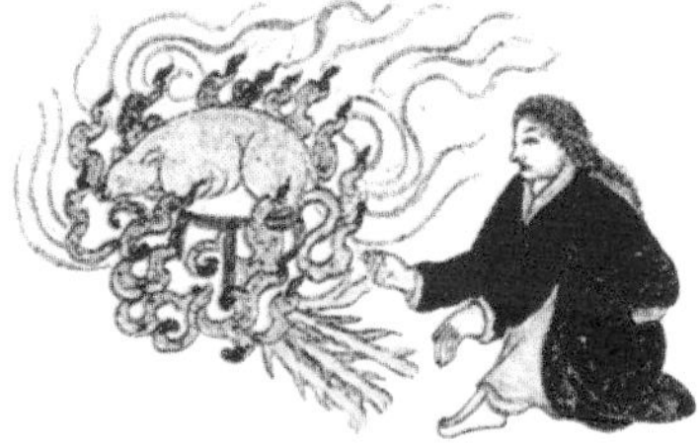

Do not roast wild animal meat with barberry wood.

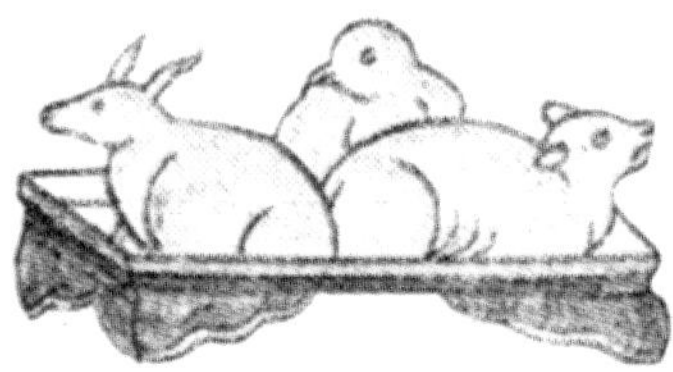

Don't eat rabbit, chicken and lion meat together.

After administering glauberite, mushroom and dandelion should not be eaten until the glauberite has been digested, or poisoning will occur.

Do not drink cool water right after eating melted butter.

Do not put fresh meat, *rtsam pa*, yoghurt and butter in the same container.

Do not cover the container of hot food if the steam hasn't dissipated.

If meat has not been thoroughly digested, do not take the next meal.

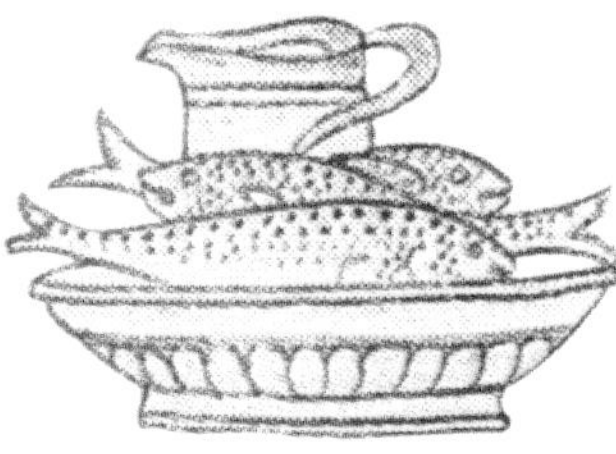

Do not take fish and cow milk together.

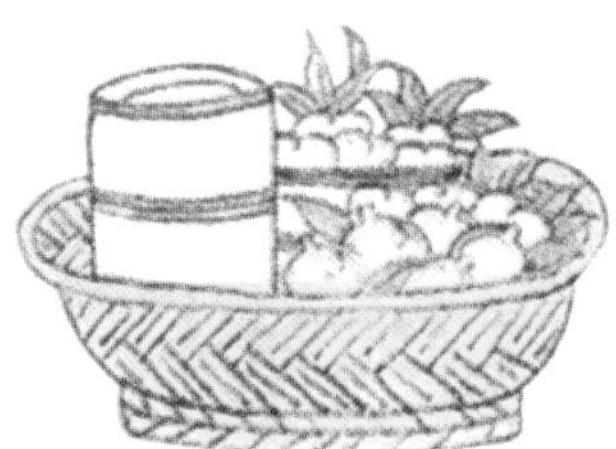

Do not take fruit and cow milk together.

Do not take eggs and fish together.

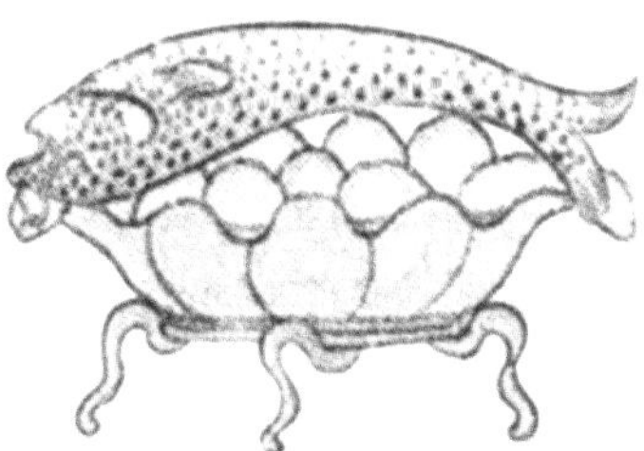

Do not eat mushrooms right after taking glauberite.

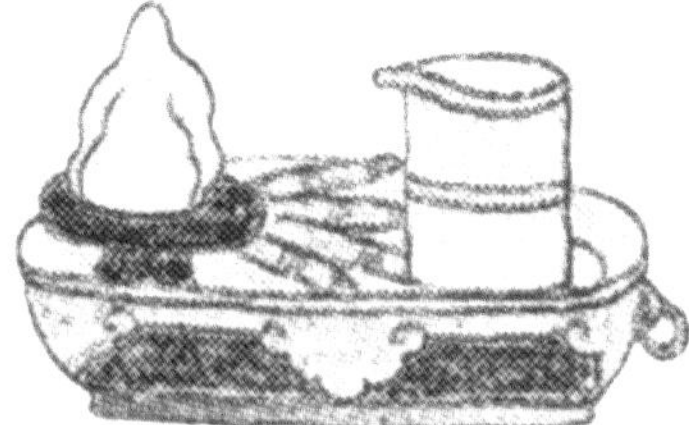

Do not drink cool water right after taking melted butter.

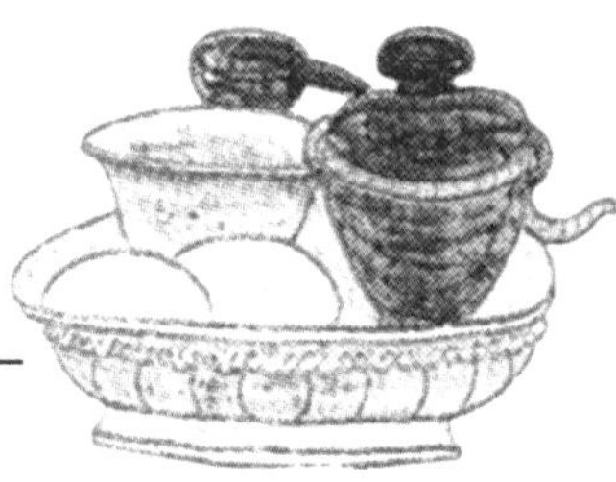

Do not put fresh meat, *rtsam pa*, yoghurt and butter in the same container.

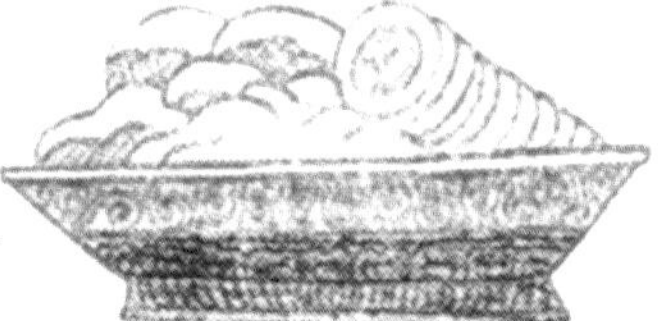

When boiling meat, do not cover the container before the steam has dissipated.

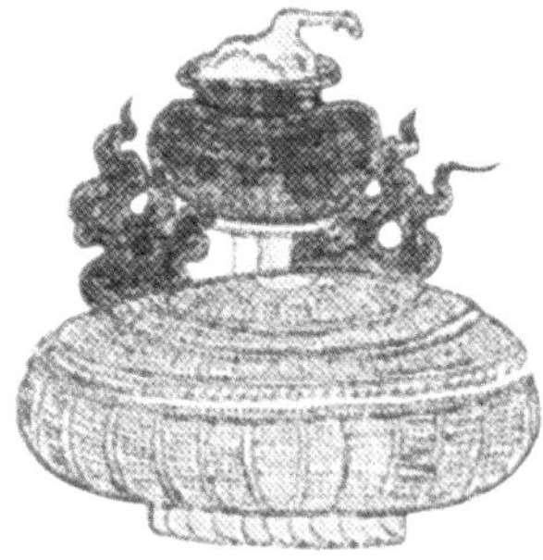

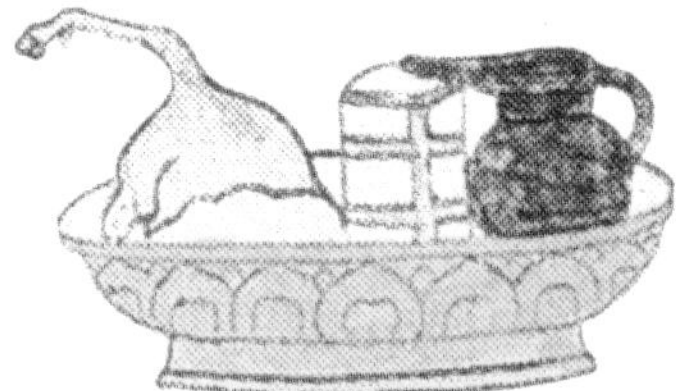

Do not eat cow milk and sour food together.

These taboos must be given attention in daily life in order to cultivate good habits. If bad habits have already been established, they must be gradually checked and corrected. If stopped suddenly, *rlung*, *mkhris pa* and *badkan* diseases will occur. If one is willing to cultivate health, good dietary habits are important. Eating well and understating how to eat are very important. Health cultivation can only be practiced by understanding how to avoid poisonous foods, and what foods are incompatible.

Based on the heavy or light nature and the strength of the stomach fire, half of the stomach space is for food, one-quarter for beverages, and the remaining quarter for *rlung*, *mkhris pa* and *badkan*.

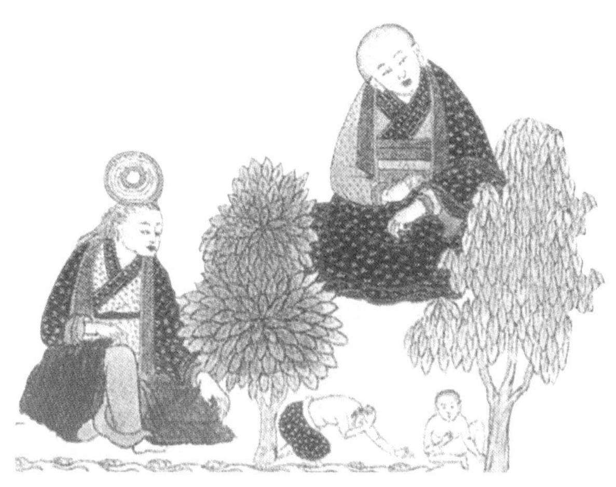

རོ་ཙ།

CHAPTER 6 HEALTH CULTIVATION THROUGH SEX

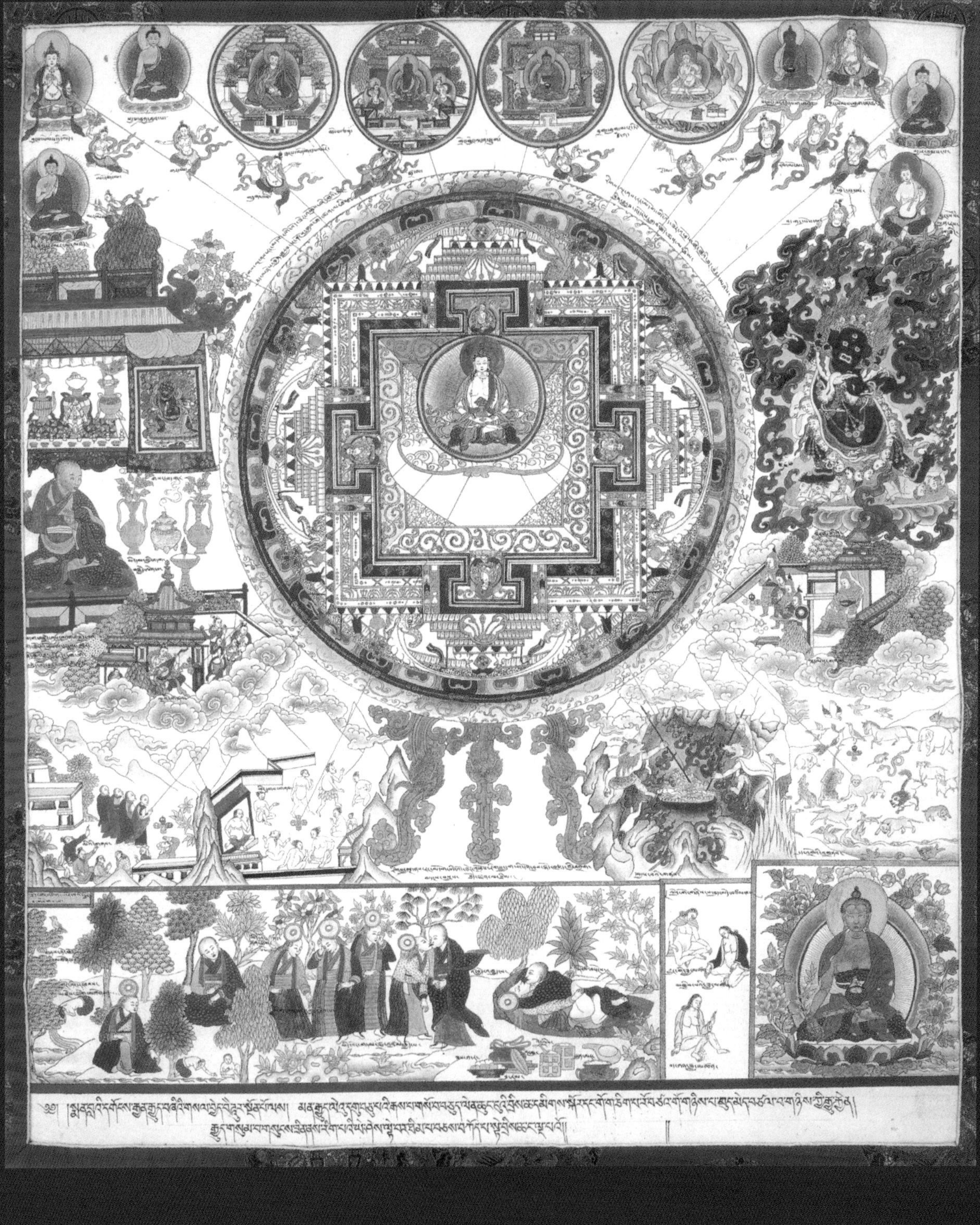

Methods of health cultivation, from *Thangkha* fifty-five in the *Sman thang* series of *The Four Medical Tantras*.

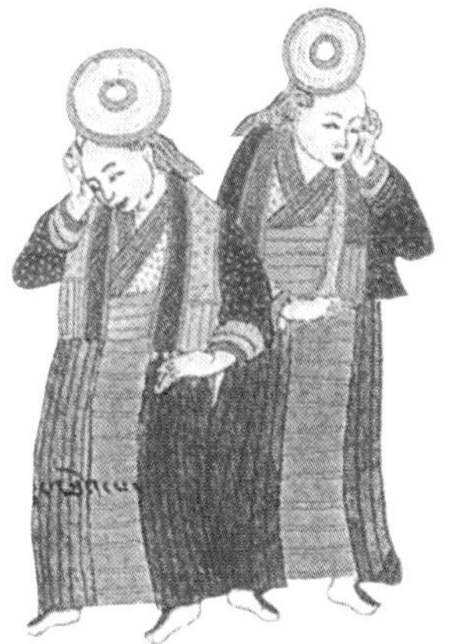

Tibetan medicine doesn't demand abstaining from sex.

The "descending *rlung*" is responsible for male semen and female blood, is in charge of sexual behavior, and is an important part of the life process. Tibetan medicine says that adequate sexual activities are beneficial to health, whereas inadequate sex is detrimental to the body's health. Healthy sexual activity is stressed, and sexual taboos, sexual diseases, and nurturing methods are all explained.

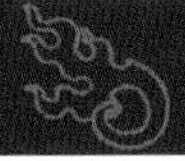
General Knowledge About Sex
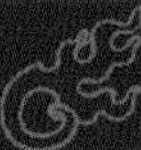

The seven essences of life (the essence from food, blood, muscle, fat, bone, marrow and semen) are successively formed. Semen is divided into spirit and dregs. It makes the body lustrous, and is the root of health and longevity. The dregs refer to male semen and female blood. It is clear that adequate sexual activity has a direct influence on the overall health of life.

The different genders

The period from fertilization to the differentiation of a male and female fetus is called the sex differentiation period. Tibetan embryology holds that after the conjugation of the paternal semen and the maternal blood, if semen is predominant, this will give rise to male fetus; if blood is predominant, a female fetus; and equal amounts to a hermaphrodite. During the 4th week of pregnancy if the fetus is a hard mass, it will be a boy; a soft loose mass means a girl; if it is an oval mass, it is a hermaphrodite.

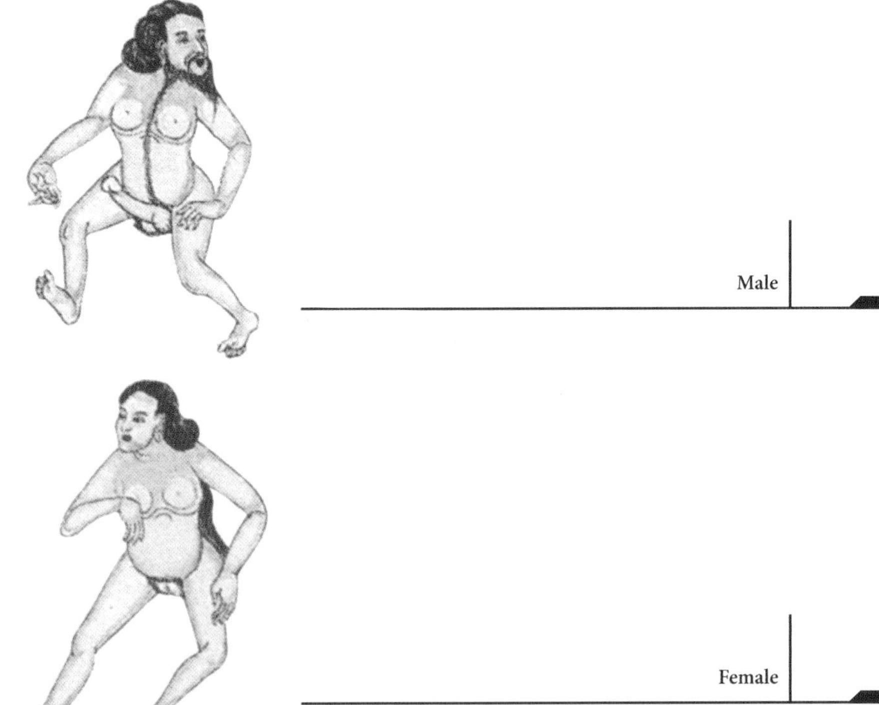

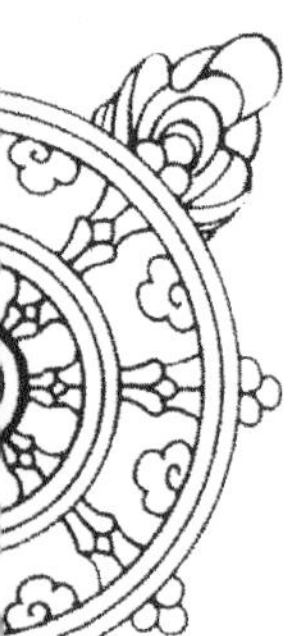

Tibetan medicine recognizes three genders, male, female and neutral. The neutral type is further divided into five sorts: hermaphrodite, asexual, envy, changeable, natural castration, and stony female. A hermaphrodite has the genitalia of both a male and female; an asexual doesn't have any genitalia and even though sexual desire exists, it will be unable to have intercourse; envy types are those who when witnessing other people in intercourse feel envy; changeable neutrals are when both sex genitalia are present, but appear alternately every two weeks; natural castration and a stony woman are those with incomplete genitalia.

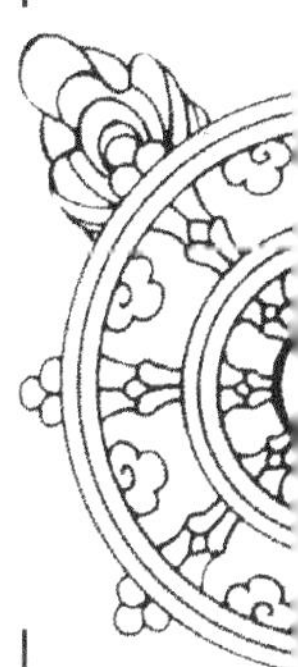

In *The Four Medical Tantras*, there is a "prescription for changing a female to a male." Before the 4th week of pregnancy, when the sex is still not yet clear, if one wishes to have a boy fetus, select a ghost date from the calendar, put many kinds of metal together and heat them until their color changes. Put this in milk with a handful of the husband's semen and let the wife drink it and then adopt the spirit of the essence of the Sun and Moon. After this, avoid intercourse for eight months. Don't sleep in the nighttime, and instead, sleep in the daytime. Don't eat food that is too pungent, sharp, or heavy. Don't strain when urinating or defecating. Don't bathe in cold water. If bloodletting is performed, a miscarriage or a still born fetus will result.

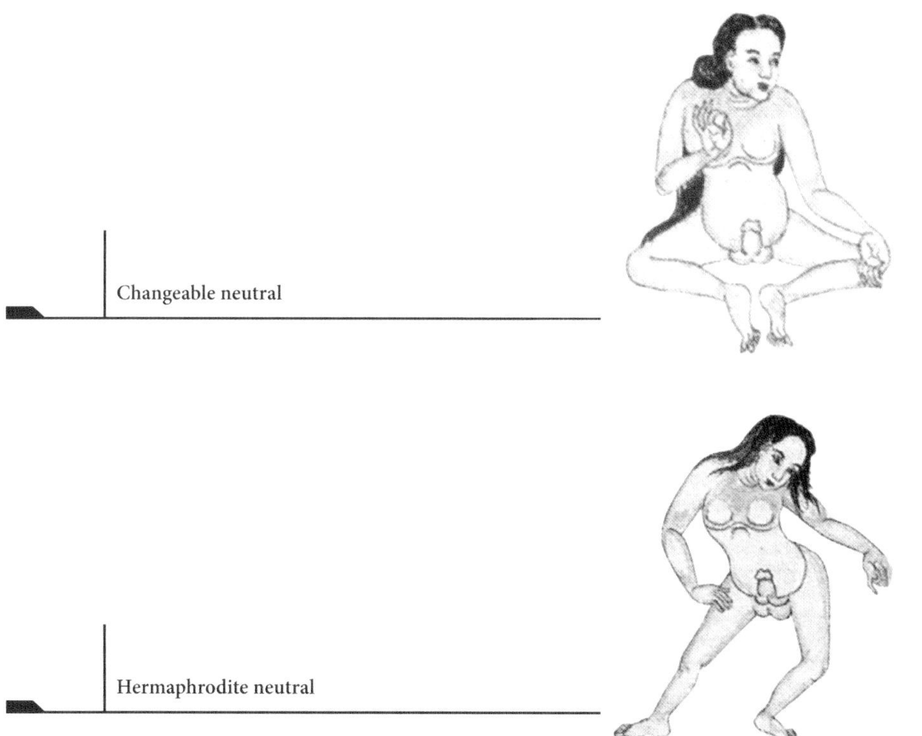

Changeable neutral

Hermaphrodite neutral

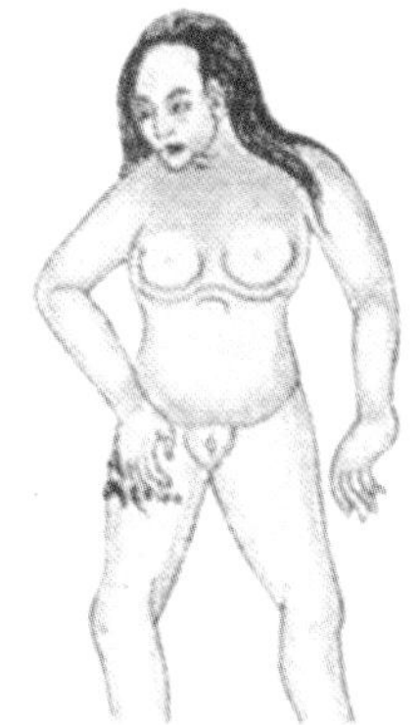

Asexual neutral

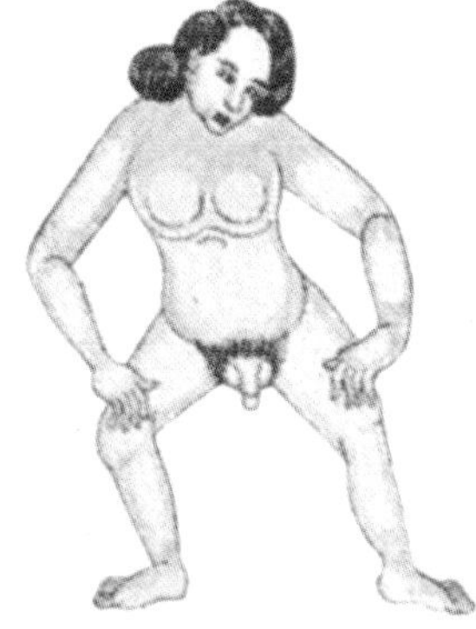

Natural castration

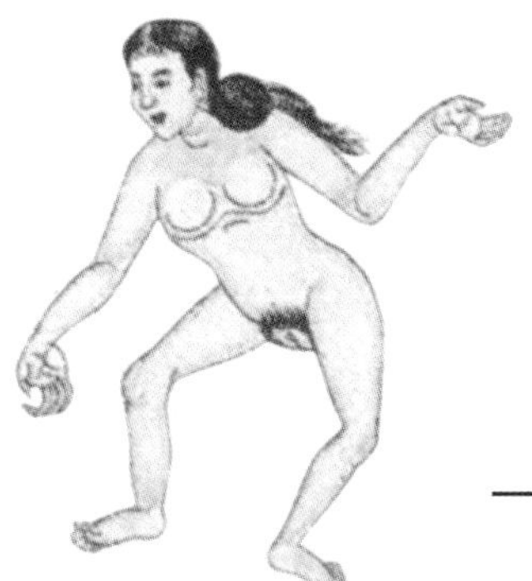

Stony girl

Hermaphrodites have both male and female genitalia; changeable neutrals have male genitalia in the first half of the month, and female genitalia in the last half of the month; an asexual neutral has no genitalia at all; natural castration and stony girls are those with under developed male and female genitalia respectively.

The basis of sex

Both males and females have three vessels that combine below the navel, forming a vessel node something like a lymph node, which is called *bsam bse'u* in Tibetan. This is the location for the storage of the essences of the five-sources, and the dregs of the seven essences, or the location where male semen and female blood are stored.

The *Sman dpyad zla ba'i rgyal po* says, "Being the site where blood and semen are stored, *bsam bse'u* is the size and shape of a hen's egg. It is situated to the left of the navel, connected to the left kidney, and through the vessels connects to the 13th vertebra and the genitals. It produces seeds with the lung and kidney... Though invisible to the naked eye, it is shaped like a new moon or full moon. The uterus in man is atrophied. When desire is strong, it is full of semen. The female uterus is empty and small and enlarges after being fertilized, connecting with the navel through a band."

Another medical classic, the *Mes po'i zal lung* also mentions the *bsam bse'u* by saying, "There are three combined vessels below the navel, forming a vessel-node like lymph node called *bsam bse'u*, which is the container for red blood and white semen. The male semen accumulates in the *bsam bse'u* through the vessels. During intercourse, when the zenith of happiness is reached, red blood and white semen flow out of the *bsam bse'u*."

Both of these quotes from the classics seem to imply that the *bsam bse'u* is actually the ovary in females and the seminal vesicle in males. During intercourse, semen enters the vagina and the conjugation of semen and blood lead to the production of an embryo.

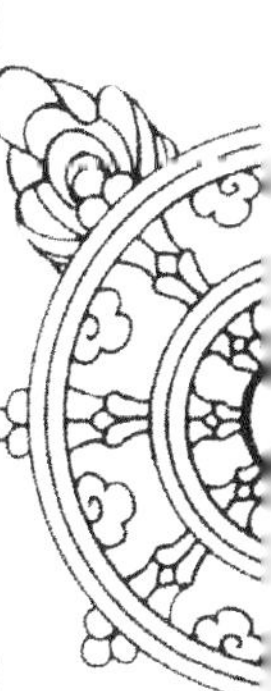

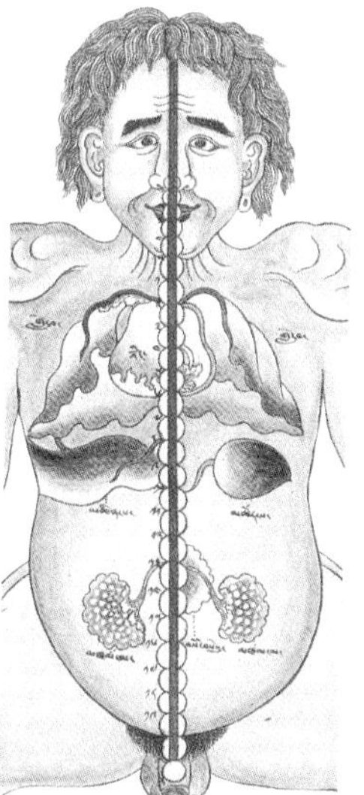

The position of the reproduction vessel among the organs.

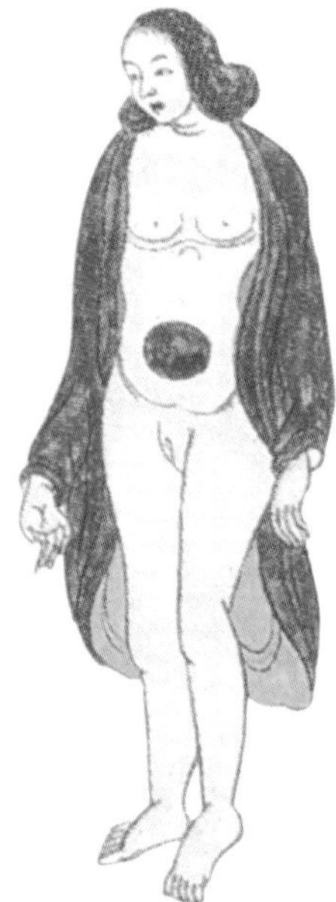

Female sexual characteristics and ovary.

Tibetan medicine refers to the location for storing male semen and female blood as the *bsam bse'u*. Under the action of the descending *rlung*, ejaculation and menstruation produce offspring.

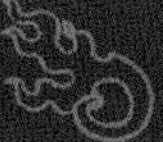 Healthy Sexual Behavior 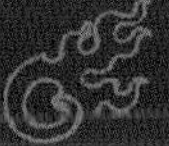

In Tibetan medicine, sex is seen as the highest of all human desires. A healthy sex life not only satisfies normal needs and sexual passion, but also makes the spirit-light active, which gives one a long life. Unhealthy sexual activity will cause a loss of spirit-light gradually or suddenly, leading to various diseases. This is closely connected to the root of health and longevity.

Surroundings

Love is the basis for the joining of the both sexes and reproduction of descendents. Surroundings are an important factor that influence sexual passion. Excellent surroundings include a house surrounded by green trees, with birds chirping, the fragrance of flowers, mild weather, breezes, and comfortable temperature. These kinds of surroundings make both partners relaxed and put them in a happy mood, full of zest. Sexual desire is thus generated.

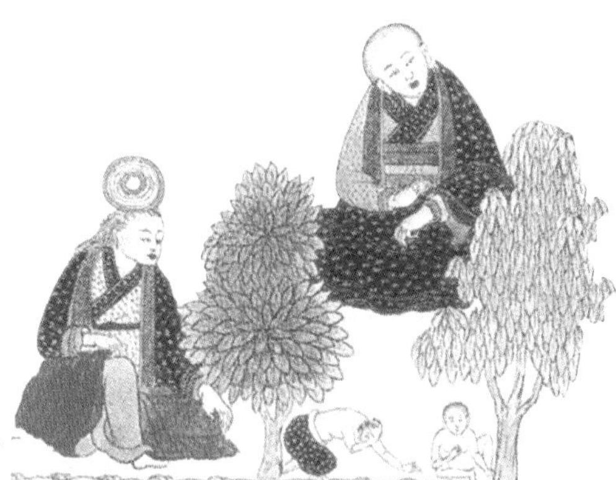

Excellent living surroundings with fragrant flowers and chirping birds.

The partner

A charming and beautiful partner who uses sweet words can arouse love and passion.

Preparations

This is a very important step, and includes rubbing of oil and bathing. This is not only necessary for personal hygiene, but also strengthens the body and helps induce a pleasant mood. The emotions of both partners become even more bright and clear.

An mild enema may also be necessary. During intercourse, if there is a desire to defecate, suppression of this desire may lead to a foul odor in the mouth, headache, spasms in the limbs, catching cold, formation of masses, blurred vision, abdominal pain and distension, and heart disease. One must be sure that during intercourse, desires of hunger, thirst, and urination do not arise. Thus, it is important that before intercourse both people have eaten, drunk water, and urinated if necessary.

Appropriate sexual activity

The amount of healthy sexual activity varies depending on constitution, age, and interest. For young people, sex can be had frequently and should be decreased gradually as age increases.

In terms of the seasons, intercourse can be frequent if the body is energetic; in summer, twice a month is appropriate; in winter people can safely engage in sex frequently; while during autumn and spring, the frequency should be somewhere between that of winter and summer. It must be noted that these recommendations are for healthy people. For the elderly and weak, the frequency should be decreased or even stopped altogether.

How can one judge if the frequency is too much? Observing the physical reaction after intercourse is a simple method. When no uncomfortable reactions appear, this shows that the frequency is appropriate, and the amount of sexual activity is healthy. If unpleasant reactions are observed, then the frequency of intercourse should be decreased.

Reasonable and adequate intercourse makes a couple even more intimate. Many partners are a similar age, but vary in interests and constitution. If the stronger partner is selfish and seeks only to satisfy themselves and ignore the other, it may hurt the passion and health of both partners.

Sexual taboos

Sexual taboos fall into two categories, moral and physiological.

Intercourse is forbidden with animals, other people's spouses, or with a partner one does not love. When one has sex with a partner one does not love, there is no love though there is sex; when one has sex with another person's spouse, there is no morality at all. When one has sex with other animals, there is neither nobility, nor love.

Sex with a pregnant woman or a woman during her menstrual period is forbidden. Having sex with a pregnant woman may affect the growth of descendents; and having sex with menstruating women will hurt both partners.

Sex is forbidden with a debilitated, emaciated, ill, or depressed person. Sex during these times will worsen the person's condition and there will be no joy in intercourse.

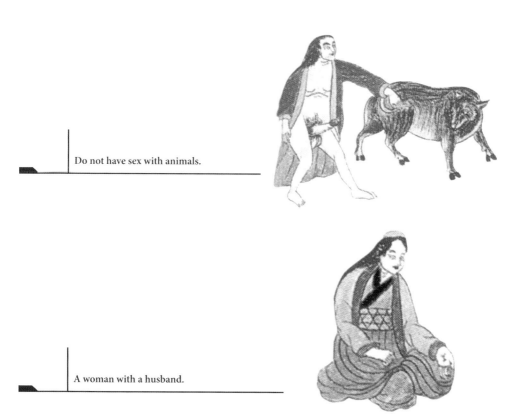

Do not have sex with animals.

A woman with a husband.

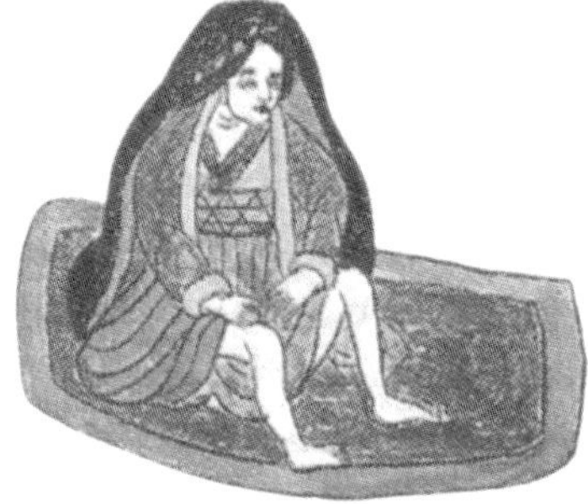

Weak woman

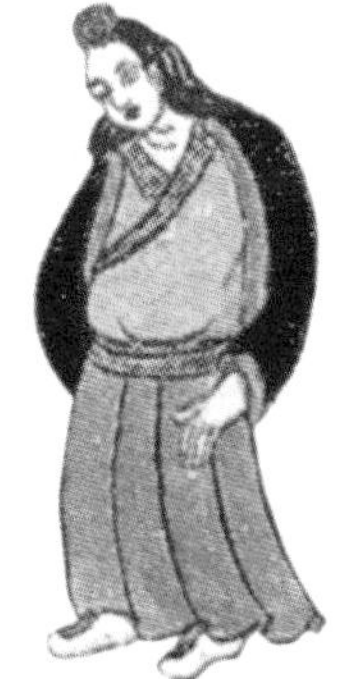

Pregnant woman

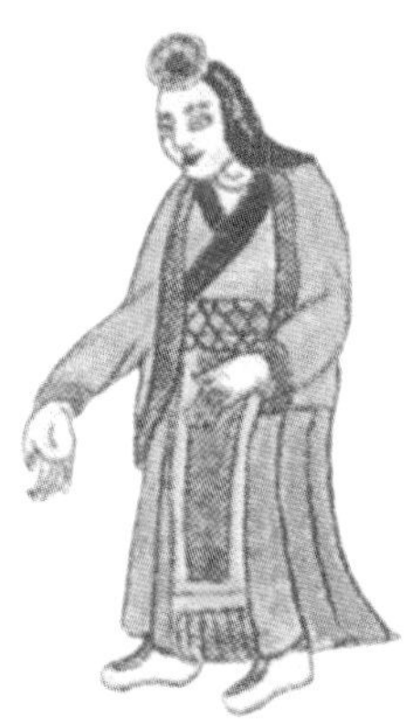

Ugly woman

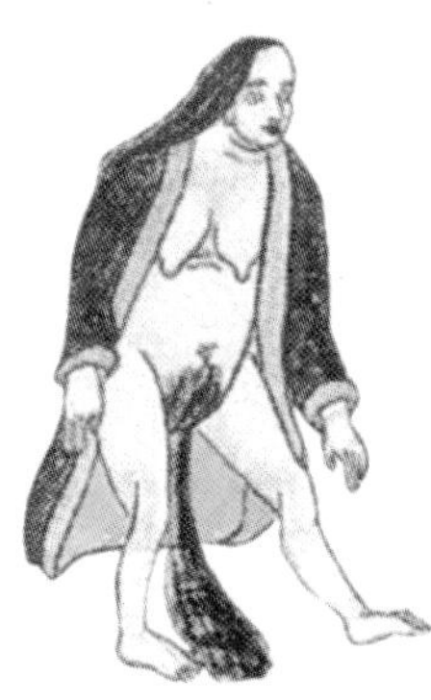

Woman during menstruation

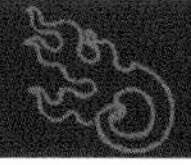 Common Male Sexual Diseases 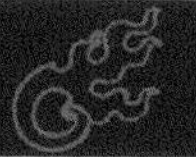

Intentionally suppressing the desire to urinate or defecate or forcedly excreting urine or stool, overindulging in sex, overstrain, prolonged constipation, overeating of sweet, sour and irritable foods, and living in a cold-wet place will lead to constipation, urethral prickles, urethral adhesions, prolonged erection, inability to retract the foreskin, and rashes of the penis.

Prickles in the urethra

Pain in the urethra like being pricked with a needle.

Treatment: boil highland barley flour and Tibetan aniseed in butter to make a paste and apply to the genitals. Repeat the compress as needed. Do not eat irritable, sweet or sour foods. Avoid vigorous movements and intercourse.

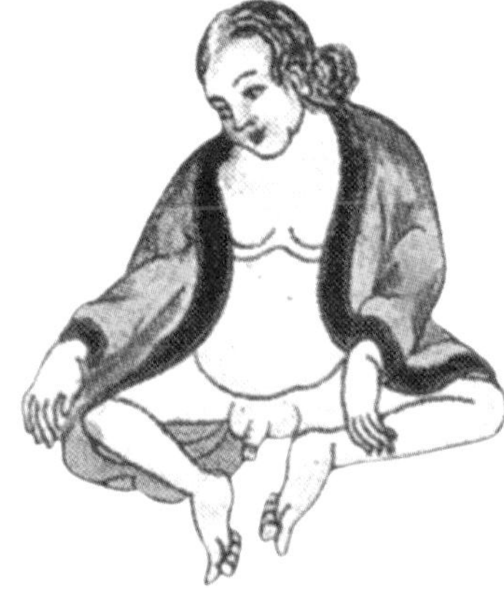

Injury by pricking.

Urethral adhesions

This is when the urethral orifice is blocked by mucus, and is characterized by bending of the urethra, inability to urinate, and is mostly caused by suppressing the desire to ejaculate, or living in a wet-cold place.

Treatment: use fine straw rubbed with oil and insert it into the urethra to expand it (avoid rough movements), bathe in a hot spring or medicinal bath. Avoid food that may induce inflammation and physical overstrain.

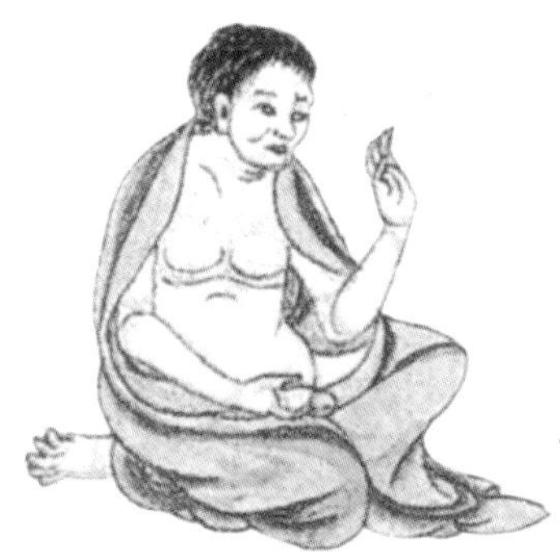

Adhesion

Prolonged erection of penis

Prolonged erection is often accompanied with swelling, rashes, itching and pain of the penis, and is mostly caused by too much intercourse or suppressing the desire to urinate, defecate, or ejaculate.

Treatment: eliminating swelling by prescribing *Chebulae Powder* plus *Five Peng Powder*, *Treasured Talisman Pill*, and *Chinese Iris Powder with Sixteen Ingredients*, followed by *Cardamom Powder with Ten Ingredients*, *Snow Frog Flesh Pill with Thirteen Ingredients*, *Areca Powder with Twenty-Eight Ingredients*, and *Pomegranate Sun Powder*. Modifications of these formulas can be made according to the individual's condition. Avoid sweet, sour and foods that can induce inflammation. No vigorous manual labor or intercourse.

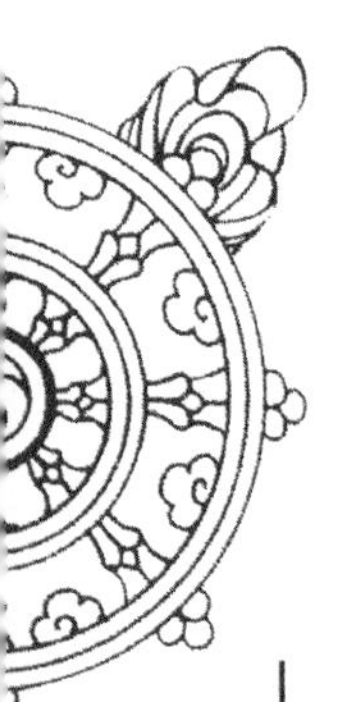

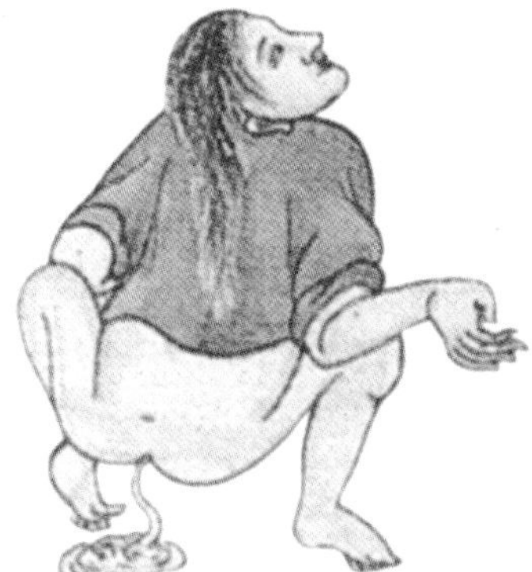

Forceful defecation and urination.

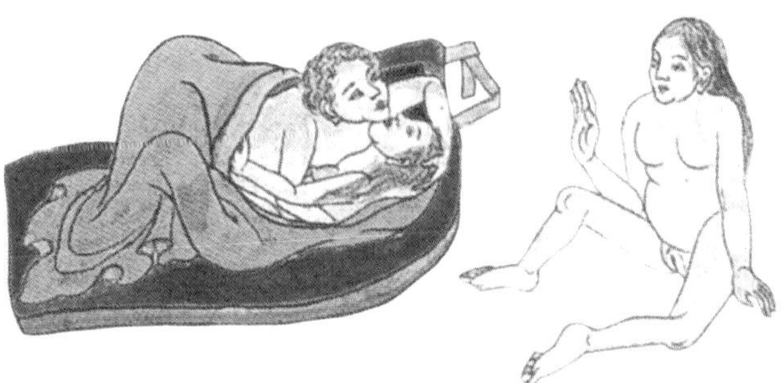

Over indulging in sex.

Inability to retract the foreskin

Characterized by a turning outward, swelling, and knotting of the foreskin like a knot, and induced by overindulgence in intercourse and non-hygienic habits.

Treatment: rub with oil and a compress of medicinal oil, followed by bathing in a medicated solution or hot spring. Follow the same dietary and lifestyle restrictions as above.

Rash of the penis

Rashes of the penis are like white mustard seeds, they are painful and itchy, and are caused by overindulgence in intercourse and suppression of desires to urinate, defecate, and ejaculate.

Treatment: puncture the rash and allow any blood or fluid to run out, rub with oil mixed with *Wine-Residue Powder with Ten (or Thirteen) Ingredients*. Medication: *Chebulae Five Peng Powder, Thirteen Ingredient Powder*, and *Chinese Iris Powder with Sixteen Ingredients*, followed by medical bathing or bathing in a natural hot spring. Follow the same dietary and lifestyle restrictions as above.

Seminal emission

This includes nocturnal emissions, urethritis, seminal emission due to prolapse of organs or a broken vessel gate, seminal emission, and cold dripping semen, and is caused by overindulgence in sex, a strong sexual desire, and over eating of sweet and sour food.

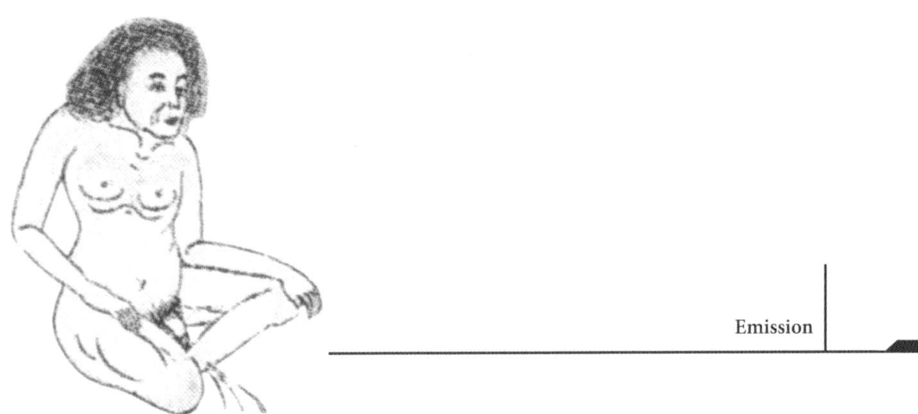

Seminal emission syndromes are of two kinds, cold and heat. In cold cases, there is seminal fluid mixed with the urine, frequent urination, dripping of blood after emission, lassitude, dizziness, a sallow complexion, low back pain, and a sunken slow relaxed pulse.

Heat emission types have hot urine, dripping urination, burning pain in urethra when urinating or ejaculating, concentrated seminal fluid mixed with blood, when pulling the scrotum upward severe pain may occur, and a hot pulse. In serious cases, the semen is mixed with blood. The semen flows out in a slender thread with severe pain, the urethral orifice is red and in the morning is sealed closed by accumulated mucus.

Treatment: at the initial stage, for either cold or heat syndromes, involves the use of *Decoction of Cluster Mallow with Six Ingredients.*

For cold emission syndrome, *Five Peng Secure the Essence Powder* and *Cardamom Powder* are used alternately, and the following medication can be selected if appropriate: *Secure the Essence Powder with Fourteen Ingredients, Pomegranate Sun Powder, Chebulae Powder with Ten Ingredients*, and *Areca Powder with Twenty-eight Ingredients*. For external treatment, moxibustion can be applied at the 13th, 14th, and 19th vertebrae, or at the tendon on the surface of the tibia. As for diet, warm food is recommended and no sweet or sour foods. Meat and vegetables should be avoided before the inflammation has vanished. Do not have sex or stay in cold-wet places.

For heat emission, use *Barberry Paste with Eight Ingredients*, and *Chebulae Powder with Seventeen Ingredients*, while inflammation still exists, use *Barberry Paste with Eight Ingredients* plus *Five Peng Powder*, and *Benevolent Heat Five Peng Stop Dripping Powder*. For emission due to downward pouring of liver fluid, *Carthamus Powder with Thirteen Ingredients*, or *Chebulae Powder with Ten Ingredients* plus three fruits, musk, crab's shell, climbing fern spore, Chinese jumper, and aconite ground to a powder and administered with warm boiled water. For severe case, bear bile and carthamus ground as powder and taken orally can be used. External treatment includes bloodletting.

In addition, emission can be classified as strong-semen emission, diseased emission, toxic emission, and emission while dreaming.

Strong-semen emission occurs in a strong person who has plentiful semen and is greedy in sex. To calm these kinds of patients, sexual intercourse is recommended or *Duck's Head Pedicularis Decoction* is recommended for oral use.

Diseased emission is caused by *rlung* disease and leads to weak kidney fire. Treatment is similar to cold emission.

Toxic emission is caused by toxicity of the kidney. Emergency treatment with biomedicine is necessary.

Emission while dreaming occurs when meeting a female in the dream. For treatment, butter from mare's milk, mixed with stool and goat hairs should be mixed and applied to the center of the sole of the foot.

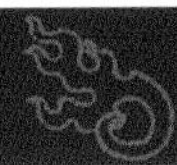

Common Female Sexual Diseases

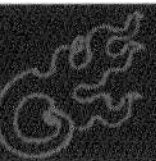

Structures and functions unique to women include the uterus, vagina, mammary glands, menstruation, pregnancy, and delivery. Under the influence of *rlung*, *mkhris pa badkan*, frequent intercourse, and inappropriate care after delivery, female diseases can occur. These include diseases of the female genitalia, the maternal blood, female wind, tumors of the womb, and worms in the womb, with symptoms such as disharmony of menstruation, pain in lower body, etc.

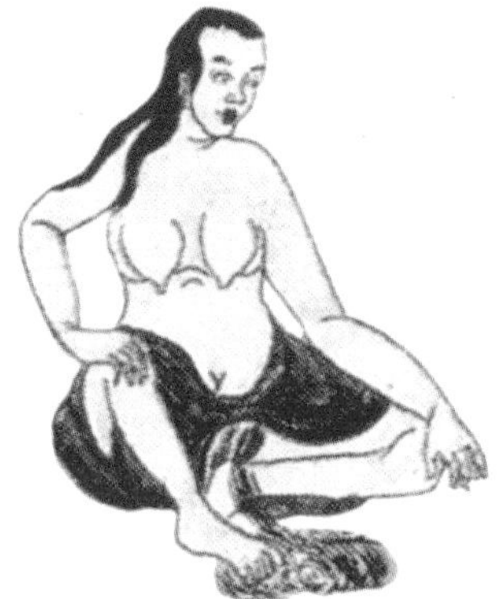

Vaginal bleeding

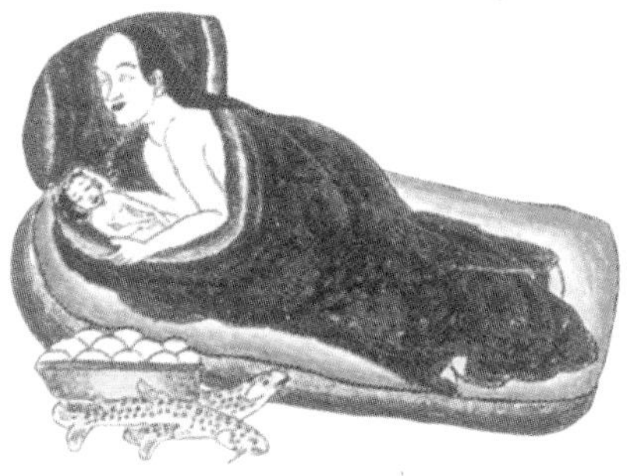

Inappropriate care after delivery.

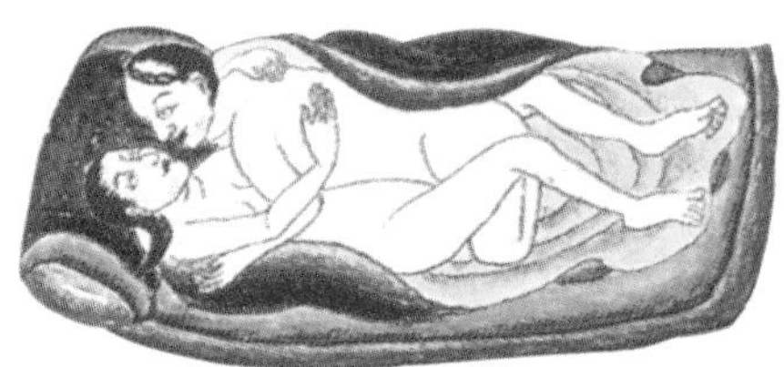

Frequent intercourse

Diseases of female genitalia

Immoderate sexual habits and poor habits during menstruation and delivery may lead to disturbance of the three factors, which in turn involves the womb and vagina in various diseases of the female reproductive system.

Diseases of *rlung*

Symptoms include dull uterine pain, a curved cervix, leaking of mucus, extreme constriction or relaxation of the uterine opening, a sensation of ants crawling in the vagina, uterine bleeding with scanty, dilute blood, foam or clots, and frequent urination.

Treatment: *Five Peng Powder* plus pea flower, hollyhock and round cadamon ground as powder and taken orally. For external treatments apply oil rubbing and warm purging. A soft paste made of butter and *Tibetan Sweetclover Powder with Five Ingredients* can be inserted into the vagina.

Diseases of *mkhris pa*

Manifestations include pus or yellowish black menstruation with a foul smell, fever and thirst.

Treatment: the basic recipe plus Yunnan swertia ground as powder taken orally. Topical treatment includes *Many Vessels Skimmia Powder with Five Ingredients* mixed with bee honey and then inserted into the womb. Take 200 g asparagus tuber boiled in water to make a concentrated solution, add milk, butter and boil again. Finally 400 g each of polygonatum, asparagus tuber, raisin, long pepper, and licorice root are added and boiled again. Add 500 g sugar and take half of the above medicine and mix it with honey to be taken orally. This is a good recipe for disharmony of menstruation, and diseases of *bsam bse'u*. Other medications are *Fennel Powder with Nine Ingredients* boiled in butter and wine and taken orally. Decoct pine resin, tribulus, and adhatoda together for oral administration. A paste made of butter and the formula *Yunnan Swertia with Five Ingredients* can be placed into the womb.

Diseases of *badkan*

Manifestations include itching, mild pain, thick and sticky vaginal discharge, and a cold lower body.

Treatment: the basic recipe plus white cardamom, ground as powder for oral administration. A powder made of *Bibo with Nine Ingredients* mixed with honey can be placed into the womb. Taking brown sugar, wine and honey mixed with *Long Pepper Powder with Three Ingredients*.

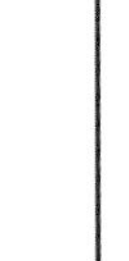

Blood diseases

This is mainly dripping menstruation. Treatments include administering the basic recipe with modifications and mild purging.

For those with any disease, the diet should be warm and soft. When *rlung* predominates, avoid sweet and sour food, sex and physical overstrain.

Tumor of the uterus

When rlung congregates with the menstrual blood and yellow fluid in the womb a tumor may appear. Its symptoms are similar to pregnancy, with a hard and solid abdomen, sometimes with distending pain, and dripping yellow fluid. There are nine sorts of such diseases.

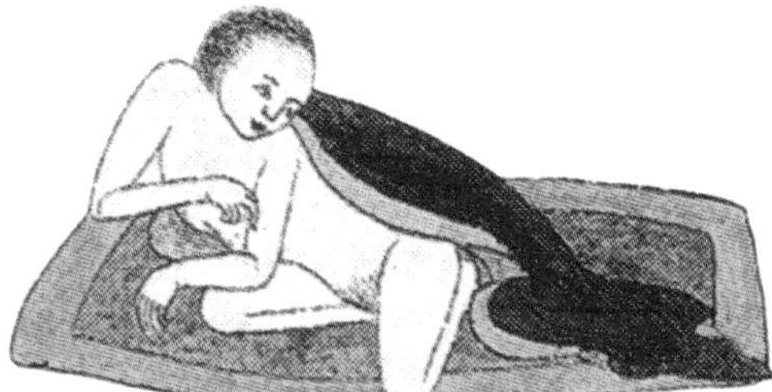

Tumor of the uterus

Tumor due to overindulgence in sexual intercourse

Manifestations include the accumulation of filth, a sluggish lower body, heaviness of half of the body, emaciation, rough breathing, and uneasiness. This tumor occurs mainly in young people.

Numb tumor of the uterus

Manifestations include twisting of the cervix, the essence in the womb changing into yellow fluid and leaking out, a binding sensation in the lower abdomen, inability to urinate, pain in the waist and coccyx, distended epigastrium, and poor digestion. This disease occurs in young girls that have sex with many males.

Uterine tumor caused by seminal fluid

Manifestations include tearing pain in the muscles and marrow, and is caused by impaired seminal fluid, which, unable to fertilize, collects in the womb.

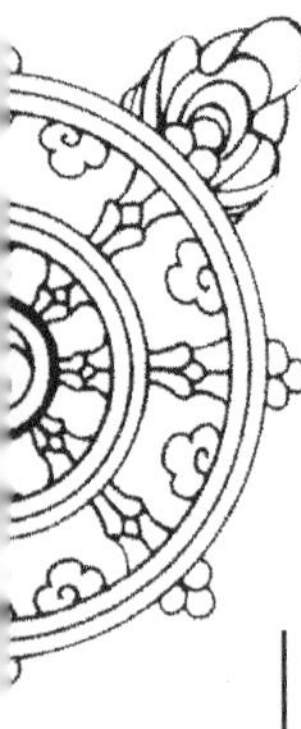

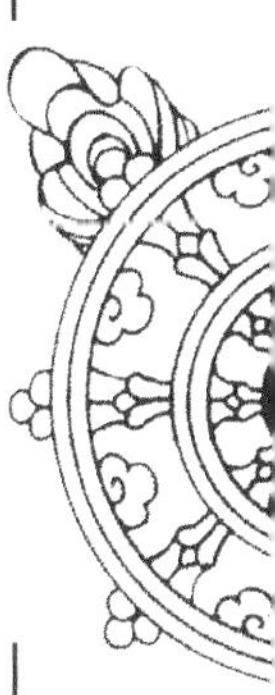

Blood tumor after delivery

Manifestations include changes in the color of the flesh, swelling of the joints, and numbness. This kind of tumor is caused by blood clots retained in the womb. At the terminal stage, leprosy may occur.

Broken button blood tumor of the uterus

Manifestations include hardening of the womb, dripping of mucus blood, abdominal distension, noises in the intestines, and infertility. This is caused by a dead fetus in the womb.

Benign tumor of the uterus

This type of tumor is mainly characterized by aching pain in the muscles. This is caused by a rupture of vessels inside the uterus.

Uterine nodules

When a young girl is raped by a strong young man, the vagina and uterus are ruptured. This may lead to swelling of the lymph nodes, a dripping of black blood, frequent and painful urination, and a weak lower body.

Hard uterine hematoma

This is caused by a failure of the uterus to expel bad blood that then coagulates. The tumor is hard, and the patient experiences paroxysmal pain in the lower abdomen.

Blister tumor of the uterus

When a blister mass appears in the uterus it often manifests as a dripping of yellow fluid, a leaking of yellow menstrual blood, and distention of the lower abdomen.

General treatment: immerse a mixture of flowers in wine or boil grain and rub the liquid over the whole body, especially the lower abdomen and coccyx. A mixture of dried ginger, salt and butter used to rub and massage the body, together with *Three Dose Pill* taken orally drastically disperses the tumor.

Initial stage: *Pure White Powder with Six Ingredients* plus snake flesh, sal ammoniac and sea buckthorn ground into a powder and taken orally. One can also administer orally *Sea Buckthorn Powder with Nineteen Ingredients*, and *Ably Dispersing Clever Remark Powder with Eleven Ingredients*. For chronic cases give *Break Blood Tumor Diamond Pill*. For severe case, use *Break Blood Tumor Diamond Pill*, *Carthamus Pill with Seven Ingredients*, or *Chuzhan Juba Pill*, swallowed with a decoction made of rhubarb and snake flesh.

Parasite diseases of the uterus

Caused by trichomonads, it is characterized by severe itching of the vagina and uterus. There are two sorts:

Severe itching of the uterus

Manifestations include itching of the coccyx and genitals with a foul smell, enlarged breasts, vexation, insomnia, desire to meet with men, and emaciation.

Treatment: *Musk Deer's Coccyx Powder with Eight Ingredients* plus musk, white thorn fruit and vermilion. Topical treatment: a compress made with grain, fresh flowers, and molsa.

Severe itching with yellow fluid (enraged parasite disorder)

When the parasites are active, and the patient doesn't engage in intercourse with her husband, then itching will get worse. To relieve it, the patient masturbates and irritates the parasites. This will result in a hardened and painful uterus, yellow fluid from the vagina and itching.

Treatment: oral administration of *Mercury Recipe with Ten Ingredients*, together with a douche of *Molsa Decoction with Eight Ingredients*.

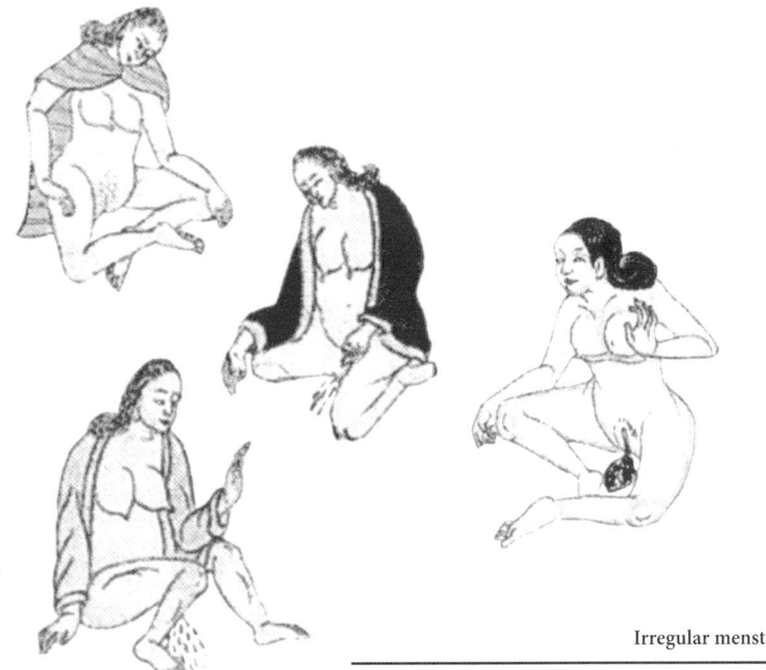

Irregular menstruation

Female wind diseases

Wind diseases are mostly caused by yellow fluid, which is spread by rlung pathogens to the vessels and internal organs. Manifestations include a contracted urethra, vaginal discharge, spotting menstruation, steaming pain in the joints, pain in the muscles, heart palpitations, unpleasant dizziness, cold sensations in the head, mania and forgetfulness, and general edema.

General treatment: nourishing methods should be used, giving the patient nourishing food and medicine, including nutritious meat recipes, nourishing wines, and nourishing medicinal formulas. An example of a nourishing meat recipe is to use the meat from a two year old male sheep. While boiling the meat, add fresh milk, fresh butter, cinnamon and nutmeg. This dish can be eaten three times a day. Also the patient should be careful not to catch a cold.

There are six groups of female wind diseases

Kidney female wind

Manifestations include steaming pain in lumbar vertebrae, worse after being exposed to cold, and a pulling sensation below the waist.

Treatment: use the kidney of a male goat, ox, and a male horse. Cut up all the kidneys and put them into a sheep's stomach, add three fruits, white sword bean, cnidium fruit, long pepper, dried ginger, cinnamon, coriander, chebule and cook until the meat is done. Then mix the dish with mutton, and eat it at dawn.

Small intestine female wind

Manifestations include a binding sensation in the lower abdomen and irregular menstruation.

Treatment: take the blood of a three year old sheep, add cinnamon, dried ginger, long pepper, pepper, round cardamom, chebule, white sword bean, coriander, angular salt, and cnidium and mix with rice powder and then put the mixture in a sheep's small intestine and cook. Take at dawn.

Stomach female wind

Manifestations include paroxysmal upper abdominal pain and poor digestion especially when eating cold food.

Treatment: alternately use *Pomegranate Powder* and *Areca Recipe with Seven Ingredients*, taken with marmot meat and snow chicken. For external treatment, use heated earth blocks as a hot compress. If the pain is serious, take garlic oil or *Turquoise Pill with Thirteen Ingredients* and *Sea Buckthorn Pill with Nineteen Ingredients*, given alternately in the morning and evening. Moxibustion can be performed on the stomach point on the back.

Bone female wind

Manifestations include steaming heat, chilliness, and numbness in the joints and coccyx.

Treatment: eat soup made with the tail bone of a three year old sheep and the flesh of the tail. Add dried ginger, long pepper, pepper, the outer skin of new bamboo, red and black madder root, licorice and cook well. Drink a bowl at dawn.

Heart female wind

Manifestations include unconsciousness, madness, fainting, dizziness and tinnitus.

Treatment: take a monkey heart, bear heart and a marmot heart. Slice and place the meat into a sheep's stomach. Add cinnamon twig, cinnamon bark, wild spiny jujube seed, chebule, nutmeg, cardamom, and purple sal ammoniac. Cook all the ingredients in water and then mix the liquid with mutton and eat at dawn. *Aquilaria Powder with Eight Ingredients* and *Costusroot Powder with Twenty-one Ingredients* can also be given.

Head female wind

Manifestations include eye screens, pus from the ear, dizziness, and tooth or cheek pain.

Treatment: use a 3-year-old sheep's head for treatment. Boil the sheep's skull in water, with sheep brain and mutton. When cooked, place in a sheep's stomach. Pour the soup over the head to eat. Butter, wine or three fruit medicinal wine can also be used. When life-preserving *rlung* is predominant, take *Aquilaria Powder with Eight Ingredients* and give moxibustion on the fontanel point, hundred meetings (at the vertex) and the posterior fontanel points.

Female blood diseases

These diseases are vessel diseases and are due to a disruption of menstruation, yellow fluid and rlung. Manifestations include dripping menstruation, steaming heat in the lower body, afternoon fever, pain, burning heat in the lower abdomen, back, and diaphragm, blisters, and a tense pulse. Treatment includes the application of heat and cold alternately. There are ten types of female blood disease.

Coagulation of uterine blood syndrome

Manifestations include a heavy body, aversion to movement, downward pulling pain in the lower abdomen, and paroxysmal pricking pain.

Treatment: use deer horn, purple sal ammoniac and achyranthes root mixed with wine to be taken orally. Topical treatment includes hot compresses with salt or grain. Bloodletting can be performed at large intestine transport (two fingers lateral to the fourth lumbar vertebrae) and the inner ankle vessel. Eating warm food is best.

Kidney female blood syndrome

Manifestations include vaginal pain and itching, steaming heat and burning pain in the lower body.

Treatment: use wine made with juiced cinnamon. Add achyranthes root, antelope horn, and Himalaya mirabilis for oral administration. Bloodletting at the ankle vessel, the taking of a powder containing polygonatum, asparagus tuber, and tribulus and moxibustion at the 14th vertebra can also be performed.

Breast female blood syndrome

Manifestations include swollen breasts with pricking or severe pain.

Treatment: oral medication of a decoction prepared with white flowered gentian, adhatoda and chebulae, followed by grain oils. A powder of bovine bezoar, musk, mercury, bear bile, and crab; or *Carthamus Pill with Seventeen Ingredients* can also be given. Topical treatments: bloodletting at the six meetings vessel at the back of the palm, or application of a paste made of musk, aconite, arcorus, gentian, madder, stone essence, and lac (a resinous substance secreted by the insect kerria lacca). Moxibustion can be given over the 3rd and 7th vertebrae.

Milk female blood syndrome

Manifestations include dripping menstruation like water, pain in the urethral orifice, nausea and vomiting, vexation and heart palpitations.

Treatment: oral administration of a recipe containing cinnamon, tribulus, Chinese pine root, dried ginger, high mountain gentian, and brown sugar. Topical treatment: hot compress with grain then rub the body with salt and butter.

Small intestine female blood syndrome

Manifestations include burning pain or paroxysmal cutting pain in the intestines.

Treatment: oral administration of sheep lung, dried ginger, and old butter; or a decoction of chebule and rhubarb for mild diarrhea. Topical treatment: bathing with *Manna Bath with Five Ingredients*, or a hot compress with manna. Moxibustion can be given at the 17th vertebra.

Spleen female blood syndrome

Manifestations include pricking pain of the spleen, upset stomach, and pricking pain of the lower abdomen.

Treatment: purging with knoxia, cinnamon, and white sal ammoniac, followed by *Pomegranate Powder with Eight Ingredients*. Topical treatment: moxibustion over the 1st vertebra.

Gallbladder female blood syndrome

Manifestations include weakness, lassitude, thirst, dry mouth, cough, and yellow skin.

Treatment: wash with a decoction of chebule, herpetospermum, and sun spurge, followed by oral administration of *Swertia Powder with Eight Ingredients*. Bloodletting at the gallbladder vessel point and moxibustion at the 10th vertebra can also be employed.

Liver female blood syndrome

Manifestations include red or yellow eyes, pain in the liver, and headache.

Treatment: purging with a recipe consisting of carthamus, cinnamon, long pepper, and chebule, followed by bloodletting at the short angle point, oral administration of *Carthamus Recipe with Seven Ingredients* and moxibustion at the 8th vertebrae.

Lung female blood syndrome

Manifestations include frequent coughing, a swollen face, a pricking pain over the upper body, and numb limbs.

Treatment: mild purging of the small intestine, bloodletting at the six neck points. Oral administration of *Sandalwood Powder with Eight Ingredients* or *Bamboo Sugar Powder with Seven Ingredients* plus grape and licorice, followed by medicinal oil containing madder and areca leaves. Finally, moxibustion at the 4th and 5th vertebrae can be given.

Heart female blood syndrome

Manifestations include pricking pain on the upper body and burning and cutting pain in the lower abdomen.

Treatment: after purging with a decoction of chebule, crystal salt, and asafetida, *Aquilaria Powder with Eight Ingredients* and *Antelope Horn Powder with Fourteen Ingredients* should be given alternately in the morning and evening. Moxibustion over the 6th and 7th vertebrae followed by oral administration of three-fruit medicinal oil should finish the treatment.

Obstetric diseases

These diseases, ranging from pregnancy to delivery, include abnormal reactions to pregnancy, abnormal fetal positions, difficult delivery, retained placenta, postpartum hemorrhage, postpartum paroxysmal pain due to blood stasis, prolapse of the uterus, and postpartum toxicity.

Abnormal reactions to pregnancy

Manifestations include laziness, irritability, nausea, vomiting, loss of appetite, cravings for certain foods, and relapses of old diseases.

Treatment: if a serious disease relapses, biomedical treatment is indicated. Let the woman eat what she likes. Keep her home dry. She shouldn't sleep in the day time, eat horse meat, donkey meat, or poultry. Avoid overstrain, but don't be immobile either, and avoid catching colds.

Abnormal fetal position

For reversed head and feet or breech presentation, hold the pregnant woman's feet high and shake them, then press the fetus with fingers, and pat the breeched fetus in order to return the fetus to a normal position.

Difficult labor

If the baby is alive, promote delivery with medication. Use a powder of antelope horn taken with wine, or take the finely ground powder of antelope horn and red bean. Or give *Ably Dispersing Clever Remark Powder with Six Ingredients* or *Ably Dispersing Clever Remark Powder with Eleven Ingredients* orally. External treatment: hot compress on the abdomen with earth from a marmot cave that faces eastward.

For cases when the fetus is dead, use antelope horn, tail hairs from a bat, knoxia, and brown sugar with wine for oral administration.

Retained placenta

Oral administration of antelope horn, sal ammoniacum, wild rabbit dung, and scorched genital hairs taken with wine, *Ably Dispersing Clever Remark Powder with Six Ingredients* or *Ably Dispersing Clever Remark Powder with Eleven Ingredients.*

Postpartum hemorrhage

Take sugar wine, cane sugar wine, or orostachys wine orally. Also bee honey, sugar, leather ash, and ashed snow chicken feathers can be fried together and taken with sugar wine and bone soup. Topical massage and fumigation can also be used. When the lower body feels cold, treat with bathing methods and moxibustion at the 16th vertebra.

Postpartum pain due to static blood

Oral administration of zanthoxylum, wine, bee honey wine, or cane sugar wine. Fumigate the body with earth from a marmot hole. If this is ineffective, use the dregs of wine mixed with salt as a hot compress along with bloodletting at large intestine transport (two fingers lateral to the 4th lumbar vertebrae).

Prolapse of the uterus

Wash the area with warm water and milk. Insert a bamboo syringe into the anus and blow, or push the uterus back in place with the hands while inducing hiccough with zanthoxylum. If treatment is still ineffective, hold the uterus with a blanket and then push it back with sal ammoniac. At the same time, hold both feet upward and shake them. Fumigation of the perineum should also be done. Avoid sitting up and walking. Lie on the stomach with the buttocks raised.

Postpartum toxicity

Manifestations include lassitude, severe thirst, red saliva, pain in the upper body, a fine-rapid pulse, and is mostly caused by a sudden increase of *mkhris pa* due to overstrain, sleeping in the daytime and eating old butter or old meat.

Treatment: use a solution of chebulae and rhubarb and give bear bile plus *Carthamus Powder with Seven Ingredients* orally. External treatment involves bloodletting short angle point, hollow organ vessel, gallbladder vessel, and large intestine transport. As far as medicinal and dietary therapy are concerned, hot and cold should be applied alternately and appropriately. Improve the nutrition and eliminate the cause of the disease.

Women have a uterus, vagina, breasts, menstruate and deliver children. *Rlung*, *mkhris pa* and *badkan* can produce blood disorders. Frequent intercourse and inappropriate care after delivery can cause other female disorders. Tibetan medicine pays special attention to female health.

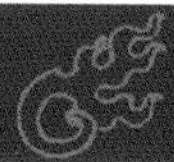

Infertility and Strengthening Yang

In Tibetan medicine, it is claimed that pregnancy happens on the basis of internal and external factors. Intercourse between the father and mother is the external factor; while the interaction of the semen-blood with the five-sources is the internal factor. Paternal semen and maternal blood are the roots. Any disorder of either party may lead to infertility.

Male infertility

Only normal seminal fluid can yield a proper fertilization. Seminal fluid with disorders of *rlung*, *mkhris pa*, *badkan*, blood, or a mixture of any of the above two or three factors will lead to an abnormal state and pregnancy will not occur. This is male infertility.

Normal seminal fluid is heavy, pale-white in color, like lustrous nectar, astringent, sweet and plentiful. Seminal fluid affected by *rlung* disease is rough, black, and pungent; that with *mkhris pa* disease is yellow, sour, and smells of putrid blood; that with badkan disease is sticky, cool, grey, and sweet; that affected by mixed *rlung-mkhris pa* disease where *mkhris pa* prevails due to *rlung* action is scanty and dry; that of mixed *badkan-mkhris pa*, under the influence of greasy *badkan* and moist *mkhris pa* is knotted and in small fragments; that of mixed *rlung-mkhris pa-badkan* becomes a feces-like material.

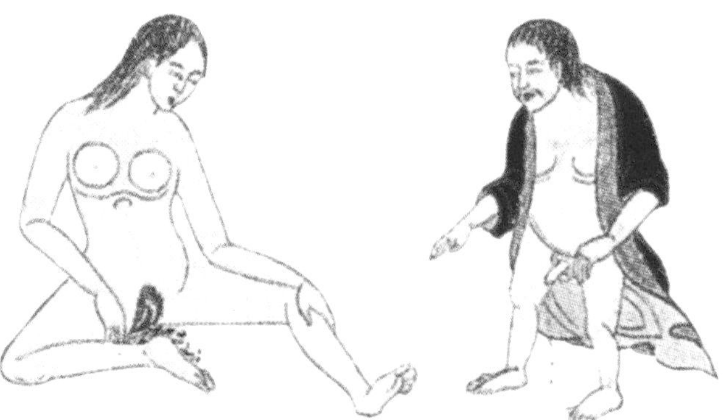

Healthy semen and blood leads to pregnancy, and also can be used as medicine.

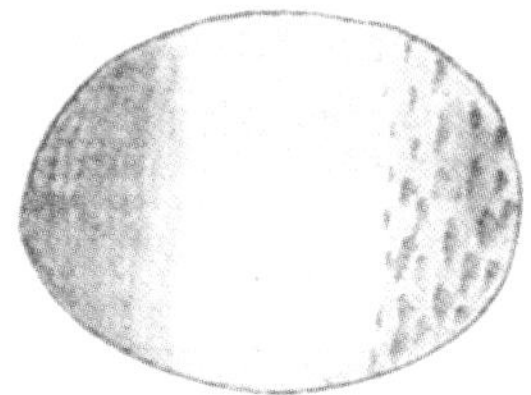

Semen-blood with *rlung* disease is black in color, rough, and tastes astringent.

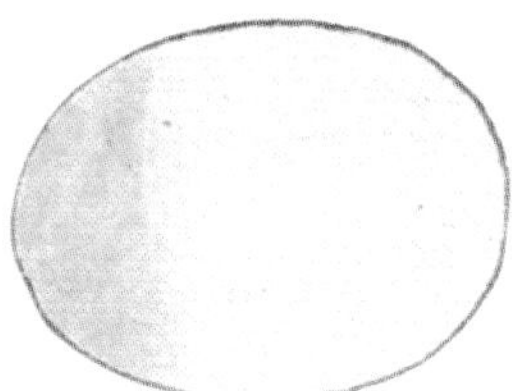

Semen-blood with *mkhris pa* disease is yellow with a foul smell.

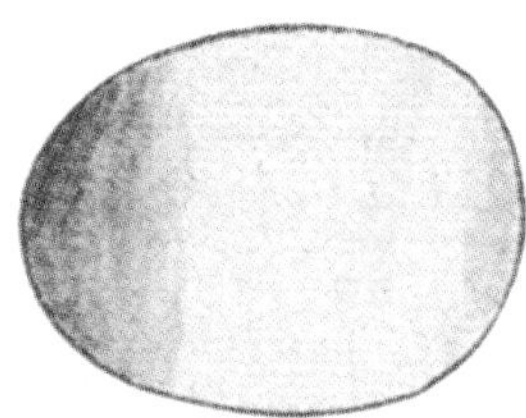

Semen-blood with *badkan* disease is light in color, sticky, cool, and sweet.

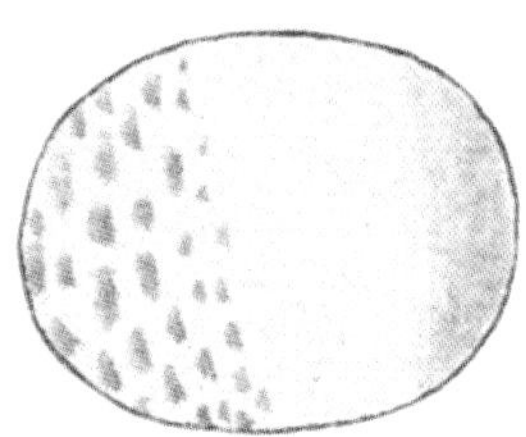

Semen-blood with a blood disorder has a putrid smell.

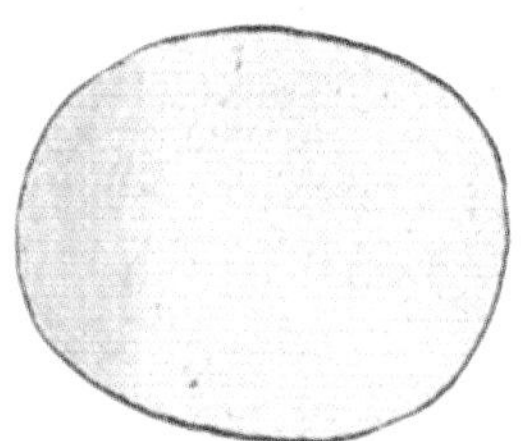

Semen-blood with a mixed blood-*mkhris pa* disease looks like pus

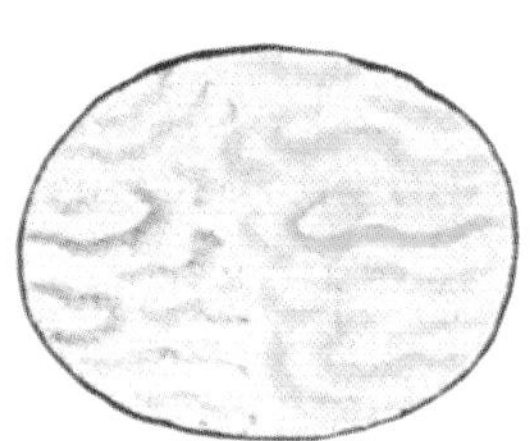

Semen-blood with a mixed *mkhris pa-badkan* disease coagulates in fragments.

Semen-blood with a mixed *rlung-mkhris pa-badkan* disorder looks like stool.

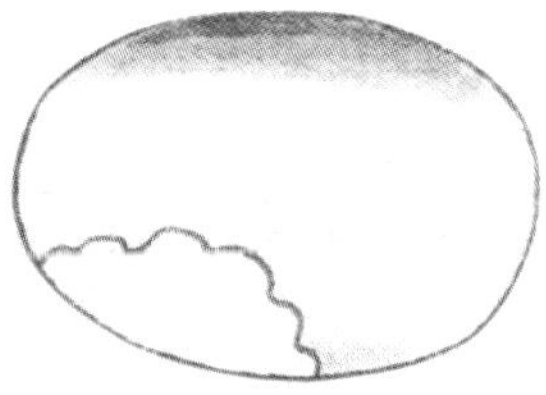

Semen-blood with a mixed *rlung-badkan* disease can't be conjugated.

Semen-blood with a mixed *rlung-mkhris pa* disease looks dry.

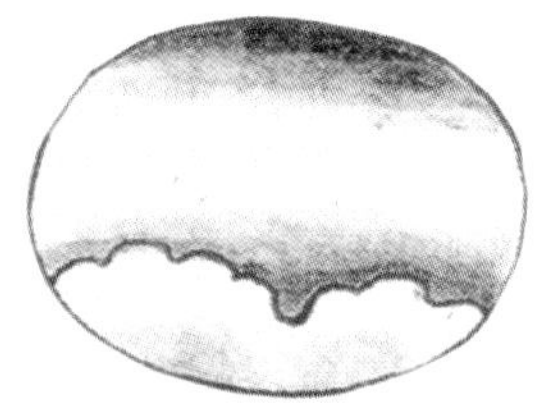

If the five-sources in semen-blood are incomplete this can also cause male infertility. With a lack of water, semen and blood can't conjugate because water is sticky and coagulates; with a lack of earth, semen-blood is hard and the female can't become pregnant; with a lack of wind, the embryo is unable to develop; with a lack of fire, the embryo is unable to mature because fire controls growth and maturity; with a lack of space, the growth of the embryo is blocked because there is no room for its growth. Therefore, normal fertilization needs all five sources. Lack of any of them can hinder fertilization.

Reproduction relies on semen-blood, which relies on the body. The body relies on food and medicine, so the treatment of infertility relies on food, medicine, and other approaches to supplement the injured semen-blood. Biomedical treatment can also be used to supplement Tibetan medical treatment of infertility.

Infertility may be due to numerous causes. The selection of food with all six tastes and medicine to supplement semen-blood is the basic treatment approach.

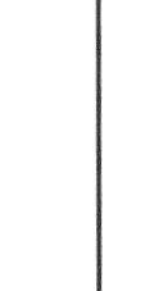

Female infertility

Infertility in females usually occurs because of a disturbance of the three factors and diseases that occur after the delivery of a child. They primarily cover three aspects:

Disturbances of *rlung*

Manifestations include yellow menstrual blood, irregular menstruation, sometimes with amenorrhea, and a sensation of opening of the gate of the womb or a swelling sensation of the lower abdomen.

Treatment: fresh ginger solution administered in the morning and evening. External treatment includes hot compresses on the lower abdomen. Moistening medicine can be put in the womb. To treat disorders that simultaneously relapse use nutritious formulas consisting of meat, wine or butter to strengthen and cultivate the body's vital qi.

Disturbances of *mkhris pa*

Manifestations include menstrual blood like tobacco juice or pus and burning pain in the lower abdomen.

Treatment: use a *Major Vessel-Moistening Recipe* to clear and drain. For topical treatment, steam the body with flowers soaked in wine. Moistening medicinals can be placed into the womb to eliminate any relapses. Nurture the body with meat, wine, and butter.

Disturbances of *badkan*

Manifestations include cold menstrual blood like flowing water or cheese scum.

Treatment: similar to that of *mkhris pa* disturbances.

Postpartum disorders

These disorders include a deceased fetus that remains in the womb, blood stasis of the uterus, and uterine tumors due to bleeding at the uterus gate. Manifestations are similar to pregnancy, sometimes with burning pain in the lower abdomen, waist pain, and pain in the 14th vertebrae.

Treatment: dried ginger solution taken morning and evening. *Chebulae Decoction with Three Ingredients* plus *Confucius Knoxia Powder with Five Ingredients* taken before breakfast. Spray wine on welted thistle and bryophyte which are then stir-fried and used as a hot compress on the lower abdomen. Lastly, use *Major Vessel-Moistening Recipe* to clear and drain, followed by nutritious meat, wine, and butter recipes, and tribulus wine to strengthen the body. Treatment of any diseases that may relapse is essential. Pay attention to daily habits and keep warm all year.

Strengthening yang

Strengthening yang is beneficial to health cultivation. After middle age, a man's sexual function declines gradually as his age increases. Strengthening yang at this period may delay the advent of impotence, increase semen, and prolong life. There is a main body and a branch for these techniques. Males are the main focus for strengthening yang. When a man has no sexual desire, no matter how many females are around him, intercourse will not occur. When a man's semen is normal and has a strong sexual desire, a female can produce descendents. Females are the branch of strengthening yang, because they are the foundation where the seed is accepted and developed. However, when a woman is not strong enough, or she can't accept semen, it is like barren earth where no sprout from a seed may grow. Hence, strengthening yang is important for both parties.

Techniques for strengthening yang come from diet, daily life, medicine, and external therapies.

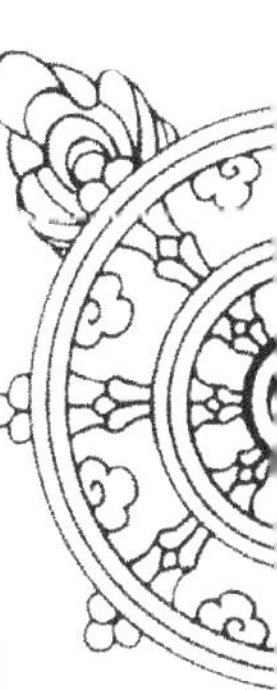

Diet

Food like brown sugar, bee honey, white sugar, broth, milk, cheese scum, and melted butter are recommended. Among them, fresh milk and fresh broth are highly nutritious.

Rice is moist, soft and can strengthen yang. It also stops diarrhea and removes the three pathogens. Seeds like sesame are heavy and warm, and also strengthen yang and expel rlung disease. Otter flesh strengthens yang as well. It treats cold kidney and low back diseases. Mutton is moist and hot, it increases body strength, generates primordial qi, and helps digestion. In addition, frequently eating melted fat can produce fire, remove internal disease, quickly produce primordial qi, increase body strength, cause the body to glow with the luster of health, and make the elderly strong.

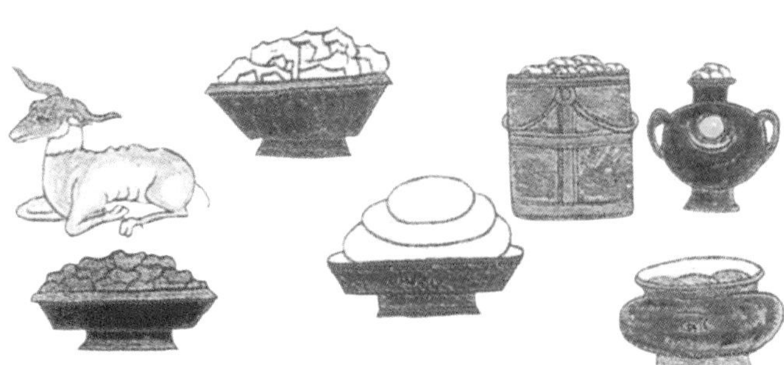

Mutton, brown sugar, bee honey, broth and milk can be consumed frequently.

Daily life

First of all, one should have fortune and a happy family, and the husband and wife should love each other. This makes both parties comfortable and energetic. All these things benefit semen and strengthen yang.

Before making love the couple should cast amorous glances, talk sweet to each other, and hug each other. Kissing also benefits and strengthens yang.

Next, ones must also guard their desire. Indulging in sex doesn't strengthen yang, but actually injures it.

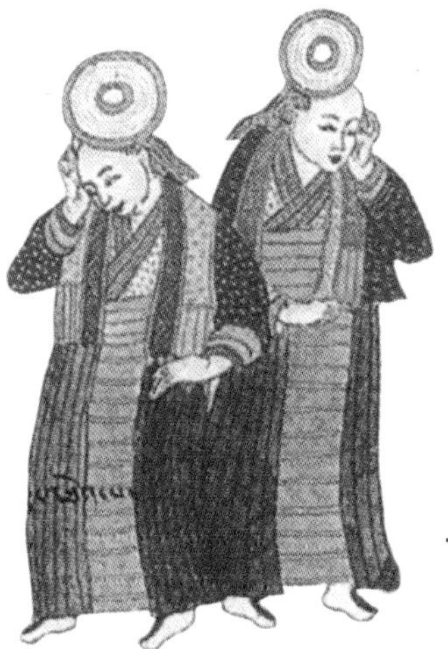

Casting amorous glances and talking sweet with each other.

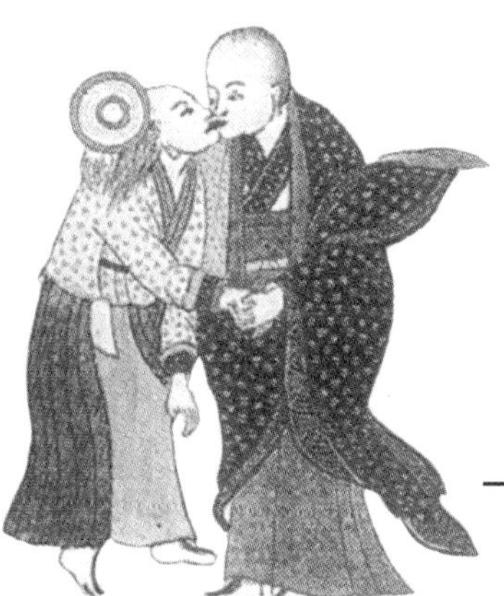

Hugging and kissing each other.

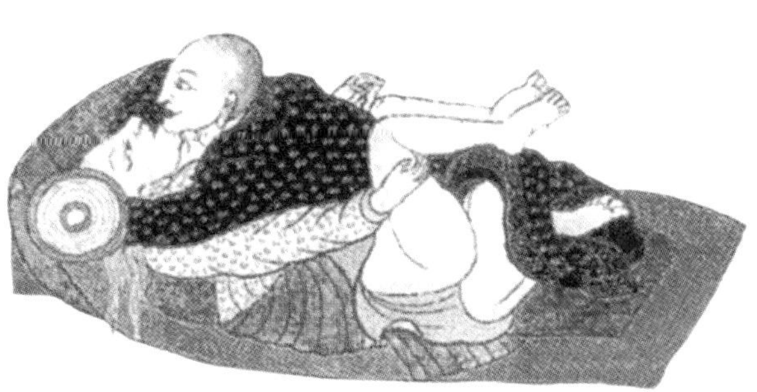

Comfortable intercourse with nourishing medication.

Medication

Snow toad, also called Tibetan toad, is an excellent medicine for benefiting semen. It is claimed that snow toad rapidly transforms into semen. Below are some recipes that use snow toad.

Snow Toad with Five Ingredients: grind red glauberite with cow's milk and mix in yellow snow toad, purple snow toad, fragrant orchid, sparrow head, henbane and brown sugar. Take it as snack or nibble frequently with wine.

Snow Toad with Nine Ingredients: grind purple snow toad, nutmeg, human coccyx, cat's tail, otter tail, glauberite, sulfur, stone essence and henbane together and put them into a sparrow's body. Sew up the body with a silk thread and fry it in butter. Add brown sugar and dry meat and take a spoonful as a snack.

Snow Toad with Thirteen Ingredients: purple snow toad, yellow snow toad, otter meat, stony lizard, chicken flesh, pigeon, sparrow's head, mountain sparrow's head, flesh from a thick-lipped fish, fragrant orchid, henbane, glauberite, asparagus tuber, and brown sugar are ground together and taken orally. It is said that this formula can increase semen quickly, and make one energetic enough to have sex with a hundred females in one night.

Another snow toad recipe: put purple snow toad, black sesame, white sesame, and snow toad flesh into a sparrow's body and sew it shut. Fry it in butter and then dry it in the shade. When it is dry, grind it to a fine powder. Mix the powder with butter and brown sugar and eat. Or use snow toad, five roots, three fruits, purple snow toad, cat's eye spurge, sheep's testes, milk, and butter, boil to concentrate, then add long pepper, dried ginger, cane sugar, a little nutmeg and take orally.

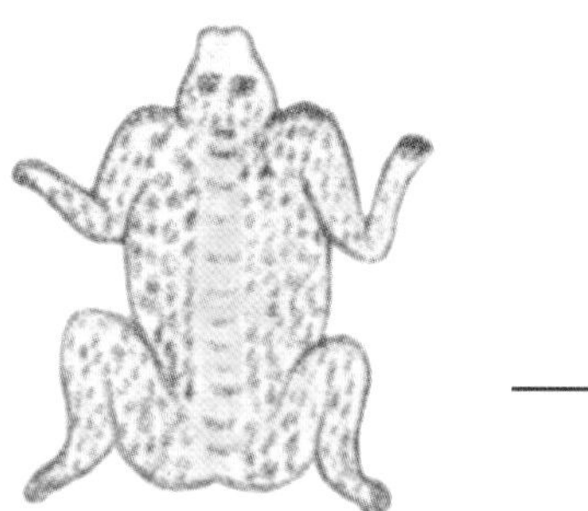

Frog

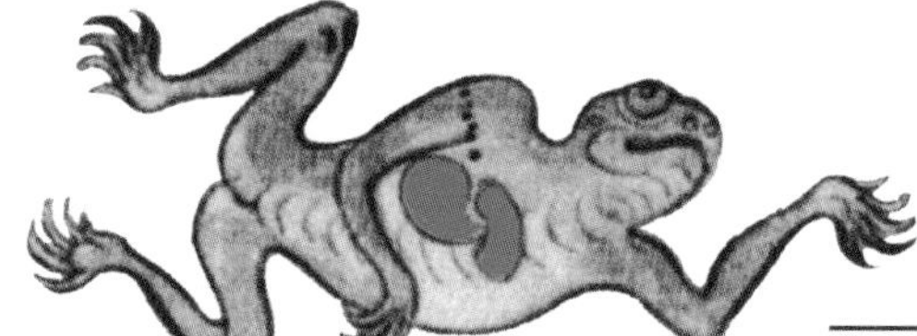

Meat of a Frog

Snow toad is excellent at strengthening yang. Common recipes include *Snow Toad with Nine Ingredients, Snow Toad with Thirteen Ingredients,* and *Snow Toad with Five Ingredients.*

Sheep's testes recipe

Boil the sheep's testes in cow's milk. Add white sugar and sesame and eat. The effect is similar to the snow toad recipes above.

Miscellaneous

Boil long pepper and emblic together and add sugar, bee honey, butter, and take the solution with milk. Another recipe: after taking cheese scum, eat rice and white sugar.

External therapy

Rubbing oil

Rubbing butter on the whole body makes one energetic. For those with nocturnal emission and low kidney function, rub otter fat or snow toad fat on the waist.

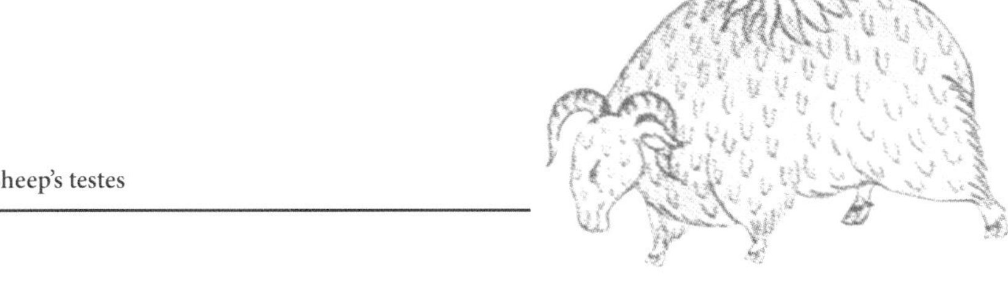

Sheep's testes

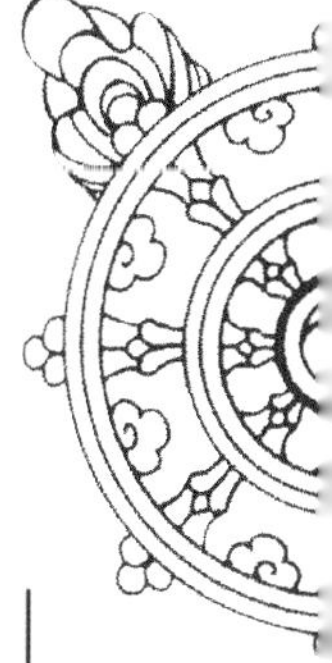

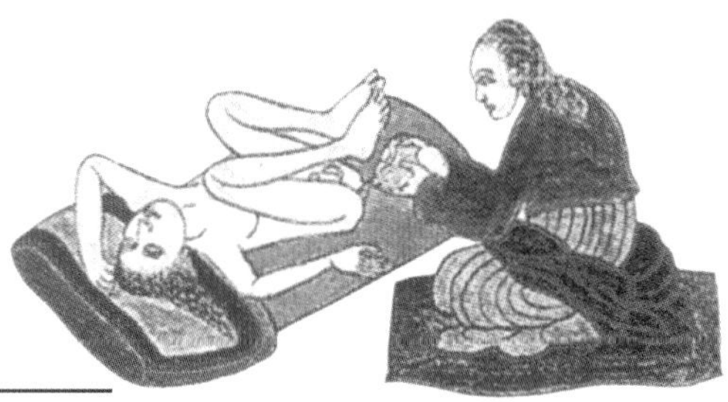

Rubbing oil on the whole body.

Mild enema of nurturing medicinals.

Warm and mild catharsis

Medicines: broth made of a land animal, goat milk, butter, long pepper, chebulae, swertia, Japanese meadowsweet, and then mixed with horse chestnut.

Administration: take a handful of the above medicine, heat it and then put into an ox skin sac or an enema bag. Lie supine and administer the medicine into the anus. Slap the center of the patient's soles slightly, then hold the toes and raise the legs and shake.

Normally, food changes to blood on the first day after digestion; changes into muscle on the second day; into fat on the third day; to bone on the fourth day; to marrow on the fifth day; and to semen until the sixth day. However, when one has sex, it can change to semen right away. When one takes food or medicine that strengthens yang, it will change to semen rapidly. This does not disturb the normal process of food metabolism. It is obvious that strengthening yang is beneficial to one's health.

Special attention must be given to the fact that strengthening yang doesn't mean indulging in sex as much as one pleases. When one steps onto this wrong path, the body is doomed to be harmed and there will be no end to the trouble caused.

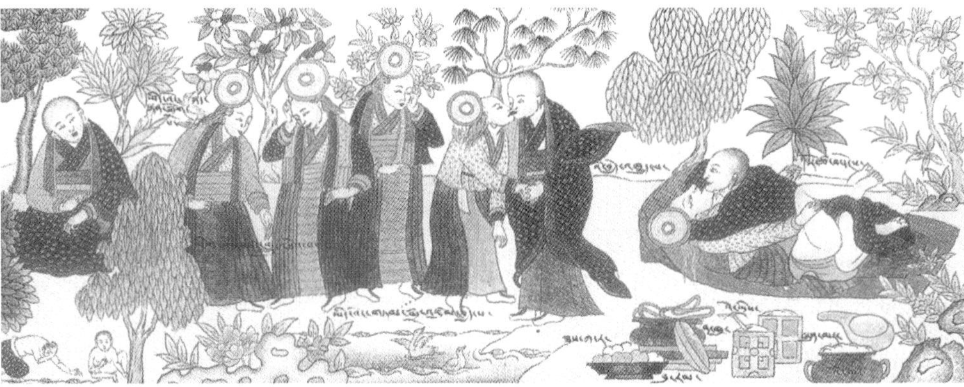

Healthy harmony between a male and a female is the root of health (part of *Thangkha* fifty-five in the *Sman thang* series of *The Four Medical Tantras*).

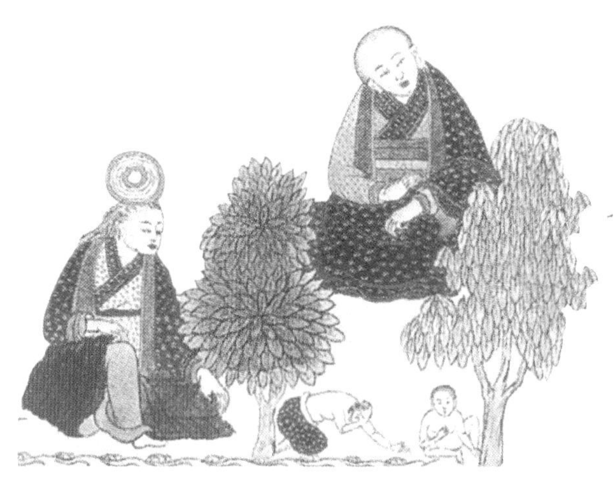

སྣུམ་ལུམས

CHAPTER 7 TIBETAN MEDICINAL BATHING

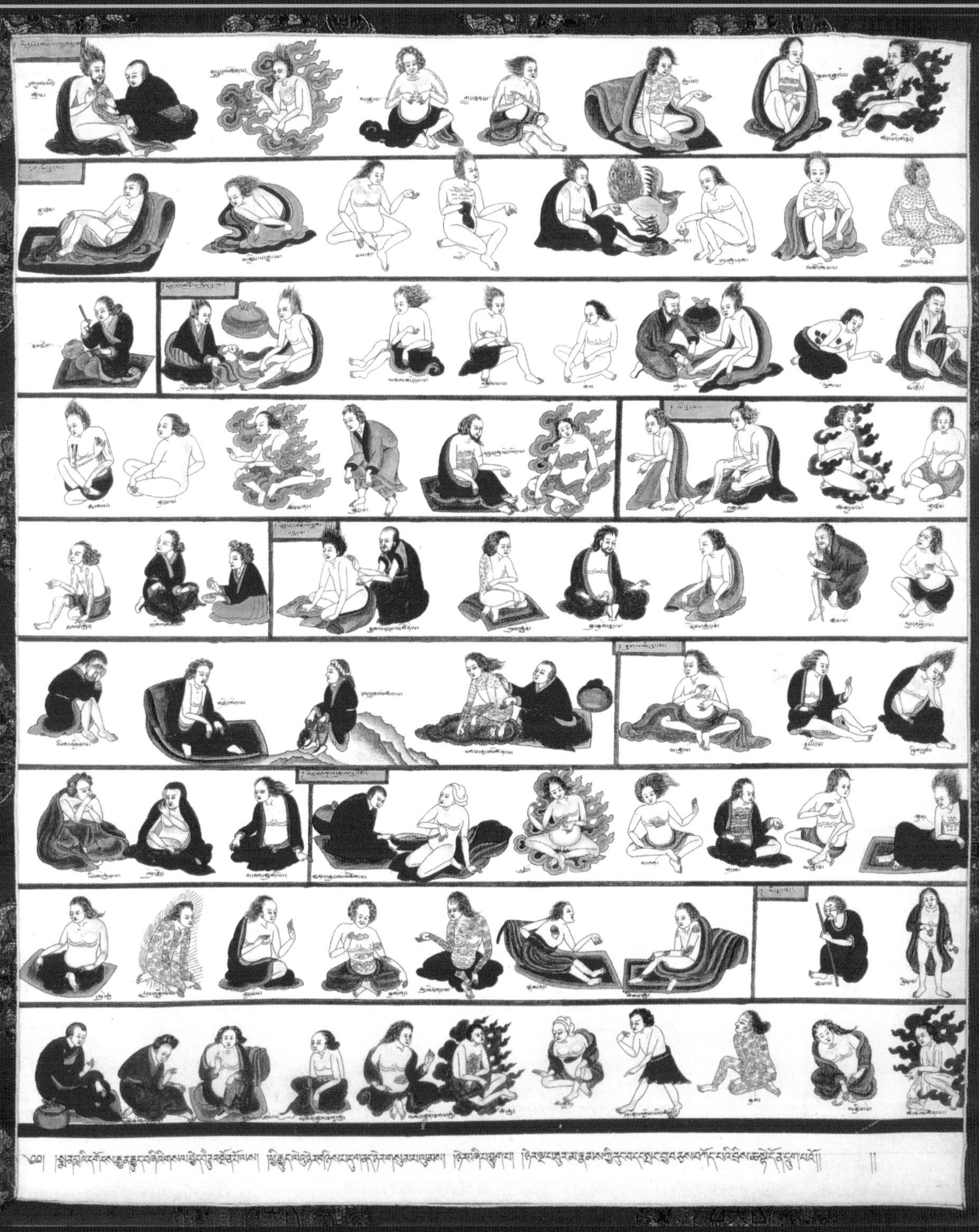

Thangkha seventy-six in the *Sman thang* of *The Four Medical Tantras*:
Medicinal bathing as an externaltherapy.

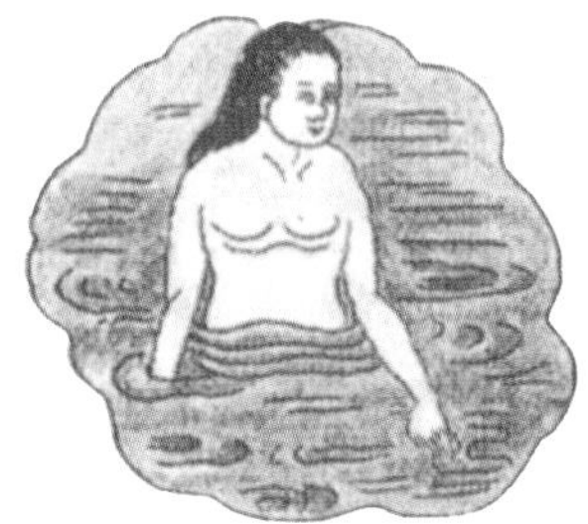

In Tibet, medicinal bathing is commonly used in daily life for disease prevention and health preservation.

There are two general kinds of medicinal baths: natural springs, and man-made baths. The former is the earliest form of medicinal bathing. However, since natural springs are not readily available everywhere, Tibetan doctors follow the principles of treatment for using natural springs to prepare medicinal solutions which have developed into the man-made baths used today. *The Five Flavor Sweet Dew Decoction* is the most famous basic recipe for medicinal baths, on the basis of which modifications can be made according to the syndrome, constitution, season or disease manifestations. It yields good results in both prevention and treatment of disease.

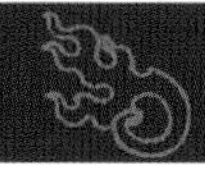

The Origin of Tibetan Medicinal Bathing

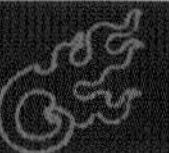

Living among the natural springs of the plateau since ancient times, the Tibetan people realized long ago the health benefits of bathing in the springs. Based on the unique geography, climate and different environmental factors of Tibet, doctors created medicinal baths, and use theory to apply them. The 25th chapter of the *Conclusion Tantra* of *The Four Medical Tantras* titled "Five Instrumental Bathing Methods" is the earliest known record. It is a very complete record and has led scholars to believe that the true origins of medicinal bathing came much earlier. There are three theories concerning its origin.

Derived from the folk customs of the Tibetan people

According to Tibetan folklore, when water passes through starlight it becomes sweet dew. Tibet has a long winter and a short summer, and spring and winter are generally very cold. The water that rushes down the mountains in spring and winter is muddy. Therefore, the best time for bathing is summer and autumn. According to the Tibetan calendar, when the Sun moves to the 10th star at 43 degrees, or during the communicating festival in August, the vesper star appears and all water becomes sweet dew with the power of medicine. Bathing in this water can eliminate disease. It is recorded in *Tibetan Records*, "On the 13th of June, build a hut along the river bank, and call all relatives and friends together to swim in the river until the 5th of August. This will do away with all disease." This is a festival to bathe, swim, and wash clothes, linens, and quilts in the river. Enjoyment and play at this "bathing festival" naturally promotes health. This is also called "The Medical Water Festival" and has been going on in Tibet for over 700 years.

There are also numerous legends on treating diseases during this bathing festival. One, which is related here, concerns a god of medicine. The story is told by Liao Dongfan like this:

Long, long ago, there were no doctors in the mortal world. All the doctors were sent from heaven by the god Dbangpo Byedqin. There was once a doctor called Sman-lha who was highly respected by the people. His name literally meant "Medicinal God." Once when he was back in heaven, there was a serious epidemic and many people lost their lives. The people knelt down to pray and ask heaven to send the Medicinal God to save them. The Medicinal God was also anxious to be able to rescue the suffering people. He went to ask Dbangpo Byedqin for permission to go, but was told that there are strict rules in heaven. If someone

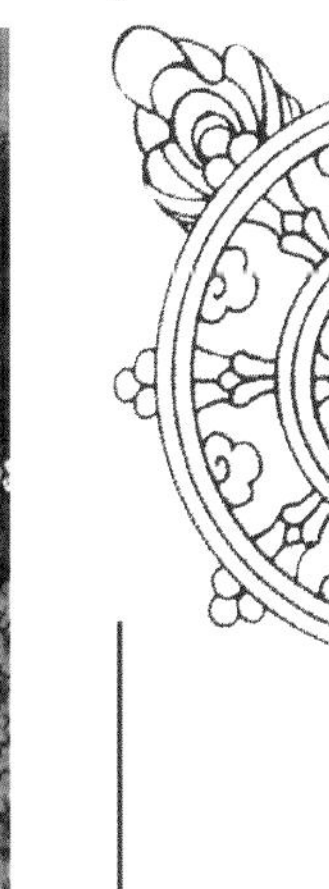

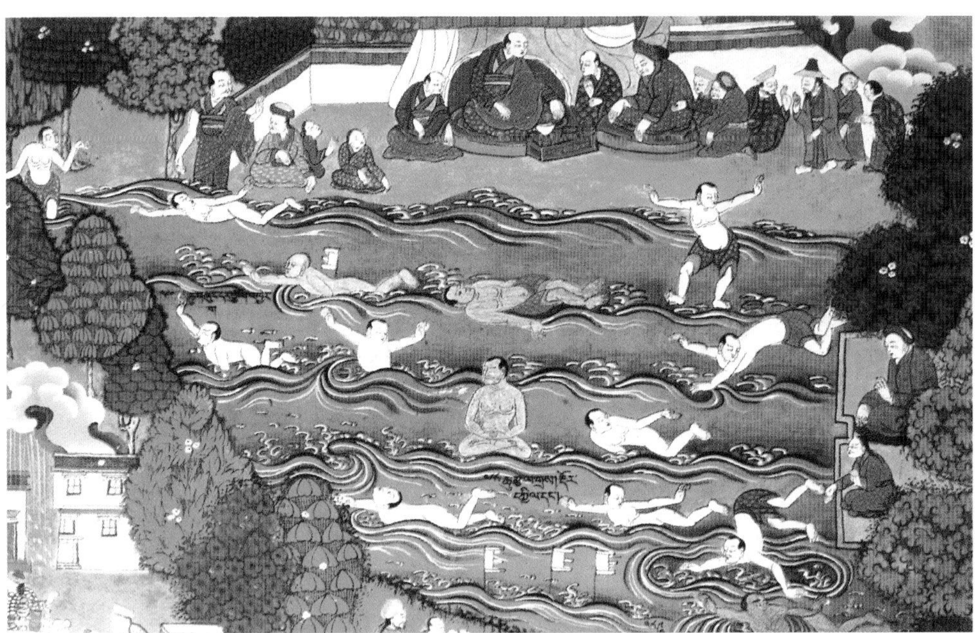

People enjoying swimming (part of a mural in Potala Palace).

has traveled once to the mortal world, they were not allowed to go back again. However, since the Medicinal God was very sincere and highly skilled in the medical arts, he was granted permission to go and rescue the Tibetan people, but only for seven days. If any longer, he would be punished. The Medicinal God knew that seven days was not enough time for him to save all the sick people who lived along the Yalutsampo River. To solve the problem, he turned himself into a star and used the light of his body to shine down and benefit the mortals with his compassionate love and great medical skills.

That very night a mortal woman suffering from disease dreamt of the Medicinal God spreading healing to the world from top of the Precious Bottle Mountain. Affecting the springs on the mountain, the river water that flowed off of the mountain became medicinal water. When she woke up she struggled and crawled to the river and submerged herself in the water. In no time at all, she was cured. Upon seeing how this woman was cured, all the sick made their way to the river, bathed there, and the epidemic was ended. The patients who had been freed from misery paid their respects to the Medicinal God, asking him to prolong the healing light of the star year after year. Since then, the Dkama Duipa Star (Abandon Mountain Star) has appeared in the sky over the Precious Bottle Mountain in early autumn each year and then reluctantly disappeared seven days later.

Derived from Buddhism

The influence of ancient Indian culture and science on Tibetan culture was realized through the transmission of Buddhism. However, by browsing the Vedic classics, including *Susruta samhita*, Vagbhata's *Astangahrdaya samhita*, Ravigupta's *Sidhasara*, and *Sman tsho ba'i mdo*, no record of medicinal bathing can be found. Nevertheless, it is natural that the bathing customs of India must have had an impact on Tibetan bathing customs through the transmission of Buddhist rituals.

In fact, bathing plays a significant role within many religions in India. Jains, for example, should bathe the god Puwapuri in a fragrant solution made of milk every twelve years, while the Brahmins also have a tradition of bathing their gods. The social custom of bathing portraits of sages was very popular in India in the pre-Buddhist era. Since the advent of Buddhism, the festival of bathing the Buddha has been practiced on the birthday and day of his enlightenment. The Tibetan regions where Lamaism prevails have similar customs of bathing the Buddha and other bathing customs as well. Based on Buddhist teachings, there are eight features of the water of early autumn: sweet, cool, soft, light, clear, without a foul smell, not irritable to the throat, and not harmful to the stomach. Autumn is thus the best season for bathing.

Another legend also reveals the relationship between bathing customs and Buddhism. It is said that once upon a time, a plague was raging over the plateau in autumn claiming numerous lives. In response, the Bohdisattva Avalokitesvara dispatched a goddess to carry some magical water from the Jade Pool and pour it into the lakes and rivers. That night all the Tibetan people dreamt of a sick girl bathing in the Lhasa River. She was not only cured, but became very beautiful as well. When the people awoke the next morning and shared their dreams they soon went to bathe in the river, ending the epidemic. Based on this legend, it is clear that Buddhist bathing customs and the tradition of bathing the Buddha strengthened the existing bathing customs of the Tibetan people, and promoted further exploration on the health benefits of bathing.

Derived from imitating natural springs

The experience of humankind generally follows the evolution from spontaneity to conscious process. It is speculated that medicinal bathing is very likely an imitation and application of the effects of natural springs. In the precivilized era, ancient humans possibly found by accident that bathing in a natural spring could relieve and even cure some diseases. Slowly people began to test the healing effect of natural springs consciously. It is recorded at the beginning of the *Root Tantra of The Four Medical Tantras* that, "There is a Malaya Mountain to the west of Lta-na-sdug. Six kinds of magical medicines are produced there. Besides, there are also five kinds of glauberite for treating all diseases, five kinds of *Brag zhun*, five medical rivers, and five hot springs." The importance of natural springs in Tibetan medicine can be thus seen.

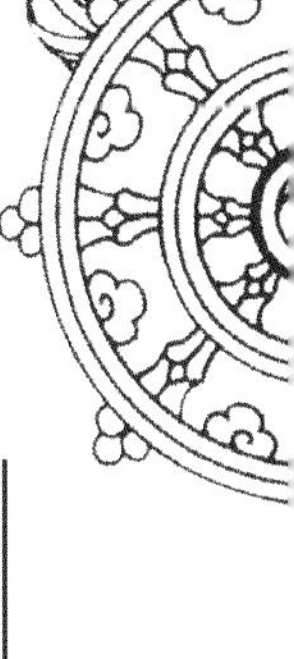

However, natural springs are generally located in remote areas that are difficult to reach, while verified therapeutic springs are even more difficult to find. There is a story told in the *Biography of Gyuthog Gonpo* about how Gyuthog Yontan Gonpo sought the Sweet

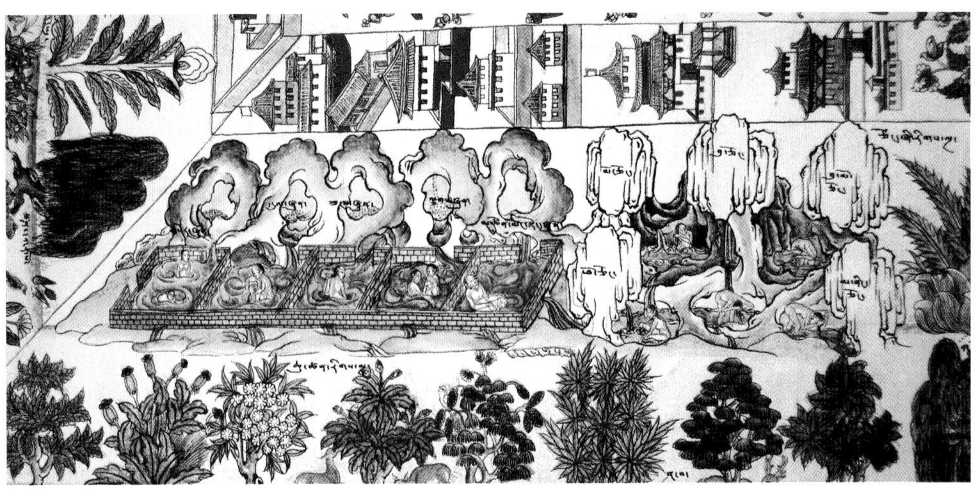

According to *The Four Medical Tantras*, medicines for treating all kinds of diseases are produced on the west side of Lta-na-sdug.

Dew Cave under the instruction of a red-robed man when he was staying in the city of Gonpo sman long. The text relates the painstaking process of locating the spring that was able to treat disease. He finally found in front of the mountain 108 springs from the eight branches of the river. For the benefit of all beings, he prayed for the everlasting existence of these springs. Then, he said, "Since these springs possess the capacity of 700,000 kinds of medicine, they are capable of tackling 700,000 kinds of disease. Hence, they will be called the Spring of 700,000 Functions. The eight branches of the river are wide, clear, with water neither too hot nor too cold, and without any scum. Its water tastes sweet, is not harmful to the stomach, and treats all disorders."

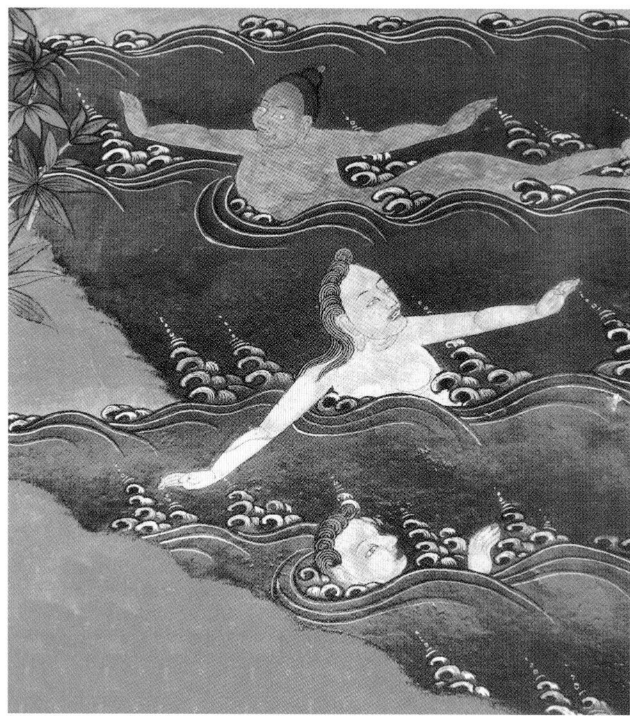

People playing in the water from a Tibetan mural.

Actually, natural springs used medicinally were very popular in Gyuthog's age. *Five Flavor Sweet Dew Decoction* was also often used clinically for medicinal bathing. Presently, the use of medicinal springs is highly respected by contemporary Tibetan doctors. It can be speculated that the origin of the methods of man-made medicinal bathing must have been rigorously researched since natural springs were painstakingly sought by early Tibetan doctors. By combining the experiences gained from the treatment principles used in the application of natural springs with the understanding of the nature and taste of medicinal substances, Tibetan doctors were able to create recipes for man-made medicinal baths of great sophistication through long-term practice.

Studies on the origin and evolution of medicinal baths are rather rare. However, it can be sure that there is no single root from which medicinal bathing is derived. Rather, it developed gradually from multiple factors based on the bathing customs of the Tibetan people.

As a mild external therapy of Tibetan medicine, medicinal bathing consists of natural springs and man-made baths. The basic solution used is called sweet dew. Man-made baths are given using complex compound recipes.

Natural Springs

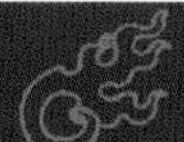

In the western region of Yadong in Tibet, there is a famous Kampo Magical Spring which is composed of twelve hot springs, each with its own therapeutic effect, all situated quite near to each other. These include the Goddess Pool that helps people recover from strokes, Ngakan Pool for arthritis, Nga gru Pool for skin diseases, Eagle Pool for bone diseases, etc. Nearby are two small hills that are made of discarded crutches that were used by people before being cured by the springs. It is said that the twelve hot springs are capable of curing over one hundred ailments. Villagers from near and far come to soak in the hot springs after working hard with their bodies. Legends have it that the hot springs are protected by twelve goddesses and the springs are located in pure earth that was hidden by Padmasabhava (the Lotus Born Buddha) 1,300 years ago. In fact, Tibet is very rich in natural springs, having a total of 677 locations throughout the country. *Shel gong shel phreng* lists 101 springs, each with its own special minerals, smell, taste, color, effect, and disease it can treat.

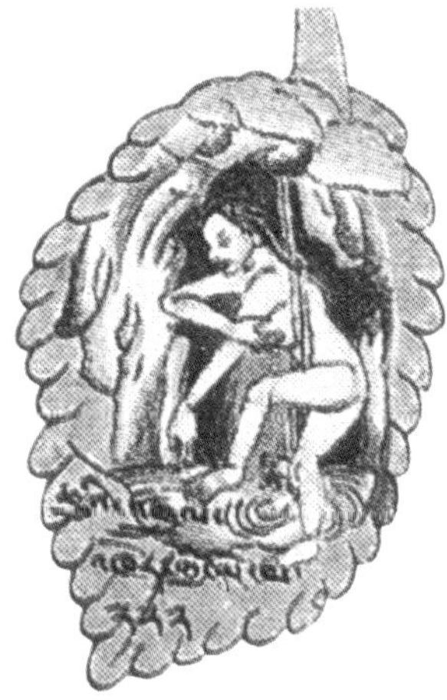

Bathing in natural springs is the basic form of medicinal bathing.

The five types of natural springs

In traditional Tibetan medicine, all five types have typical features, diseases they can treat and shortcomings. The springs are differentiated into five different kinds based on the predominant mineral in the water:

Sulfur spring: the water is yellow, bitter, has a sulfuric smell and sulfur crystals surrounding the spring.

Glauberite spring: the water is clear and colorless, and has no special smell. When added to tea or wine, its color remains unchanged. There are glauberite pebbles nearby.

Alum spring: the water is blue and turbid with a metallic smell.

Stone essence spring: the water is purple, bitter, with stone essence crystals around.

Limestone spring: water is especially clear, bitter with a scorched smell, with grayish-white pebbles nearby.

Spring (main constituent)	Features	Indication	Contraindication
Sulfur	yellow water, bitter, with a sulfuric smell, and sulfur crystals nearby	sores and ulcers, yellow fluid disease, leprosy, carbuncles	*rlung* disease
Glauberite	colorless, odorless, with glauberite pebbles around	purple *badkan* disease in the abdomen, toxicity, old fevers	
Alum	greenish-blue water, turbid, a metallic odor, with metallic stones around	tuberculosis, hardened lymph nodes, urinary stones, sores and carbuncles, abdominal masses, chronic stomach disease, iron-filth phlegm	
Stone essence	purple water, bitter, with a fragrant smell, with stone essence crystals around	purple *badkan* in the abdomen, rheumatic arthritis, difficult urination, gout	
Limestone	clear and bitter water, with a scorched smell, with limestone around	deficiency cold of the stomach, poor digestion, cold-type lumps	

Main minerals in traditional springs

The main minerals contained in the solutions of the five traditional springs are sulfur, alum, glauberite, limestone, and stone essence. In addition, there are also coal and realgar in many springs.

Stone essence (Tibetan: *Brag zhun*)

Experts still debate as to what exactly stone essence is. Some claim that it is squirrel excrement while others insist it is pine resin. The *Records of Tibetan Materia Medica* say that stone essence is a kind of blackish-brown liquid excreted with the feces of a squirrel after it eats juicy food mixed with some loose stones. The substance is stone-like with a fragrant smell.

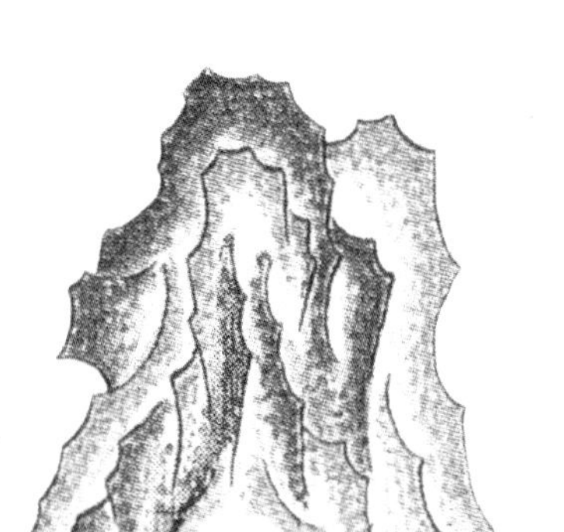

Gold stone essence

This is the feces of a species of flying squirrel found in Tibet, Qinghai, Gansu, and Sichuan provinces and is mostly found at the mouth of its cave. The material is sieved, and the sand and other waste are discarded. It is then dried in the sun for use. The animal inhabits caves in mountain cliffs. Stone essence is combined with other medicinals in formulas to treat various diseases. For instance, it is used with saffron to treat inflammation of the eyes or edema, glauberite to treat *badkan mugpo*, and nutmeg for stomach problems.

Other authorities hold that stone essence is formed by the six spirits (gold, silver, copper, iron, tin, lead) that run out from rocks facing the sun in the mountains during hot summer. What it actually is remains to be investigated.

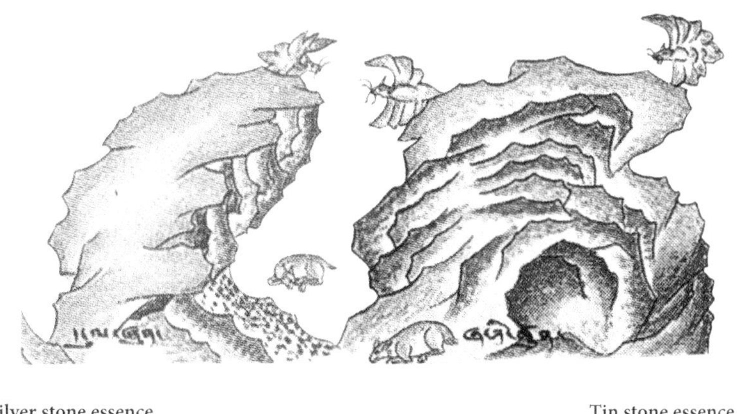

Silver stone essence

Tin stone essence

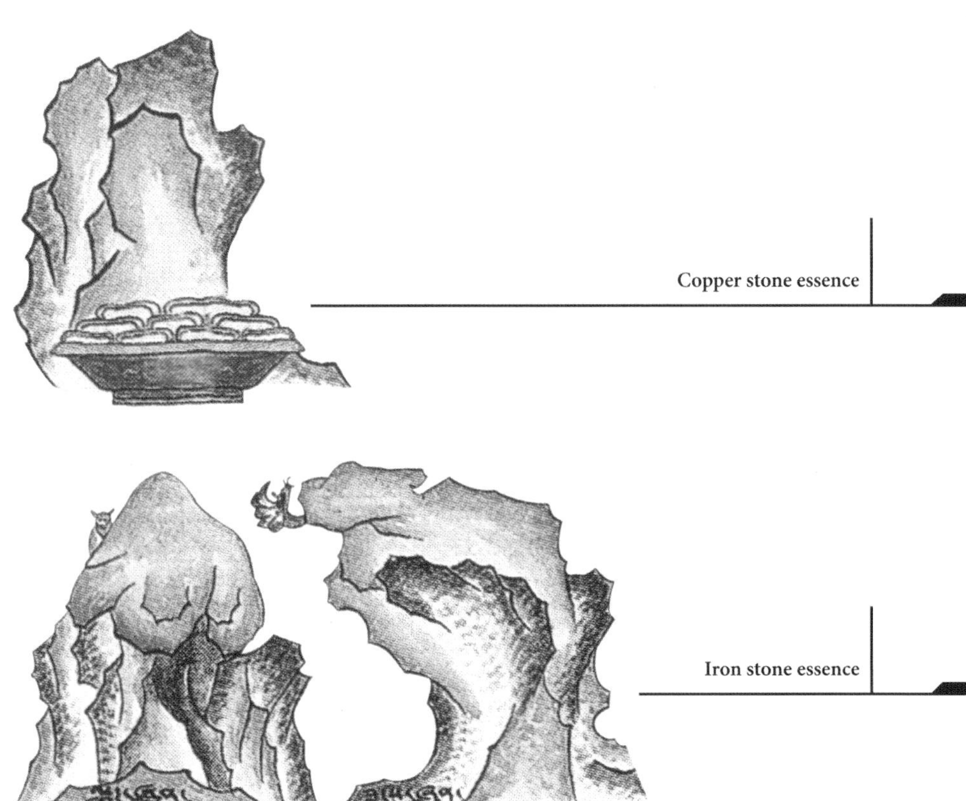

Copper stone essence

Iron stone essence

Glauberite (Tibetan: *Cong zhi*)

These are the natural crystals of sulfur ore. After being mined, the impurities are removed and it is ground to a fine powder. It is found in Tibet, Shanxi, and Qinghai. In formulas it treats abdominal distension and diarrhea when combined with Tibetan saussurea, and stomach ulcers when combined with rhubarb. Glauberite, after being scorched, can be ground as powder and applied topically for burns.

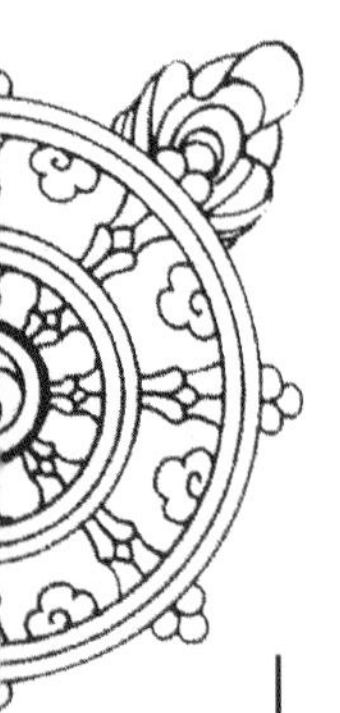

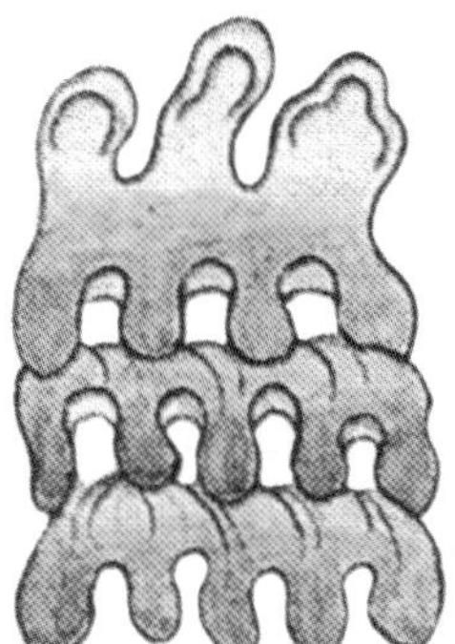

Female glauberite

Neutral glauberite

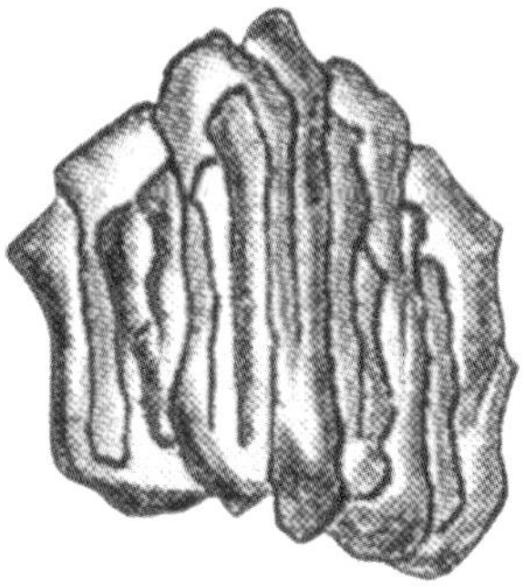

Male glauberite

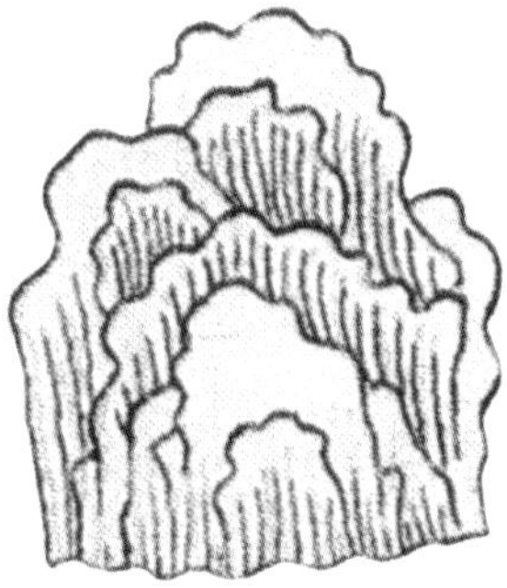

Son glauberite

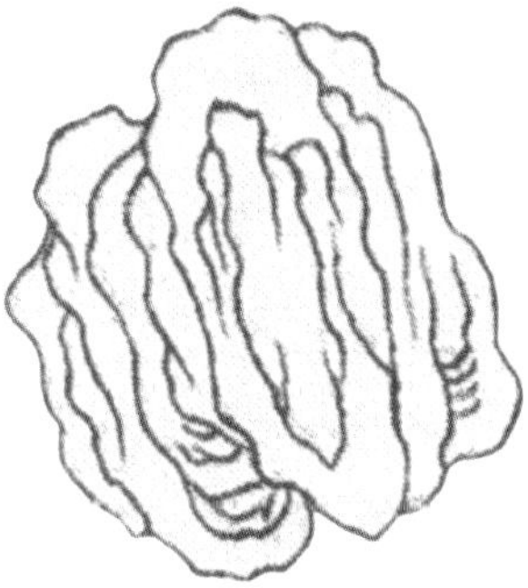

Daughter glauberite

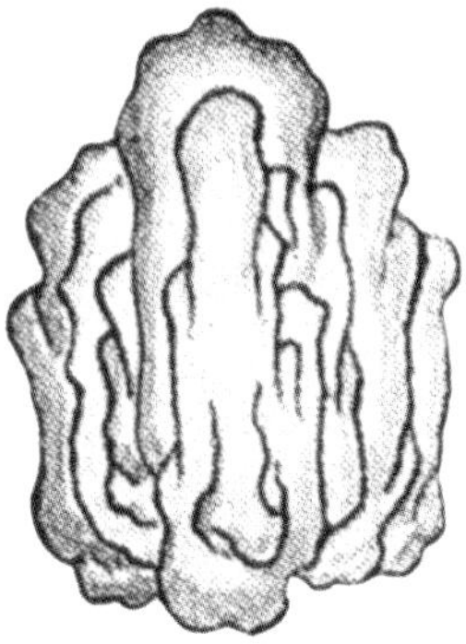

Sulfur (Tibetan: *Mu zi ser po*)

This is the natural sulfur element, commonly found in the crust of the earth. After being mined, it is heated to remove impurities or processed with sulfate salt. It is found in Tibet, Qinghai, Sichuan, Shandong, Yunnan, and Taiwan. When combined with long pepper in formulas it treats yellow fluid disease, and with frankincense it is good for skin blisters, leprosy, poisoning, and heat in the body.

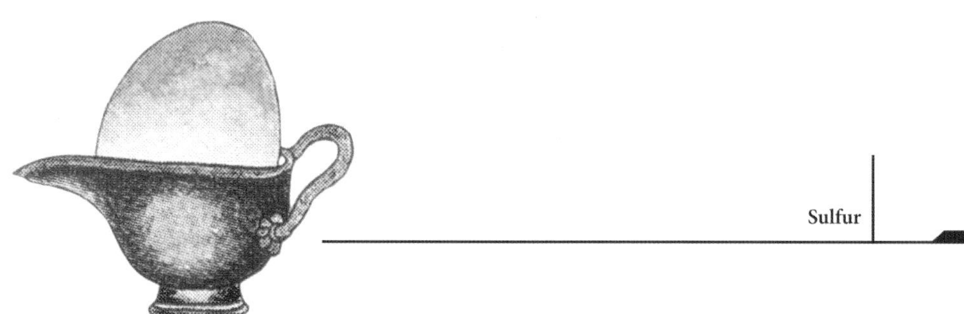

Sulfur

Realgar (Tibetan: *Ldong ros*)

This is the mineral collected from sulfide ore. Realgar is obtained after the impurities are removed. It is mostly produced in Tibet, Qinghai, Xinjiang, Yunnan, Sichuan, Hunan, and Hubei. It is mostly seen where magma from a volcano has flowed, or near hot springs, often together with orpiment. When combined with musk and areca in formulas it treats swollen gums, ulcers, and skin erosions, with chebulae it treats swollen tongue and diphtheria, with turmeric it is effective for traumas of the neck, and with the dregs from making wine for baldness and hair loss.

Alum (Tibetan: *Da tshur*)

These are the natural alum crystals extracted from minerals. It is a sulfate compound, and is mostly found in Tibet, Qinghai, Gansu, and Shanxi provinces. It is mostly formed from eroded acidic magma of volcanoes. It can be used alone to rinse the mouth to remove foul odors. It can also used together with verdigris to rub the tongue to treat erosion of the tongue. When combined with mercury, borax, sulfur and cinnabar it is used for treating syphilis.

Limestone (Tibetan: *Cu gang*)

This is the crystal of a carbonate mineral, mostly seen in limestone caves or in deposits beside springs and rivers. It is found in Tibet, Qinghai, Gansu, and Yunnan. When combined with saffron and stone essence it is effective for exuberant heat diseases, edema, and lassitude, with licorice and iron for heat in the lung and liver, and with saffron for intestinal inflammation and diarrhea.

Coal (Tibetan: *Do sol*)

Found in layered deposits in the earth, it is found in widely throughout the world. After being mined, it is washed and the impurities are removed. For medicinal bathing, the water used is often filtered by coal before being used. It is mostly used to treat nosebleed or if bad food is eaten.

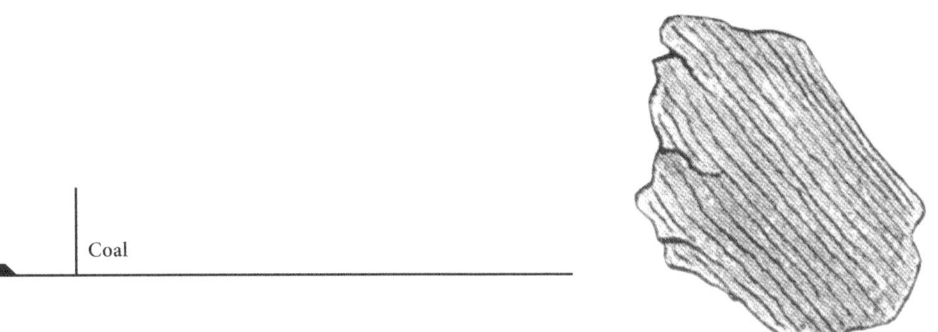
Coal

Main characteristics and effects

Naturally, each individual spring will always contain multiple minerals, enhancing its action. Based on the amount of the most predominant minerals, natural springs are divided into single springs, double springs, triple springs, quadruple springs, and so on. All types of springs can relax the tendons, facilitate the joints, expel wind, remove dampness, moisten the skin and muscles, encourage urination, disperse swellings, dry dampness, and expel pus.

To take advantage of the functions of each spring, all factors must be taken into consideration, including the individual's condition and the season. When a person is ill, an appropriate spring is selected according to his physical constitution and disease. The minerals must be suitable, so that the bathing is beneficial, or there may be harm. Natural springs are always changing their ingredients. Springs are usually more therapeutic during dry seasons than during the rainy season. In Tibet, late winter, spring, summer, and autumn are the best times. Boiling springs are best when the steam ascends. The end of autumn or spring is the best time and yields the best therapeutic effects.

Modern scientific research reveals that the therapeutic effects of natural spring bathing influence many systems. This includes regulation of nervous function, protein metabolism, the metabolism of water and ions, the immune system and histamine levels.

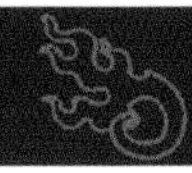

Man-made Medicinal Baths

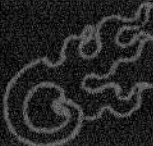

According to tradition, by imitating the treatment principles of treating disease in natural springs, early Tibetan doctors developed man-made medicinal baths that are based on knowledge of medicinal substances. Eventually, the basic recipe for *Five Flavor Sweet Dew Decoction* was formulated.

The ingredients of *Five Flavor Sweet Dew Decoction*

Being the basic recipe for medicinal baths, *Five Flavor Sweet Dew Decoction* with modifications constitutes all bath recipes. As recorded in *The Four Medical Tantras*, it is composed of savin, Tibetan ephedra, sweet wormwood, rhododendron, and myricaria. Their actions for the ingredients are as follows: savin is indicated for kidney disease; rhododendron for disturbing phlegm pathogens; myricaria for clearing internal toxins; ephedra for clearing heat in the liver and spleen; and sweet wormwood for clearing and dispersing swelling of the extremities. The decoction's combined action is to expel phlegm, remove damp, clear heat, resolve toxins, activate blood circulation, eliminate stasis, and benefit the kidney to strengthen the lower back.

Yin sweet dew – Tibetan ephedra

The above-ground parts of Tibetan ephedra are used. It is mainly found in Tibet and the south slopes of the Himalaya Mountains, from 3,300-4,600 m (10,800-15,000 ft.) above sea level. When combined with dandelion it is used for heat *mkhris pa* disorders like liver heat, spleen heat, new or old heat diseases, bleeding, and depression. More specifically, when used with dandelion it treats lung abscess, coughing and coughing of blood due to lung heat, and with saffron and notopterigium it helps stop bleeding due to wounds.

When used in medicinal baths, its action is to clear liver heat, relieve the surface and penetrate blockages. There are four kinds of ephedra used in Tibetan medicine, namely those grown on cliffs, on slopes, in the hills, and in water. The kind grown on cliffs is the type mostly used in medicinal baths.

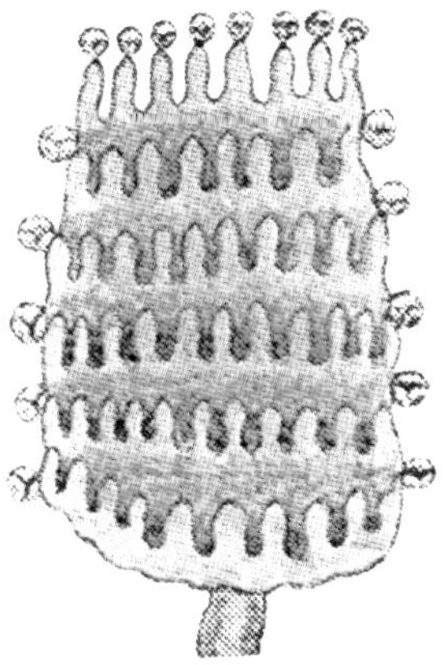

Tibetan ephedra

Yang sweet dew - savin

This includes several kinds of plants of the family Cupressaceae, such as *Sabina tibeticum*, *Sabina wallichiana*, *Sabina saltuaria* and *Sabina przewalskii*. The branches and leaves are mostly used, though sometimes the fruit is. It is mostly found in high mountains of western China. When combined with rhododendron and asteris, it is used to treat kidney disease, anthrax, ulcers, and abscesses. Its fresh specimen can be used topically. Its fruits can be used to treat heat of the liver and gallbladder and joint pain.

Earth sweet dew - sweet wormwood

The entire sweet wormwood plant of the family Compositae is used. It is found throughout Tibet and rest of China. It is mostly used alone when fresh to treat malaria, or used with other medicinals for malaria, summer-heat (summertime flu), or to quench deficient fevers. Folk recipes use it to effectively keep mosquitoes away.

When used in *Five Flavor Sweet Dew Decoction*, it is used to remove swellings of the extremities.

There is still debate as to exactly what kind of herb should be used in the decoction. In early times, Artemisia annua was mostly used. Later, other species were also used. Even though it is not known what exact species is the genuine one used the formula, all species in common use yield a satisfactory therapeutic effect.

Water sweet dew - Myricaria

The flowers, leaves or tender branches are used. This plant is found in the western part of Tibet, growing in valleys along rivers. It is mostly used in diseases that involve toxic heat, blood fevers, yellow fluid diseases, and epidemics. When boiled alone, it is used to treat toxic heat and poisoning. When combined with drynaria and other medicinals in *Myricaria Decoction with Fifteen Ingredients*, it can treat all kinds of heat disorders caused by toxins. With sabina, asteris, and other ingredients it forms *Myricaria Decoction with Six Ingredients* to treat fever, headache, bitter taste in the mouth, joint pain, and epidemic diseases.

There are also other species of myricaria that are available and can be used, but they are seldom applied in practice.

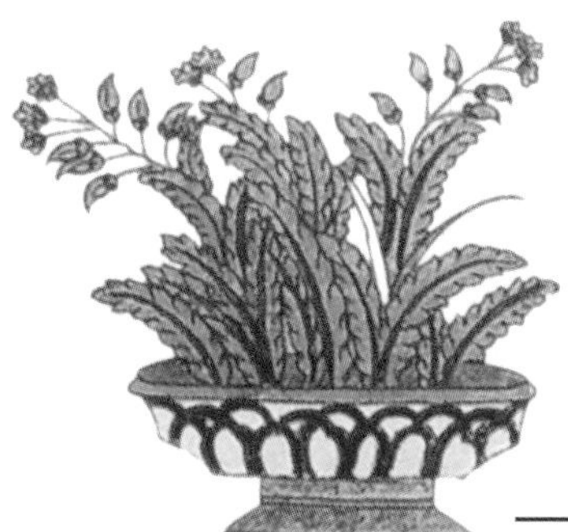

Myricaria

Grass sweet dew - Rhododendron

There are over twenty species of rhododendron used in Tibetan medicine, but only *Dali rhododendron* is used in grass sweet dew. The white type treats all lung diseases, while the black type is primarily for removing cold disease. In practice, the white one most commonly used. More specifically, the leaves of the yellow flowered rhododendron are the preferred ingredient in grass sweet dew. Although the leaves are most commonly used for medicine, sometimes the flowers are also used.

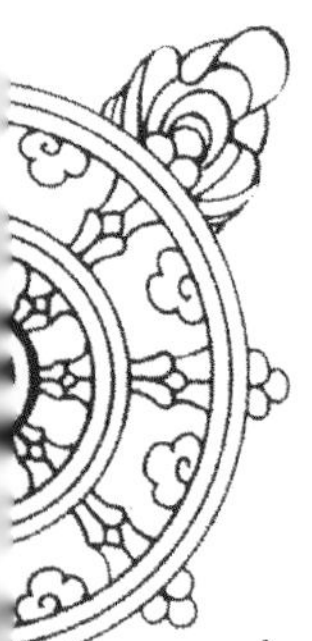

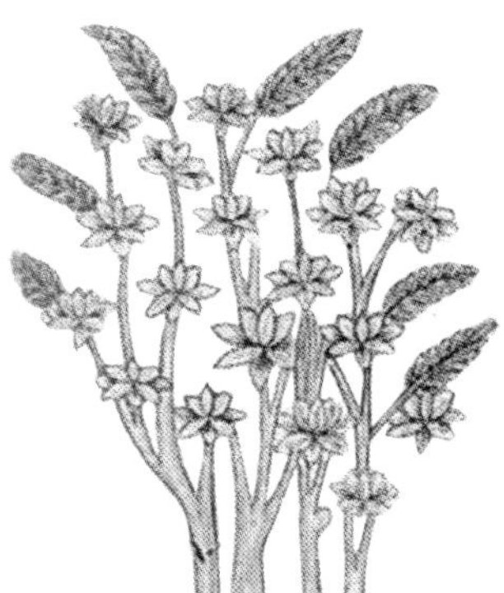

Rhododendron

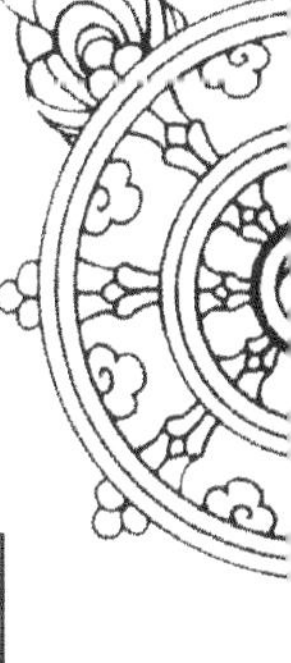

Both white and black rhododendron are found in Tibet, Qinghai, Sichuan, Yunnan, and Gansu, and grow at 3,000-4,200 m (9,800-13,700 ft.) above sea level, on shady slopes and inside bush. Its leaves are used for stomach cold, loss of appetite, coughing, and skin problems. Together with cinnamon, nutmeg, pepper, or dried ginger it treats diarrhea, vomiting, loss of appetite, stomach pain, and other digestive issues. When combined with turmeric and dandelion root it treats lumps in the stomach or intestine, and with saussurea and glauberite it treats hepatitis, inflammation of the stomach and intestines, and other digestive diseases. Patients with skin diseases can bathe in *Five Flavor Sweet Dew Decoction* directly.

Rhododendron flowers are used in cases of edema, emphysema, bronchitis, poor digestion, hoarse voice, and difficulty acclimatizing to a new environment. When combined with pomegranate seeds, saffron, long pepper, clove, and cinnamon it treats abdominal pain and distention, poor digestion, edema, dizziness, coughing, hoarse voice, and difficulty acclimatizing to a new environment. Together with sal amoniac and the three pungent medicines it is used for kidney disease and inability to urinate. It can also be used to help eliminate phlegm.

Some standard modifications of *Five Flavor Sweet Dew Decoction* include yin sweet dew, yang sweet dew, earth sweet dew, grass sweet dew and water sweet dew. Further modifications are made according to the disease and the individual.

Preparation of the decoction

There is no standardized process for the preparation of the solutions used in Tibetan medicinal bathing. The process depends on the medicinals used and the disorder that is being treated. Different doctors might also have their own process based on experience.

Ingredients

There are two main versions of *Five Flavor Sweet Dew Decoction*. One is based on The *Four Medical Tantras*, where all ingredients in the formula are in equal amount. The second one varies the ingredients based on the treatment focus in a proportion of 1:1:2:2:3. However, in practice both methods are not adhered to strictly, but are applied in a flexible way. Whatever the practitioner's methods, the amount of ingredients used should be sufficiently large to achieve a satisfactory effect.

Commonly, all ingredients are crushed and then immersed in boiling water so that the medicinals are completely covered and then left to stand overnight. The next morning, cool water is added and to the medicinals and stirred thoroughly. Simmer until all the medicinals have absorbed all of the water and are swollen and soft.

Fermentation

When the solution cools down to around body temperature, add yeast or the dregs from wine. Put it into a container and seal it tightly. Let the container stay at room temperature for three days. When the solution starts to smell like wine, with a medicinal or sour odor, it is ready. This is the most important part of the process for preparing the medicinal bath, and if it is not done properly the solution will not be effective.

If the fermenting process can not be done properly, or there is not enough time, a simpler method is available. The crushed ingredients should be wrapped in cheesecloth and soaked in water, then boiled for thirty minutes. After the solution cools down, add 500-1,500 ml (1/2 to 1 1/2 quarts) of concentrated alcohol, and add to a hot bath.

Cooking

Next, add water to completely cover the fermented material, and let it stand for one day. Strain the solution and save the liquid. Repeat this process three times, and mix the three portions of liquid together. At this point, musk and other rare drugs like saffron can be added. This liquid should be boiled to further extract medicinal properties from the ingredients. The cooking time should be three hours in spring, one hour in autumn, and the decoction is generally not prepared in summer and winter.

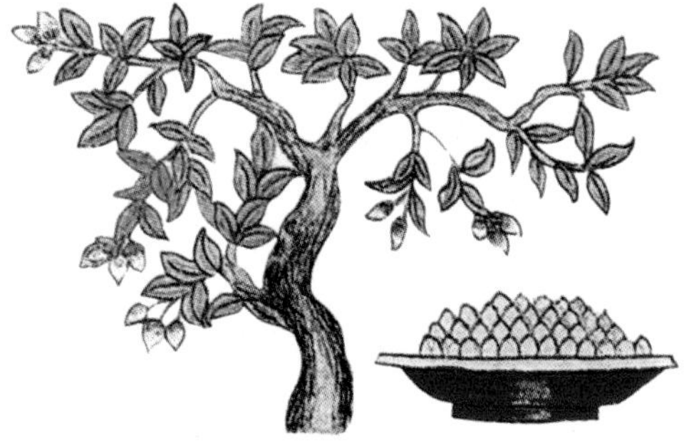

Chebule

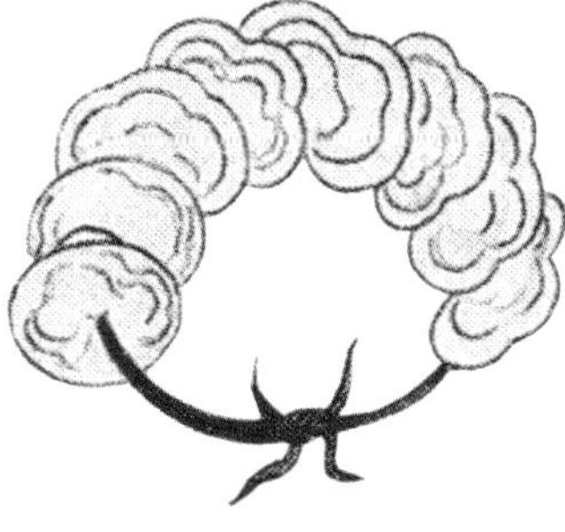

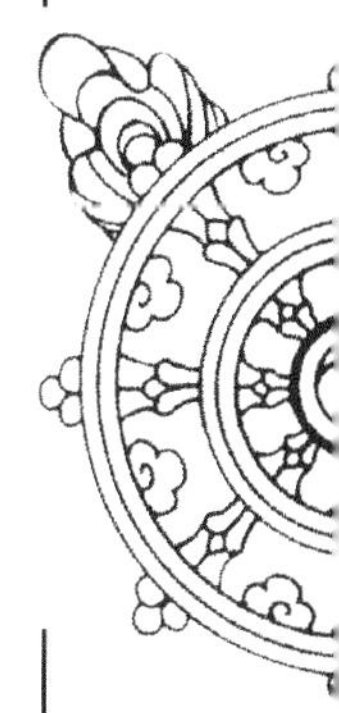

Distiller's yeast

Addition of modifications

Modifications are very extensive and include almost all non-toxic medicinal substances. Commonly used medicinals for modification are frankincense, puncture vine, the dung of a musk deer, natural alkaline, highland barley, long pepper, acorus, pearl, and iron powder. For medicinal steam baths, the recipes and preparation are basically the same, only the application method is different.

Ingredients used in medicinal baths also generally have the following features:

A dosage of around 500 g (1 lb.). Because this is an external therapy, and the formula will be diluted with water, the dosage of the ingredients should be large enough to be effective.

The ingredients are cooked after fermentation to extract to the full extent the active ingredients and to strengthen the formula's actions of relaxing the tendons and activating the vessels.

Most times it is necessary to modify basic formulas. It is essential that those making the formula have a basic knowledge of Tibetan medicinals and their natures so they can be used flexibly.

As the most important part of the preparation of the medicinal bathing solution, fermentation is closely linked to the therapeutic effect. Therefore, it is crucial that the time and temperature during fermentation should be carefully controlled.

Rare and important substances should be added at the proper time.

Do not add cool water into the prepared decoction.

Important points

Bathing with medicinal solutions

There are two basic kinds of baths, local part(s) and the whole body.

Local bathing: soak the affected body part in the medicated solution for half an hour, twice daily, 7-10 days as a therapeutic course. This is primarily for local injury and is quite effective.

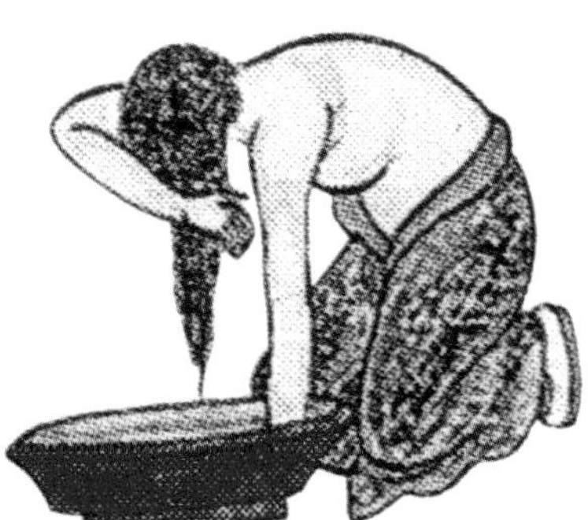

Washing the hair

Whole body bathing: lying calmly in a bath tub, the whole body up to the chest is immersed in the water. Gently move any affected body parts, or rub tender parts. Generally, ten days in succession constitute a therapeutic course, with one bath in the morning and another in the afternoon being best. The temperature and duration of the bath varies. For instance, on the first day, the temperature should be 38-40°C (100-104°F) for 20-30 minutes. Both temperature and duration can be gradually increased until 46°C (115°F) and 40-60 minutes are reached, and then the temperature can be decreased gradually until 38°C (100°F) is reached. Compress of cool towels on the forehead or head are usually necessary because of sweating and hot sensations. After bathing, have a good rest and drink plenty of water.

Through extended immersion in the bathing solution, the affected areas are well treated. Heat is cleared, toxins expelled, wind eliminated, dampness drained, parasites killed, itching stopped, and the skin will become soft and healthy in places where it was hard or injured.

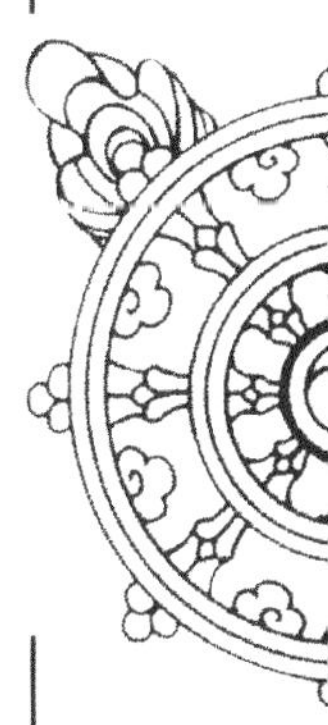

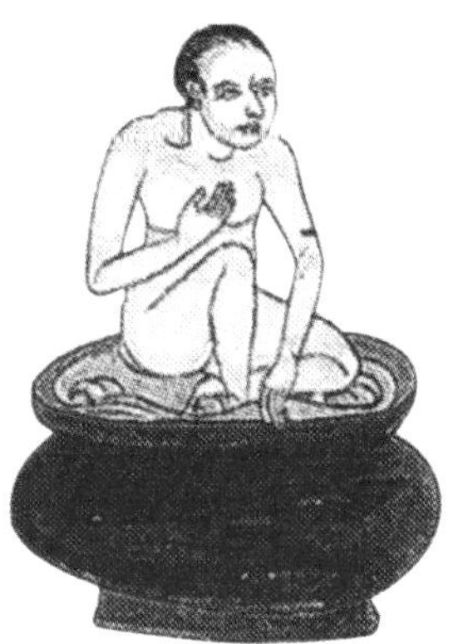

Man-made medicinal baths: another style of medicinal bathing.

- Before bathing, one should be examined by a professional, and be ready in both body and mind. In some cases bathing may be prohibited.
- The water level should be below the chest so as to avoid pressure on the heart and prevent difficult breathing.
- Bathing should not be done on an empty or full stomach, after drinking alcohol or vigorous exercise.
- The temperature and duration of medicinal bathing should be changed gradually over the treatment course, and varied with each individual. Do not bathe several times a day or go through too many successive courses.
- Pay attention to any discomfort while bathing.
- Drink plenty of water after bathing, normally beginning half an hour after bathing. Rest well, and have some nutritious food. Do not smoke, drink alcohol, or take other medication.

Medicinal steam baths

Add water to the ingredients of *Five Flavor Sweet Dew Decoction*, and boil it in a large pot that is covered with a porous wood cover. A blanket should be placed on the cover of the kettle on which the patient can lie down on. Cover the patient and the kettle with another large blanket to prevent the leaking of steam.

Closed steaming: boil the ingredients in a closed closet to make a steam room. The patient should lie or sit naked or wearing only underwear. The temperature in the room gradually increases to 40-45°C (104-113°F) and the steam bath should last for 15-30 minutes. After bathing, rest and do not wash the body. Take a steam bath once everyday or every other day, with 5-10 sessions as a treatment course.

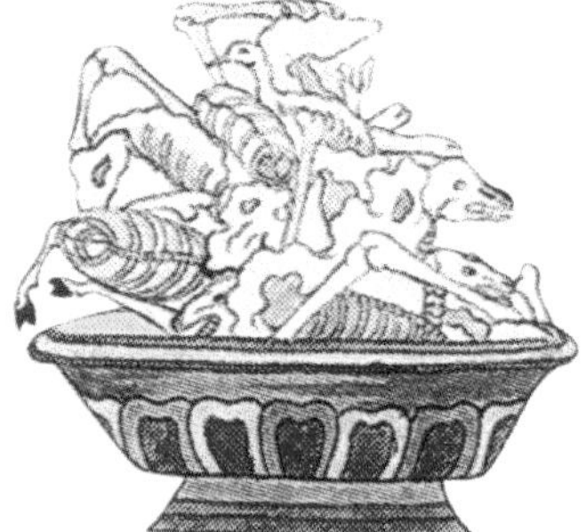

Old bones

Simple and easy steaming: pour the boiled decoction into a large container and cover with a wooden board. The patient should sit naked on the board. Cover the whole body except the head with a blanket. Steam the body.

There is another style of bathing called old-bone bathing. This involves the placement of old animal bones in a pot and boiling them in water. Bathe in the water or make a steam bath. This is good for *rlung* disease.

Local steaming: pour the boiled decoction into a container with a small opening, and hold the affected part over the opening of the container, being careful not to burn the skin. A towel can be put over the container and the body part that is being steamed so that the steam does not escape.

By allowing the steam to penetrate the body's pores, nostrils and mouth, systemic disorders can be relieved.

- An observation window should be installed in the closet, so that the conditions can be monitored, and aid given if necessary. Make the closet air-tight so that wind does not blow through the closet and cause the person to catch cold.
- When steaming a local body part, the distance between the container and the affected part can be adjusted according to the temperature of the steam, so that the patient feels comfortable, and does not get burned.
- Contraindications of steaming therapy include cancer, epilepsy, acute inflammation, cardiac dysfunction, chronic cor pulmonale, and feverish patients with a tendency to bleed.

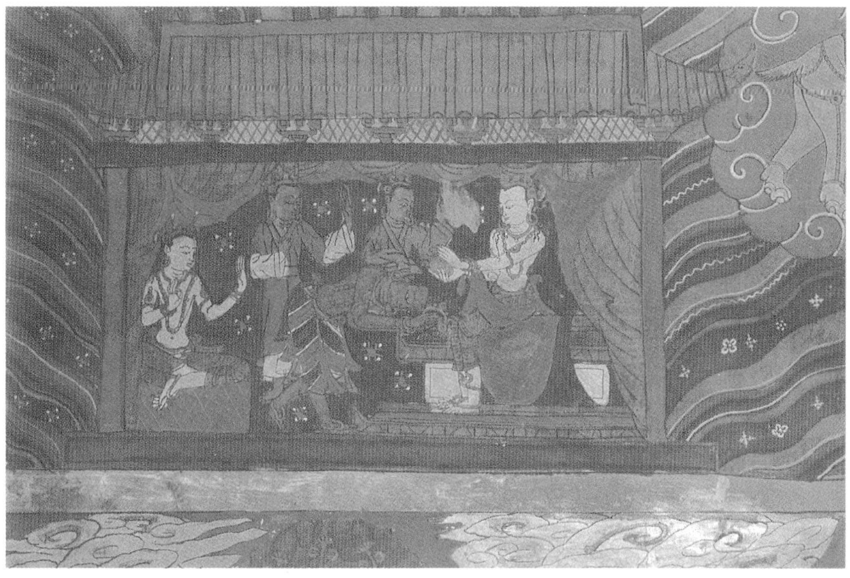

A Tibetan mural showing an adult Buddha washing hair (Tibetan mural).

Binding baths

Also called compress bathing. This is an approach in which the medicinals are mixed with water and wrapped with a thin cloth which is bound onto the affected part. It is simple and easy to apply. There are two kinds, binding baths to clear heat and binding baths to remove cold. To clear heat, the medicinals are ground to powder and then mixed with sesame oil or old vegetable oil (fresh flowers can also be used). Wrap the paste with cloth and then bind it at the affected body part. To remove cold, animal dung such as rat dung or pigeon dung is used. Bone fragments boiled in wine can also be used as a substitute. It is used on local injuries.

There are two further divisions for clearing heat:

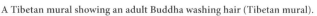

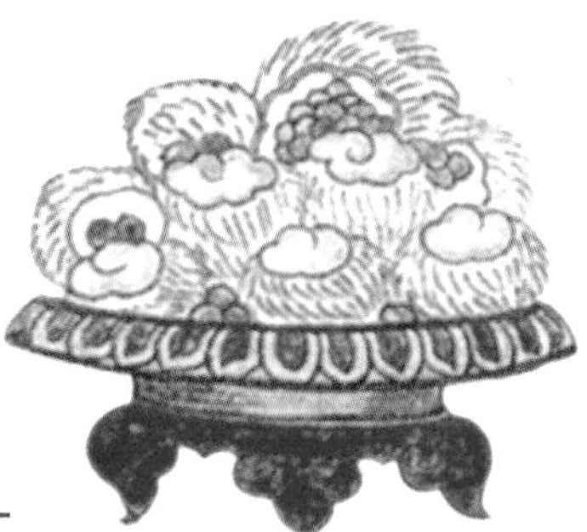
Musk

Ointment: Grind the ingredients into a fine powder and then mix it with sesame or old vegetable oil to form a paste and place it in a cloth bag, and then bind it to the affected part. Avoid binding too tightly.

Water paste: Put all the ingredients in a pot, and add water to cover them completely. Cook with mild flame. Discard the dregs and keep the liquid. Soak gauze or cotton in the solution and then fix it to acupuncture points or affected body parts with adhesive tape.

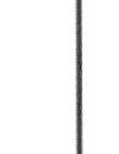

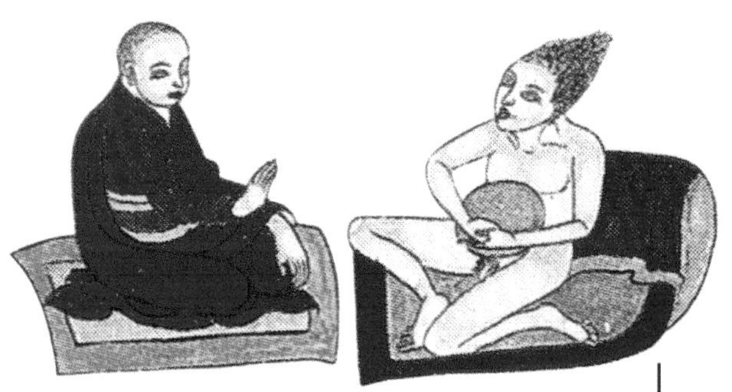

Local binding baths are a kind of man-made medicinal bath.

There are also two further divisions for removing cold:

Fry animal dung from a rat or pigeon together with assisting medicinals over a low fire. Add alcohol, and mix evenly. Wrap the result with cloth and fix it on the injured area. Another method is to crush animal bones and cook them in wine. After cooking, strain and save the liquid. Soak a cloth into the solution. Place the hot cloth on the injured area (a layer of lotion can be rubbed on the lesion first). Change the compress every 3-5 minutes. Compresses should be applied for 20-30 minutes.

- Use the correct form of binding bathing according to the disorder.
- Sanitize the injury or body part before bathing.
- Use the right temperature for compresses. Too high may cause a burn; while too low may be ineffective.
- For lesions of the sense organs, sanitization is essential. For open wounds or allergic patients, such compresses are prohibited. For pregnant women, musk is prohibited so as to prevent miscarriage. When adverse reactions like itching or exacerbation of symptoms occurs, the compress should be stopped right away.

Indications of Tibetan Medicinal Bathing

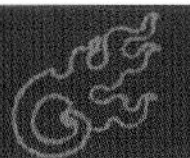

The Four Medical Tantras clearly explains indications for medicinal bathing. These indications have been substantially expanded since that time due to the accumulation of experience and discovery of useful new techniques.

Records from *The Four Medical Tantras*

In the *Conclusion Tantra*, its 23rd chapter records that stiffness or spasms of the limbs, inability to walk, skin sores, anthrax, old or new inflammation of sores, skin diseases, post-partum convulsions, hunchback, joint deformity, yellow fluid in the superficial layer, all sorts of *rlung* (wind) diseases, and especially rheumatic arthritis can be successfully relieved by medicinal baths. Contraindications include epidemic fevers, chaotic fevers, exuberant fevers, grayish edema, general weakness, loss of appetite, pregnancy, severe hypertension or heart disease, kidney disease, and active tuberculosis. Furthermore, injuries of the four filthy body parts (the two big toes and the elbows), the eyes, cheeks, testes, abdomen, and the area in front of the heart should not be bathed.

From a modern viewpoint, the above indications and contraindications are still valid. Epidemic fevers and chaotic fevers, for instance, should be treated by low temperature therapies. If the body experiences a sudden and significant change in temperature, the adaptive mechanisms of the body are mobilized and bodily substances that influence temperature such as catecholamine are secreted in larger amounts and in a shorter time than is normal. This is harmful to the body, and causes the blood pressure to elevate. It is for this reason medicinal bathing is not appropriate for weak patients. For pregnant women, the medicinal solution is able to enter her body and may affect the fetus through the placenta. For those with heart and kidney disease, sudden temperature rises may place a burden on these organs leading to increased risks of complications. Also, skin that is soft and tender is vulnerable to injury and burns. Conversely, for chronic diseases and mild disorders, medicinal bathing will not cause complications, and is thus indicated as a therapeutic method.

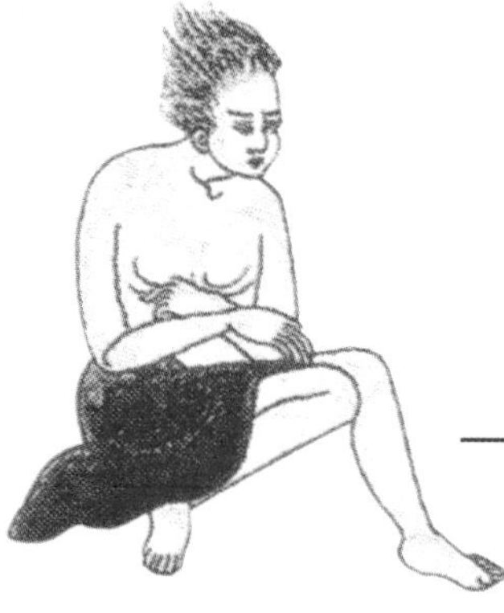

Spasm of the limbs

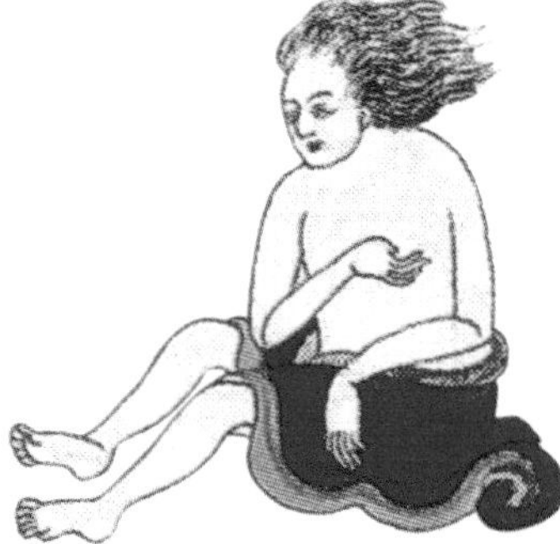

Stiffness of the limbs

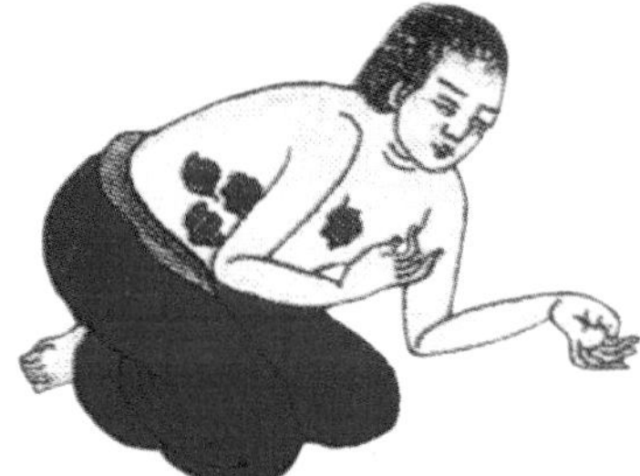

Anthrax

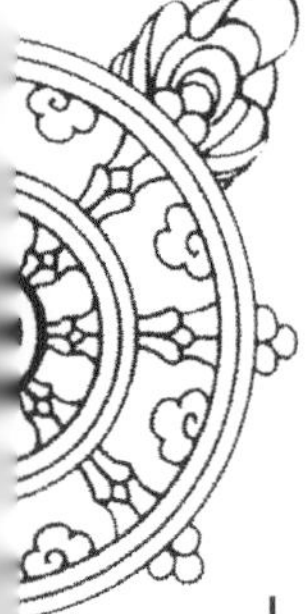

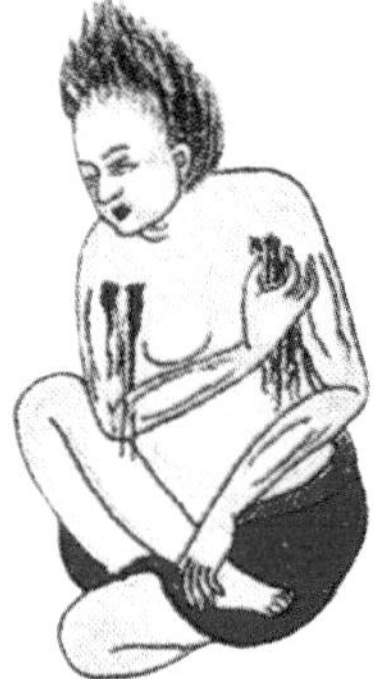

Vessel diseases

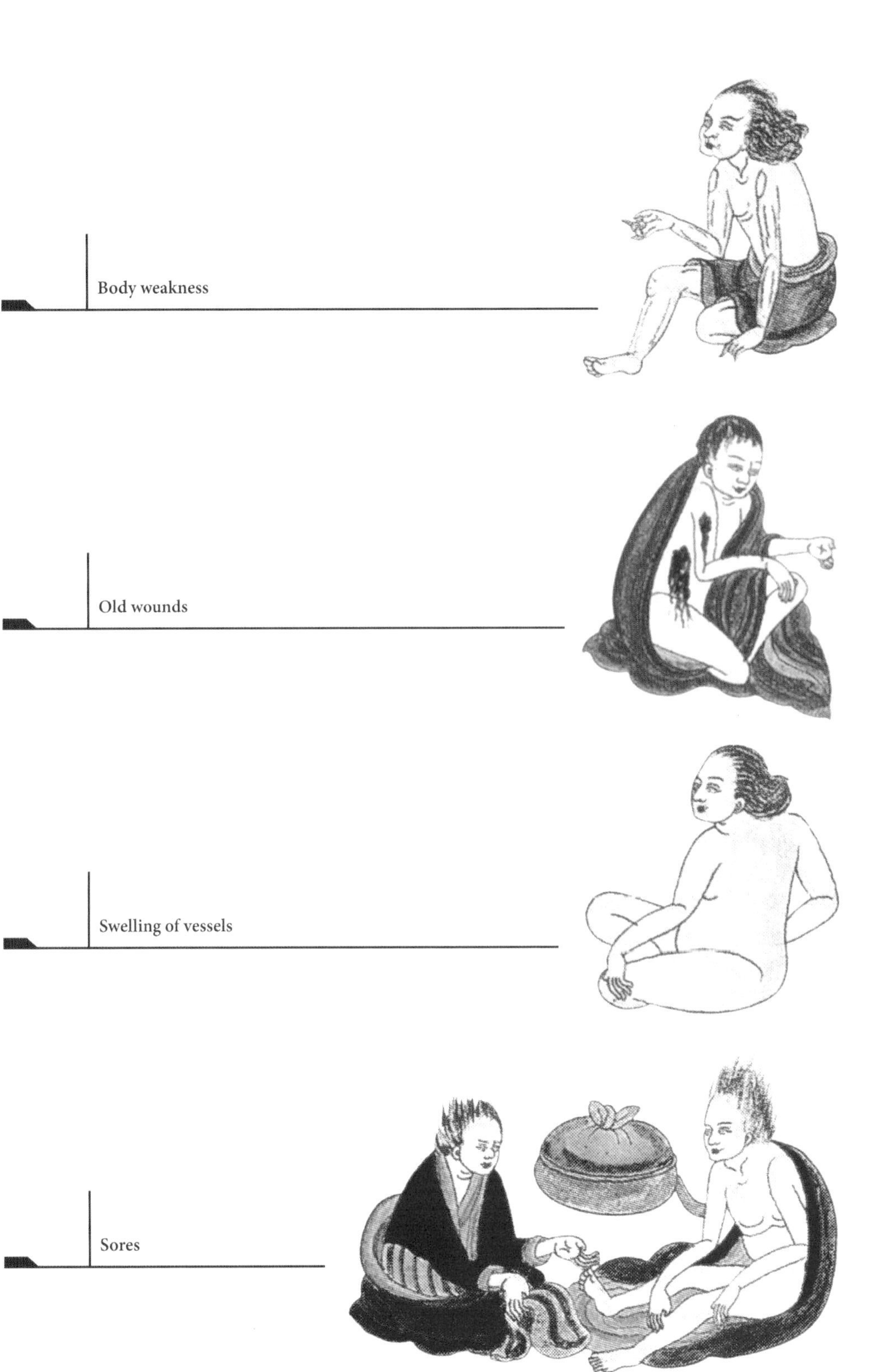
Body weakness
Old wounds
Swelling of vessels
Sores

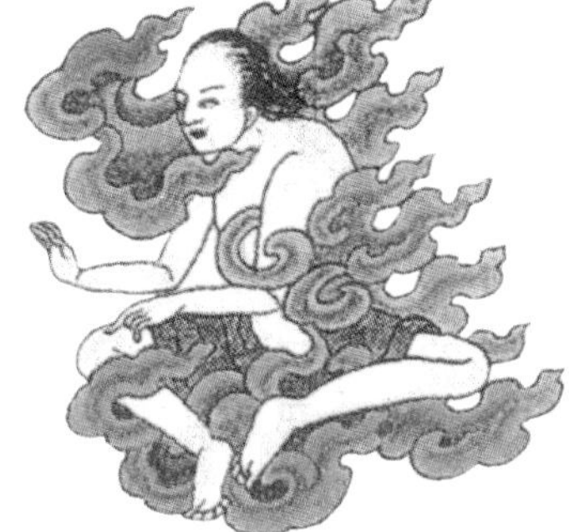

Gynecological inflammation

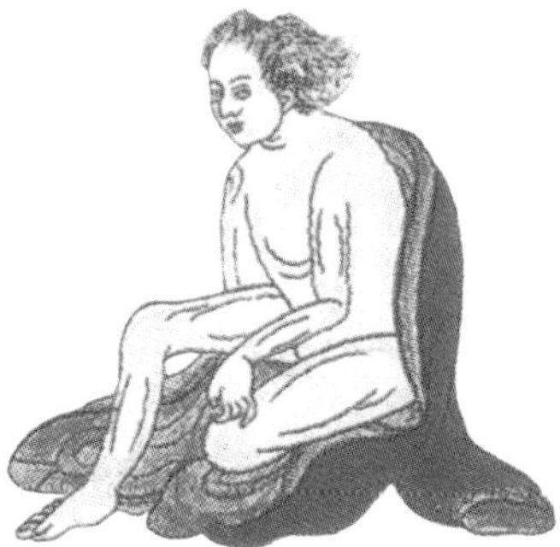

Chaotic fever

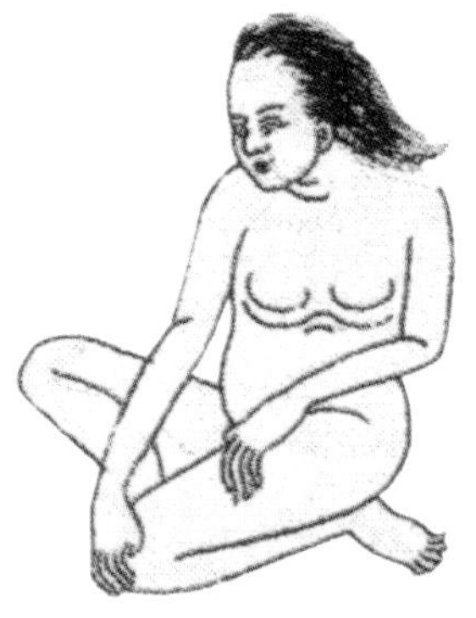

Inability to walk

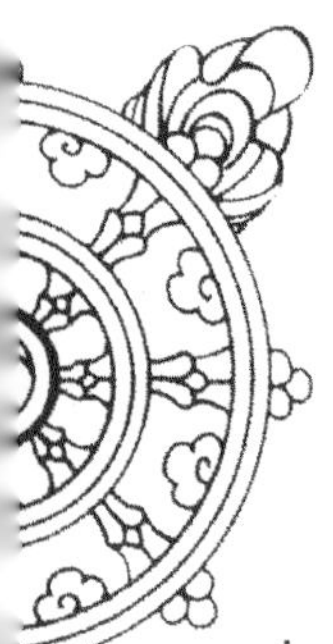

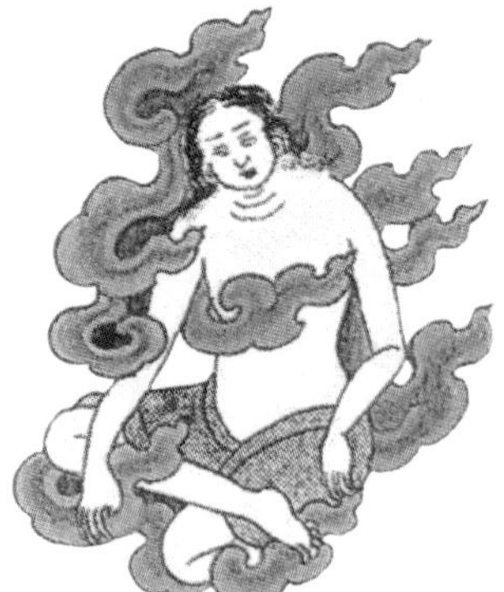

All *rlung* diseases

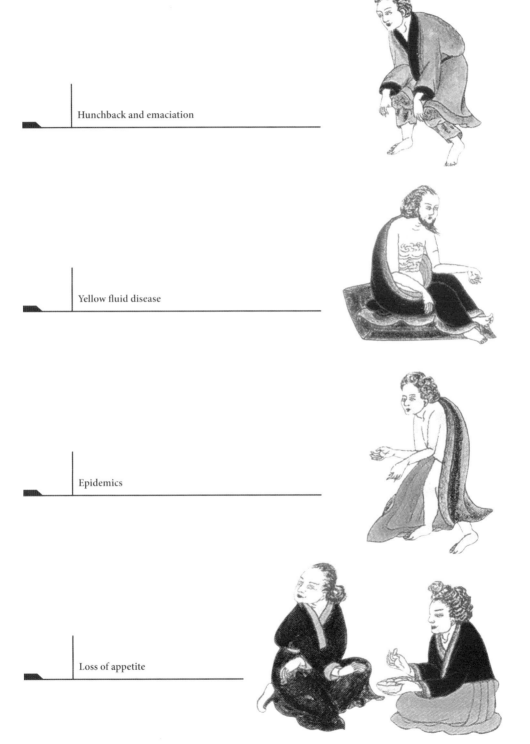

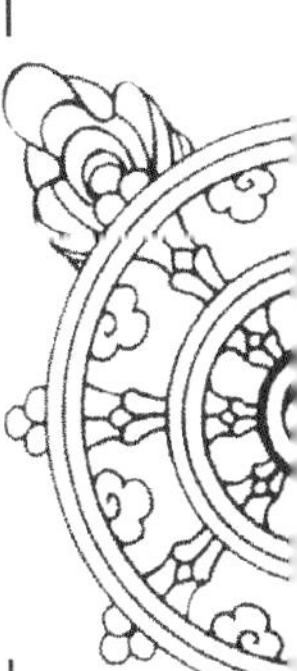

Hunchback and emaciation

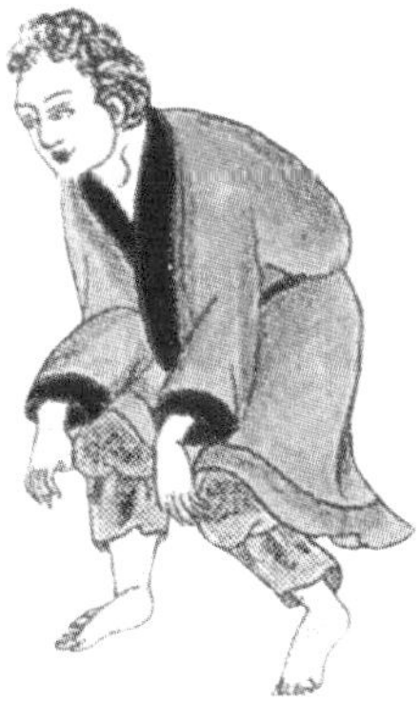

Yellow fluid disease

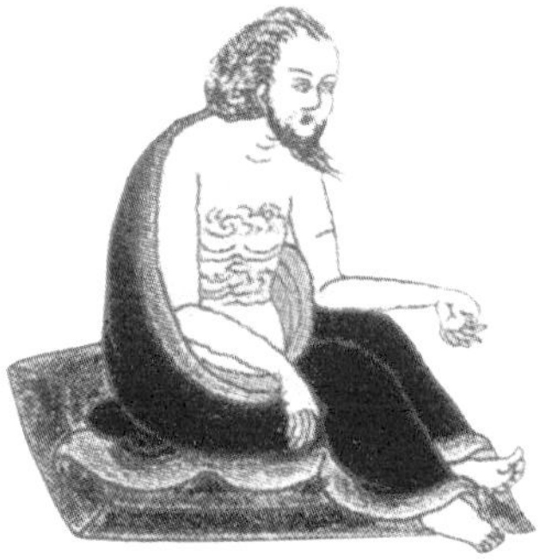

Epidemics

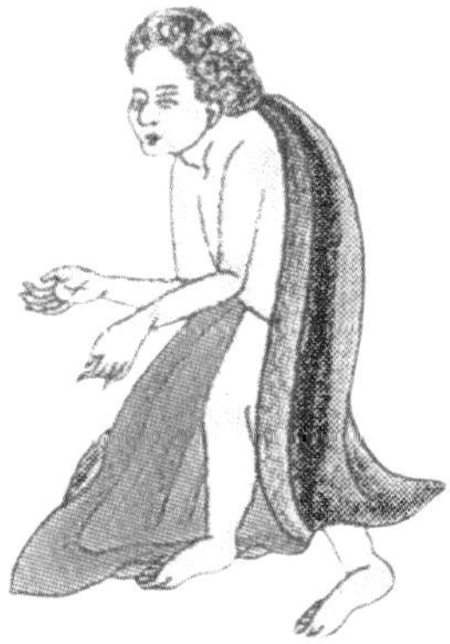

Loss of appetite

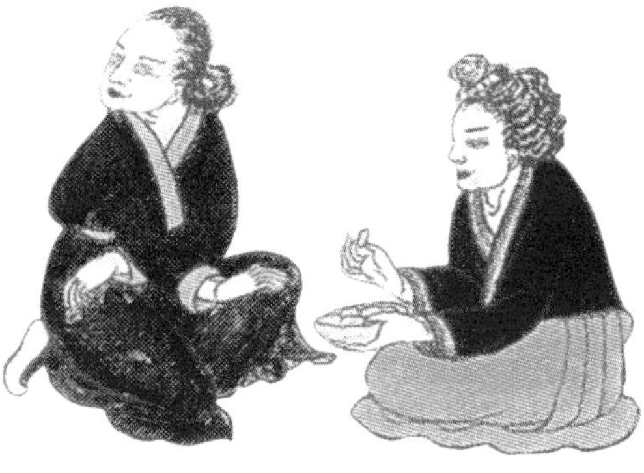

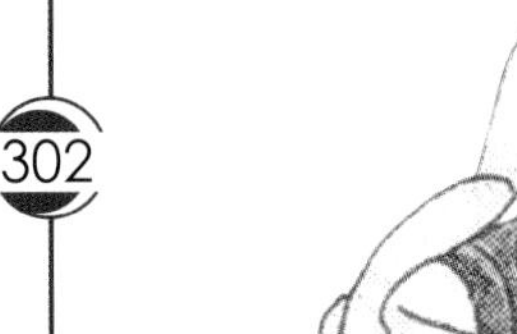

Edema

High fever

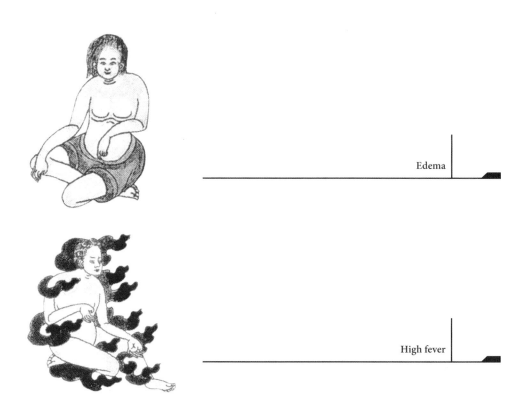

Range of indications

It is estimated that the number of diseases suitable for treatment with Tibetan medicinal bathing is over one hundred. Among them, there is one geriatric disease, one involving fertility, nineteen toxicity diseases, eight traumatic disorders, four gynecological diseases, five pediatric diseases, two types of possession by evil spirits, and seventy systemic diseases. Clinically, medicinal bathing is popular for rheumatic arthritis, recovery from strokes, skin disorders, protrusion of spinal discs, bone growths, and many female and children's diseases.

Satisfactory results are now able to be obtained in the treatment of many diseases that were contraindicated in ancient texts due to the involvement of multiple therapeutic methods. This is also mentioned in *The Four Medical Tantras* in which the following therapies are recommended: medicinals taken orally, topical therapy, moxibustion, bloodletting, rubbing therapies, acupuncture and oil therapy. Over the centuries, many new measures have been used in combination with the above, such as the improvement of bathing facilities, modification of formulas, and modern monitoring facilities that insure the safety of bathing. The combined use of modern technology, biomedicine, and many numerous traditional modalities has improved the methods and range of Tibetan medicinal baths.

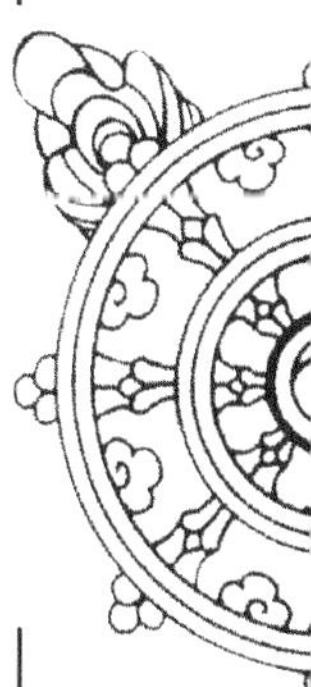

The following conditions are contraindicated for medicinal bathing:

Severe heart disease or impaired heart function

Tendency to bleeding

Physical wasting with loss of weight and muscle

Acute and chronic hepatitis or other infectious diseases

Intermediate or late stages of liver cirrhosis or functional liver problems

Critical and non-stable stages of stroke

Epilepsy and psychosis

Patients of high fever or a tendency to septicemia

Active tuberculosis

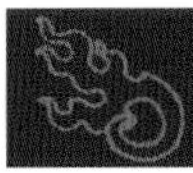

The Procedure of Tibetan Medicinal Bathing

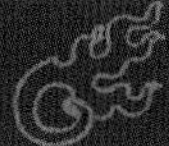

Unlike common bathing, Tibetan medicinal bathing is a special technique with a complete and strict process, which is described here.

Making a plan based on the conditions present

Differences in diseases

The condition of the patient should be first made clear, including the differentiation of internal and external illnesses, the location of disease in the upper or lower body, and hot and cold disease. Generally speaking, for diseases due to external pathogens, the temperature of the bath water can be higher, while for internal diseases a moderately warm temperature is sufficient. For disorders located in the upper part of the body, showers and washing of the head and face are important, for problems in the middle part of the body the patient should lie or sit in a bathtub, and for those in the lower part, foot washing and steaming can be employed. Severe cases should be steamed in order to expel the pathogen out of the body, or bathing of the whole body can be used. For weak patients, local bathing is better, such as steaming of the liver region for liver disease, or washing the abdomen for stomach disease. The ingredients used are varied on the basis of *Five Flavor Sweet Dew Decoction* according to different diseases. The locations for bathing are also varied based on what parts are diseased, such as washing the eyes for eye diseases, and washing the nose for nasal diseases.

The practice of medicinal bathing for various parts of the body is recorded in detail in *The Four Medical Tantras*. Generally, for patients with chronic diseases, therapy can be performed in a mild way, gradually increasing the dosage of the ingredients, the duration of the bath time, the temperature of the water, and the strength of any massage given. For acute cases the temperature of water can be higher and the bathing time can be longer. It is especially recommended that acute externally contracted diseases be treated with high temperature and strong ingredients to expel the pathogens. For chronic cases, the bathing process can be performed in several stages. For diseases with no bacterial infection, such as tinea, itching disorders, and diabetes, the method of bathing should be designed and arranged according to the characteristics of daily life and work, so as to make bathing therapy a convenient part of life that is easy to stick to.

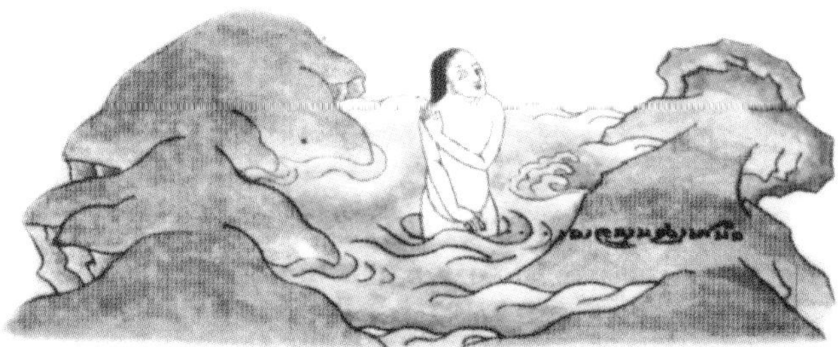

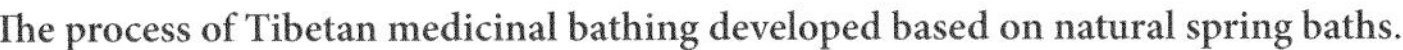

The process of Tibetan medicinal bathing developed based on natural spring baths.

Differences in syndromes

Naturally, different diseases have different manifestations, and even the same disease may have slightly different manifestations in different people. Even people with similar manifestations may actually have different diseases. Medicinal bathing must be applied according to the manifestations, including the location, nature, and changes of the signs and symptoms. For example, if a person is dizzy, medicinals with an ascending nature such as chrysanthemum can be added to the basic recipe, *Five Flavor Sweet Dew Decoction*, so the action of the formula can be guided to the head. Or for heel pain, Chinese angelica can be added to guide the action down to the heel.

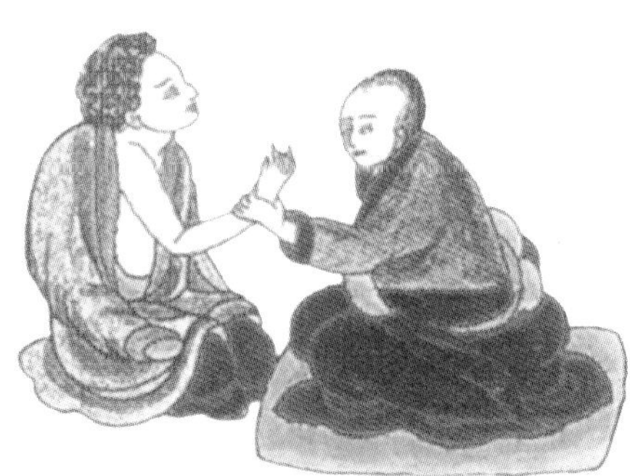

Medicinal bathing should be administered based on the patient's condition.

The modifications to the decoction should also be unique. Slippery medicinals, for instance, can be added to remove local filth. Heavy natured ingredients can make the bathing solution heavier so that local injuries and chronic diseases can be treated. Cold substances are used to treat heat syndromes, and vice versa.

Superficial syndromes of the skin should be eliminated outward through the opening sweat pores with hot substances, while astringent therapies are used to stop diarrhea. Medicinal bathing doesn't take the causes of disease into account, instead, it only considers the manifestations. Using this strategy, very satisfactory results can be achieved for local and temporary injuries.

Differences in individuals

No matter the disorder to be treated, the person is the most important factor. Since a person's surroundings, family, constitution, daily habits, sex, profession, and age will be different from one individual to the next, the task of creating a suitable medicinal bath should also vary. Considering the person's family, for instance, may reveal that they are part of a family where skin diseases are prevalent, so when bathing, sanitization is essential. Each member should have their own towel and, if possible, bathtub. Publicly used bathtubs should be strictly sanitized. For people with high blood pressure, the length of the bath shouldn't be too long, and high temperatures should also be avoided. People who work with their minds will feel relaxed in a full body bath, while cold water baths are suitable for those who work with their bodies.

Differences in seasons

The condition of the body, vessels, skin, etc. changes throughout the seasons. In the spring, yang qi ascends and the weather is warm. At this time, skin is in a state of development and bathing should be swift and mild to encourage blood circulation and the generation of yang qi. In summer, yang qi is exuberant on the surface of the body due to the hot weather and the skin is also in a state of exuberance. Bathing during summer should be rapid with heavy pressure so as to dissipate the heat energy of the body. In autumn, the weather is dry and the skin is also dry. Yang qi retracts and yin qi grows. Bathing should be mild and slow so that the blood vessels can be soft but strong, and the blood can flow without stagnation. In winter, the weather is very cold and yang qi is stored while yin qi is exuberant. Bathing in winter should be slow with heavy pressure so that yang qi can be relaxed and yin qi is not overly exuberant.

These are the general principles of bathing in the four seasons. The best seasons for medicinal bathing are spring and autumn, because the temperatures of these seasons are not extreme, and yin and yang are harmonious. Also, the quality of water available is better during spring and autumn. Despite all this, the time when an illness comes is the best time for treatment.

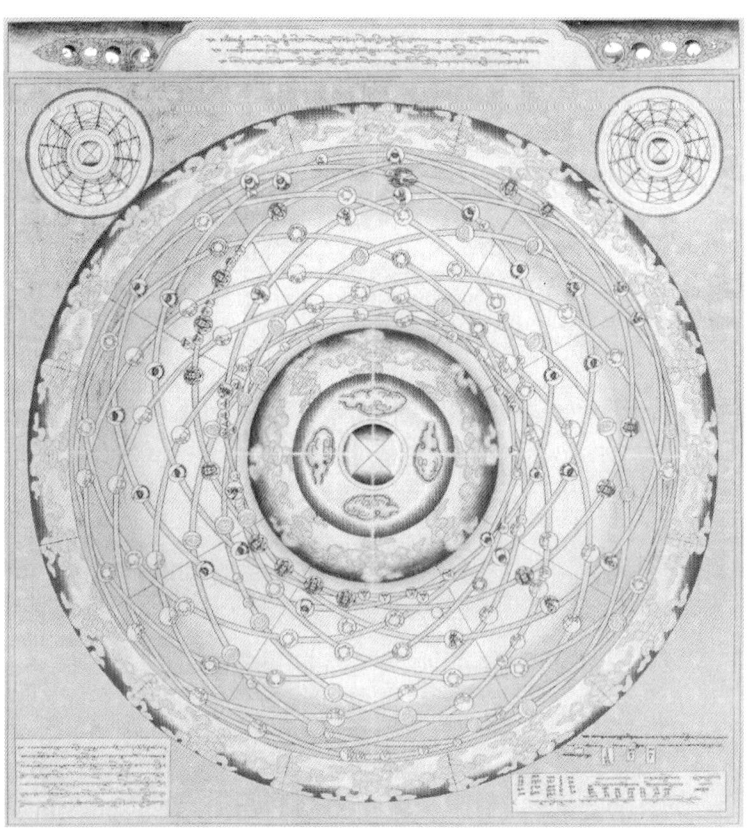

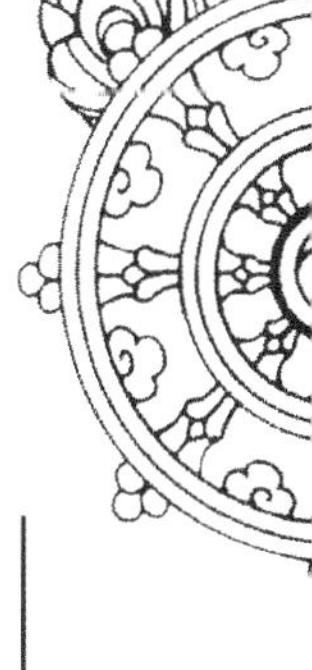

Medicinal bathing practices vary according to the different seasons. (a Tibetan *thangkha* on astrology and the calendar).

The state of qi and blood in the body vary within a day, and the principles and methods of medicinal bathing should vary as well. In the morning, when the yang qi of the body is growing and the yin qi is stored, bathing should be mild and rapid. At midday, when yang qi is exuberant and yin qi is totally stored, bathing should be rapid with heavy pressure. In the afternoon, yang qi declines and yin qi grows, so bathing should be slow and mild. In the evening, yang qi gradually vanishes, and yin qi is exuberant, so bathing should be slow with heavy pressure. In the morning when work begins, yang qi ascends to the head and face, and washing the face with hot or cold water can stimulate the mind. At midday, yang qi flows throughout the body, and bathing the whole body helps to encourage circulation. In the evening, yin qi enters the brain, and yang qi descends to the lower body. At this time, washing the feet can harmonize yang and nourish the yin, which is helpful to sleep. Though these rules here do not need to be followed strictly, they form good guidelines to consider.

Preparation for a bath

Cleanliness

Clean the bathroom, and sanitize the bathtub and all bathing facilities. Change the water and medicinal solution between bathers to prevent cross infection. The bathroom should be suitably ventilated to maintain a proper temperature and humidity. In this way, one can feel comfortable.

Pre-bath examination

Check and record the blood pressure, temperature and heart rate.

Pre-bath guidance

When someone tries a medicinal bath for the first time, they will naturally have a certain degree of tension, anxiety, or fear. Therefore, the person preparing the bath is responsible for explaining the methods and characteristics of medicinal bathing to win their confidence.

Testing the temperature

An appropriate temperature is essential. Too high a temperature may burn the skin, and too low a temperature may cause abdominal distension or even diarrhea. Generally, the temperature on the first day of therapy is 37-38°C (98-100°F), and increases to 39-43°C (102-110°F) gradually. Then, it should be lowered gradually until it returns to about 38°C (100°F) at the end of the treatment course. Different disorders require different temperatures. Skin diseases, for instance, need a temperature of 35-45°C (95-113°F); for respiratory, circulatory, nervous system, digestive and gynecological diseases the optimal temperature is 41-45°C (105-113°F); for diseases of the joints and muscles like rheumatism, rheumatoid disease, gout, sciatica, atrophied muscles, and all the different kinds of bone and joint diseases the optimal temperature is 46-50°C (113-122°F).

Remarks

Before bathing, all hormone and non-steroid antibiotic medications should be suspended for two weeks.

For weak patients and unstable conditions, 5 g of *Aquilaria Powder with Eight Ingredients* or 60 g of *Nutmeg Powder with Twenty Ingredients* can be given before bathing.

Baths should not be taken on an empty stomach or for 2-3 hours after eating a full meal.

Bathing Instructions

The bathing procedure

First put both feet into the solution, and rub the chest and the area before the heart with the solution. When the bather gets accustomed to the water, slowly lower the body into the solution, with the head and upper chest out of the water to reduced pressure which may cause palpitations, heavy feelings in the chest and shortness of breath. Move slowly, and prevent the solution from splashing the eyes, nose and mouth. During the bath, keep the water moving in order to increase its contact with the body. Gently move and massage the body, especially any painful or affected body parts. Avoid big or fast movements or rapidly stirring the solution. This may cause the medicinal action of the solution to escape, and its strength may be diminished. Do not massage the skin too heavily. For people with high blood pressure, bathing should begin from the legs so that blood circulation increases in the lower part of the body and decreases in the brain. The instructions are reversed for people with low blood pressure, i.e. starting with the upper body. This can regulate blood flow, improve blood pressure and prevent fainting.

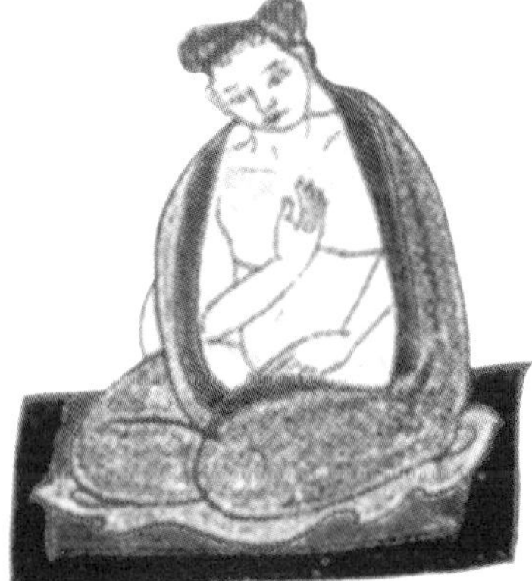

Cause the body to sweat.

The optimal time for bathing

The first session should last for about 20-30 minutes, and the duration can be adjusted according to the patient's amount of endurance. Beginning from the second day, the duration can be gradually increased until it reaches 40-60 minutes. Do not take more than two baths in one day.

Keep the bath at a comfortable temperature

When the temperature lowers after being in the bath for a while, the temperature should

be raised until it is comfortable again. If the solution is expensive or rare, it can be used over a number of days, re-heating it every day.

Possible post-bath reactions

Carefully observe the body's condition, including the complexion, expression, awareness, blood circulation, skin color, and body temperature. Avoid falling or fainting, especially with children, the elderly, and people who have had a stroke. If any adverse reactions occur, check the pulse, blood pressure, and breathing, and call a doctor if necessary.

Other hints

Don't use soap, shampoo, conditioner or other cosmetics during the medicinal bath to prevent reactions that may inhibit the therapeutic effect.

Causing a mild sweat on the forehead is good. Profuse sweating should be avoided.

Post-bath care

Sweating

Rub the body gently with a towel after bathing. Do not rub vigorously, so as to protect the layer of active medicinals that have been absorbed by the skin. Lie flat in a warm room after putting on clothes. Wrap the whole head with a towel, making a hole for the eyes and nose. Stay like this and sweat mildly for 10-15 minutes.

Taking liquid

Since a large amount of water is lost during sweating, drinking salted water is necessary. Tea is not recommended because it causes urination and will worsen the loss of fluids. Keep clothes and blankets dry and avoid catching cold.

Medicinal rubbing

After bathing, people are vulnerable to dizziness, ringing in the ears, fatigue or even vomiting due to disturbed blood and qi. Rub the body with medicinals and massage one hour after bathing in order to close the sweat pores and prevent external wind invasions. Prepare the medicine by cooking *Agui Pill* and *Aquilaria Pill with Thirty Ingredients* in butter. Rub the prepared medicine on the skin after it has cooled.

Proper self care

Diet: eat fresh vegetables and foods that are highly nutritious, high in protein, high in calories, and easily digested foods. Especially nutritious are soups (chicken, fish, or bone broths), dairy products and fruit juice. Do not eat too much greasy, spicy, cold, or raw food, or any liquor or other irritable foods. For those with of skin diseases, avoid spicy food, liquor, fish, shrimp, crab, and pork. Nearly 90% of people with skin diseases will relapse if they consume spicy food or liquor.

If someone has been recently discharged from the hospital, avoid washing the hair and bathing. Keep warm and avoid catching cold. It is especially important that people who have rheumatism, rheumatic arthritis, and sciatica avoid dampness, catching cold, and overstrain.

Exercise and strengthen the arms and legs.

Avoid sexual activity as much as possible during treatment.

Avoid bloodletting and other strong therapies.

Remarks

Avoid bathing prior to or right after meals, so as to avoid hypoglycemic reactions and digestive disturbances and causing a burden to the heart.

Do not bathe right after drinking alcohol. Since liquor makes the body warm, bathing after drinking may cause spasms of muscles or blood vessels. If the temperature of the bath is too high, it may accelerate the heart beat and blood flow, and increase the risk of cardiac or cerebral vascular diseases. People who suffer from angina pectoris, or are at risk for heart attacks or strokes may be in danger.

Do not rub the skin forcefully during bathing, or the skin may be injured and its ability to protect the body will be impaired. Bacteria and other pathogens may invade into the body through the injured skin and cause infection.

When bathing in natural springs, first get a physical exam from a professional that can help select a suitable spring for bathing. When dizziness, nausea, and palpitations occur during bathing, leave the tub immediately but carefully and rest for a while. If unpleasant reactions persist, the person may not be suited for medicinal bathing, and therapy should be stopped.

Do not bathe for too long as blood vessels in the skin may become dilated and the brain may experience a lack of blood possibly causing fainting. Those with high blood pressure, hardened arteries, or the elderly may increase their risk of stroke.

Avoid medicinal bathing during menstruation, pregnancy, and when angry. For elderly people or those with heart disease, bathe the affected parts first and then bathe the whole body. Take some fruit juice or salted water after bathing. Do not drink hot water, smoke or drink liquor. Rest after bathing and avoid direct exposure to wind.

Those with red and swollen infections should bathe first and then rub the body to improve the symptoms. For severe infections, first rub the body and then bathe so as to facilitate the absorption of the medicinal solution. For people with severe local symptoms and mild systemic ailments, steaming may be done before bathing to deal with the local symptom first. The reverse is done for severe systemic symptoms and mild local illnesses.

For people in severe pain, first massage the area to relieve pain and then bathe. For cases of mild pain, bathe first and then massage. For those with severe heat toxins, rub the body from the middle of the body outward to expel the toxins. For weak people, rub in the reverse direction to nourish the original qi.

Generally, take a break from bathing for 1-3 days after bathing for one week and then begin the next week-long bathing course. Three such one-week bathing courses constitute a therapeutic course. Whatever the purpose of bathing, either for treatment of a specific disease or for general health, persistence is essential for a satisfactory effect.

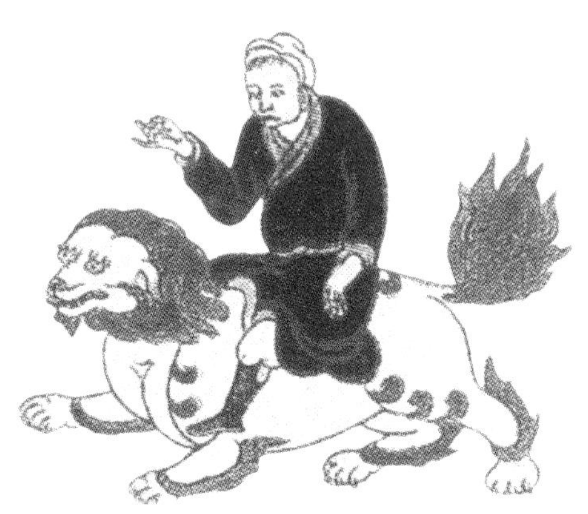

ཚེའི་སྔ་རྟགས།

CHAPTER 8 SIGNS OF LIFE

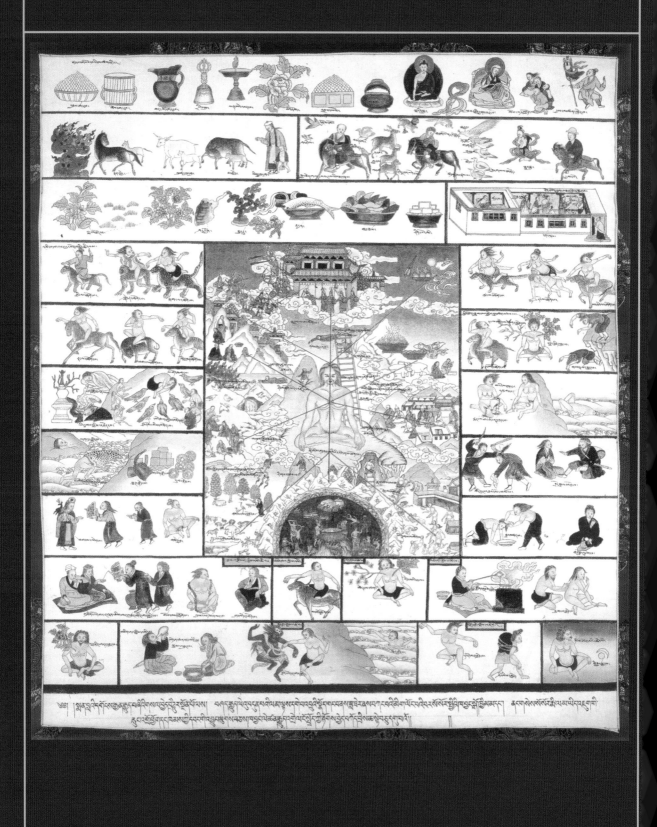

Thangkha nineteen in the *Sman thang* series of *The Four Medical Tantras:* signs of life

Just like the appearance of a flower blooming before the fruit, or clouds coming before rain, anything that happens has signs beforehand. Changes in life are no exception. Birth and growth, disease and senility, and even the end of life, all send messages to the outside world in many forms of expression during their development and maturity.

A wise man skilled in health cultivation is capable of mastering the understanding of these signs and can avoid damage. An ignorant person will turn a blind eye to the alarms life sends, thus missing good opportunities, one after another, to master his own fate. Tibetan medicine gives much importance to the external expressions of life changes. The types of signs vary, and include dreams, body signs and happenings along the road. By always paying attention to the abnormal reactions of the body, especially for those with underlying diseases, treatment and regulation can be timely and appropriate, decrease the severity of the disease, and even may save one's life. Signs can be divided into near, far, definite, and indefinite signs. Far signs can be subdivided into three types: messenger, dream, and attitude signs. This is roughly equivalent to modern physiological, pathological and psychological viewpoints.

Auspicious Signs

One dreams at night and thinks in the daytime. There are six kinds of dreams: seeing, hearing, feeling, praying, coming, and disease dreams. Seeing dreams are those where one repeats what one sees or does in the daytime. Hearing dreams are when what is heard in daytime reappears in the dream. Feeling dreams refers to those things that are felt by the sense organs reappear in the dream, such as joyful or pleasant sensations. In praying dreams, the wishes for future fortune and fate that were prayed for in the daytime appear in the dream. Coming dreams refer to visions of things that will be experienced in the future. Disease dreams are when a diseased condition happens in the dream due to unpleasant sensations in the body. The hearing, seeing and feeling dreams are all derived from instinct.

Auspicious dreams

Dreams have a certain ability to predict the future. However, not all dreams can be used for prediction. Dreams that appear in the first half of the night or just after falling asleep are liable to be forgotten, and can't be used for prediction. Dreams from the middle of the night are also not suitable for prediction. Only the dreams just before dawn which can be clearly remembered are effective for making predictions.

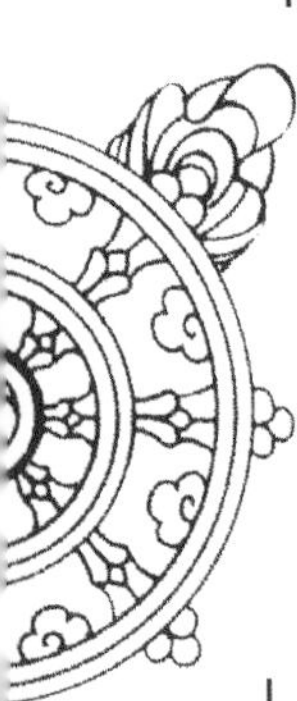

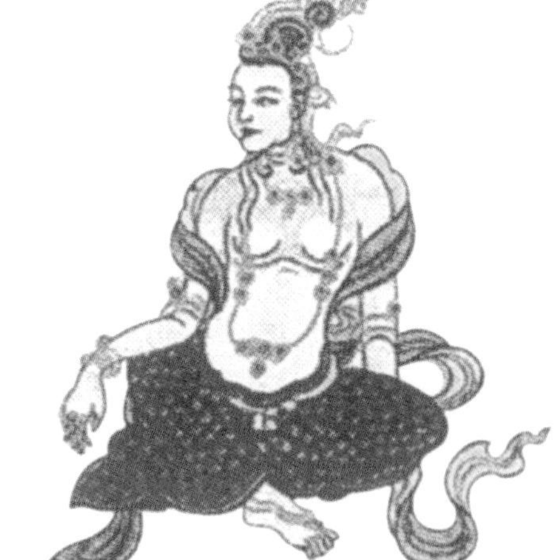

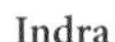

Indra

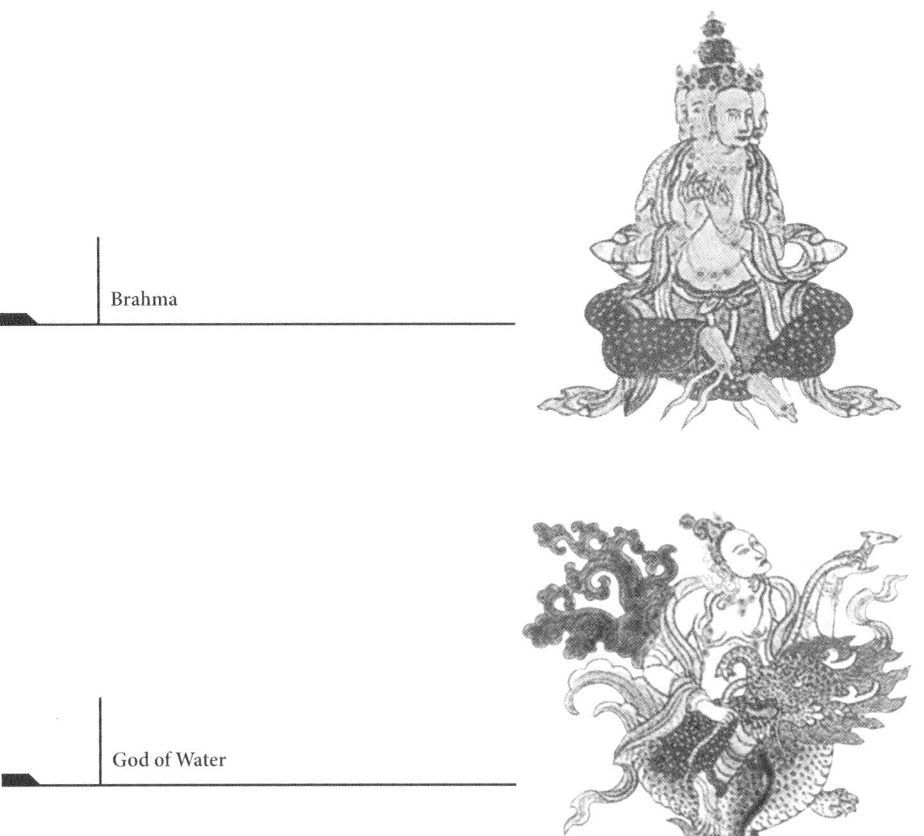
Brahma

God of Water

All of the following dreams signify health and longevity, good fortune, wellbeing or wealth.

Dreaming of gods of the secular world such as Indra, Brahma or the God of Water, especially when an elephant accompanies them for protection.

Dreams of sitting or talking with sages, famous people, kings, or ministers.

Dreaming of a humble ox wandering leisurely.

Dreaming of a tree burning in a blazing fire, or dreaming of a clear, calm, and boundless sea.

Dreaming of a man stained with blood, feces, urine or other filth, or dreaming of oneself wearing clean white clothes.

Dreaming of holding a streaming flag or a Buddhist umbrella.

Dreaming of climbing a peach, apple, or walnut tree full of fruit; dreaming of picking a fruit; or of climbing a hill or high building in a tranquil, relaxed way, calm enough to look down even when climbing very high.

Dreaming of taming a lion, elephant, horse, or ox and riding on their back, all the animals are so docile that one can ford a large river calmly and safely.

Dreaming of traveling northward or eastward.

Dreaming of an escape from a difficult condition, such as miserable labor, a dangerous cliff, or conquering an enemy in a fight.

Dreaming of praising or worshipping a god or a ritual offering.

Dreaming of respecting and being filial to one's parents so that they can be happy in their remaining years.

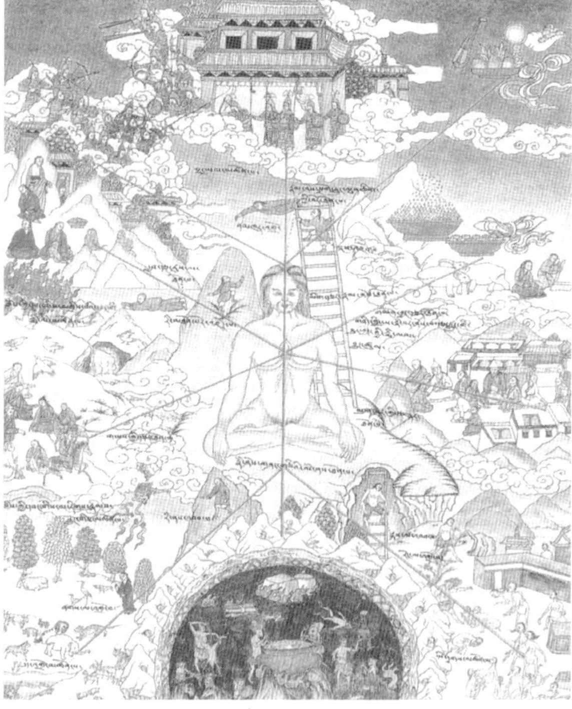

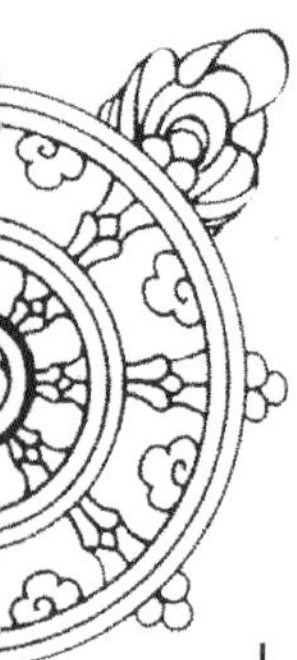

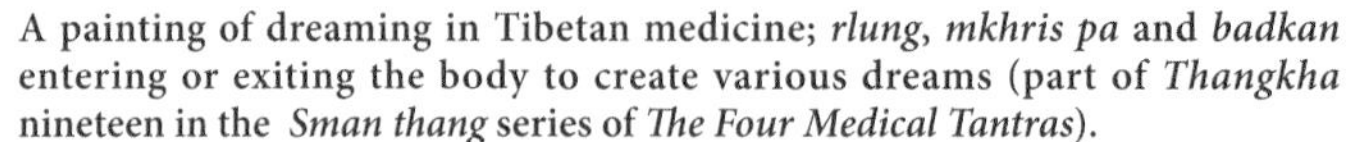

A painting of dreaming in Tibetan medicine; *rlung*, *mkhris pa* and *badkan* entering or exiting the body to create various dreams (part of *Thangkha* nineteen in the *Sman thang* series of *The Four Medical Tantras*).

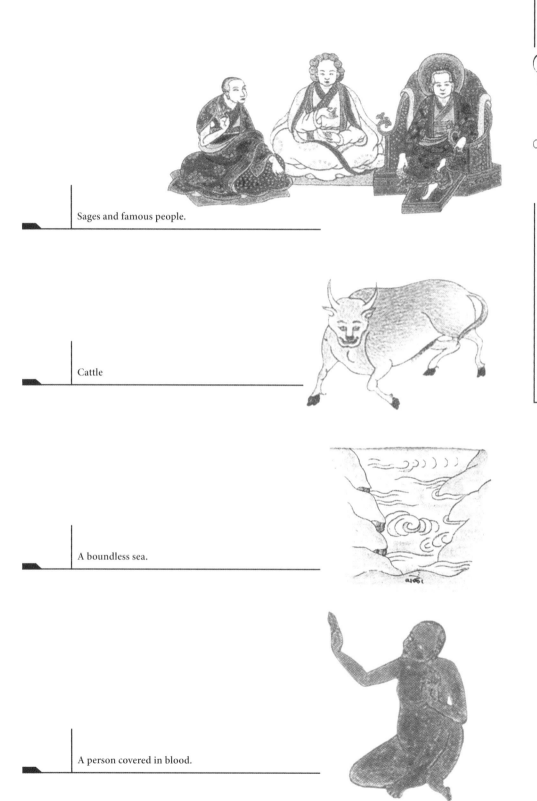

Sages and famous people.

Cattle

A boundless sea.

A person covered in blood.

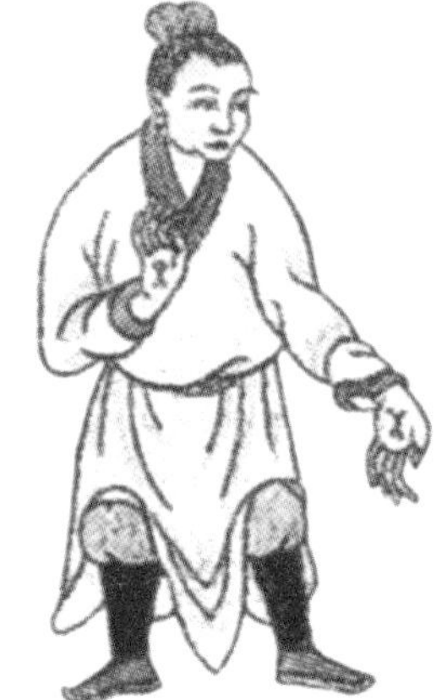

Wearing white clothes.

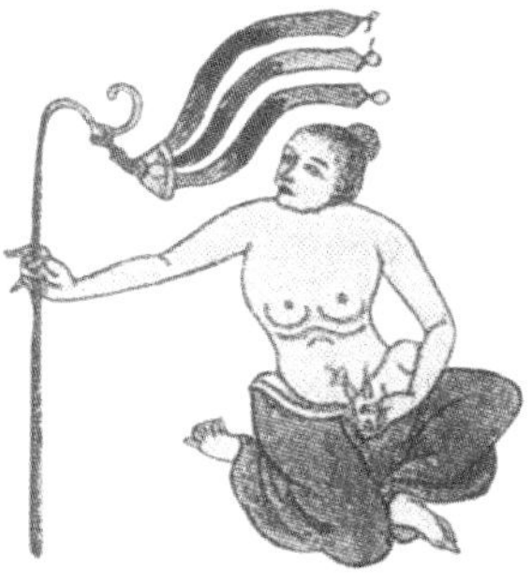

Holding a Buddhist streamer.

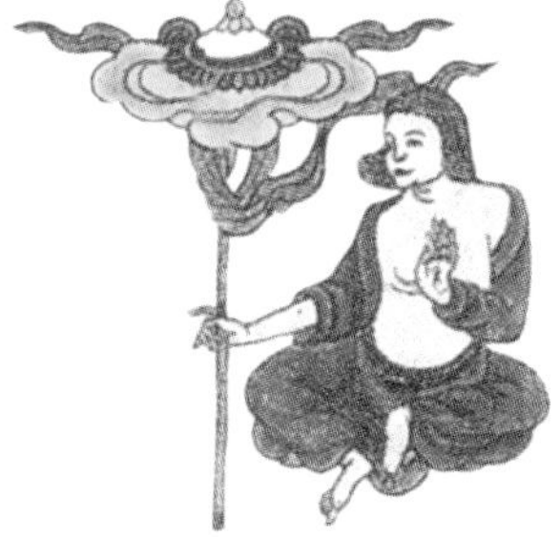

Holding a Buddhist umbrella.

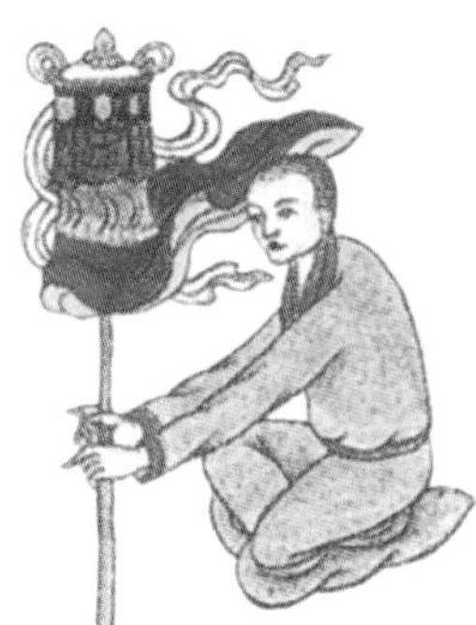

Holding a Buddhist flag.

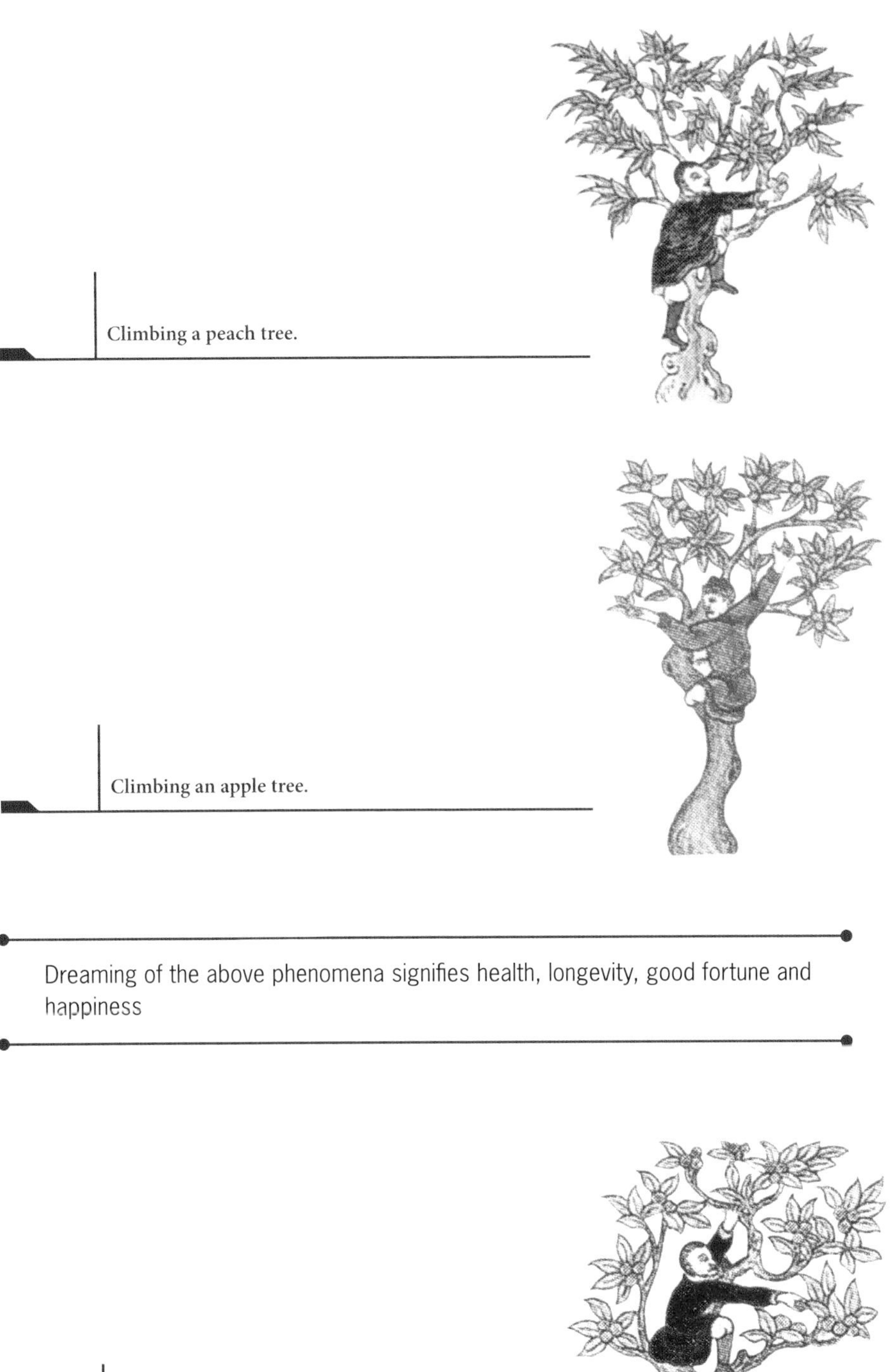

Climbing a peach tree.

Climbing an apple tree.

Dreaming of the above phenomena signifies health, longevity, good fortune and happiness

Climbing a walnut tree.

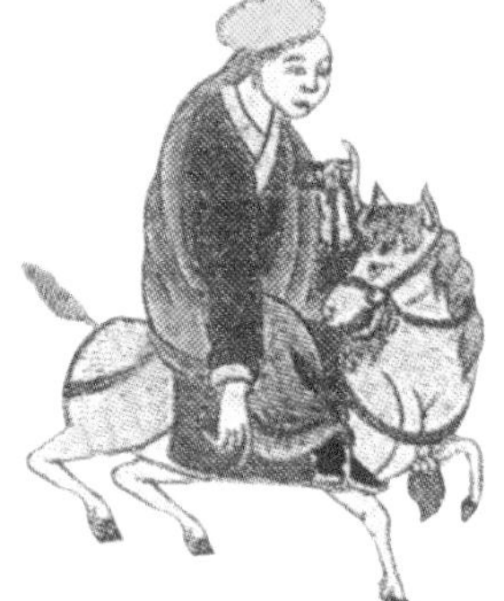

Riding on a horse.

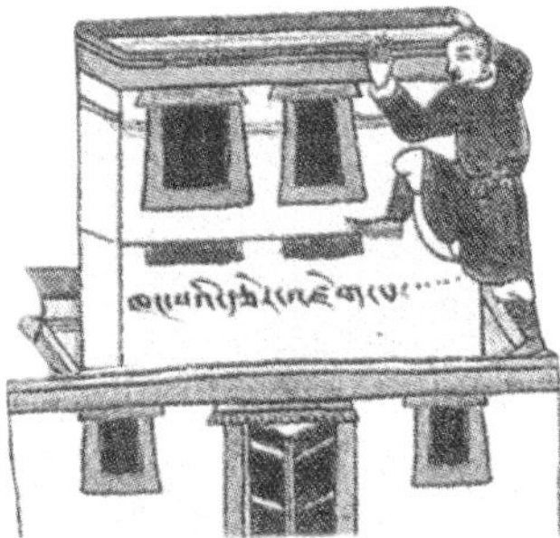

Climbing a house.

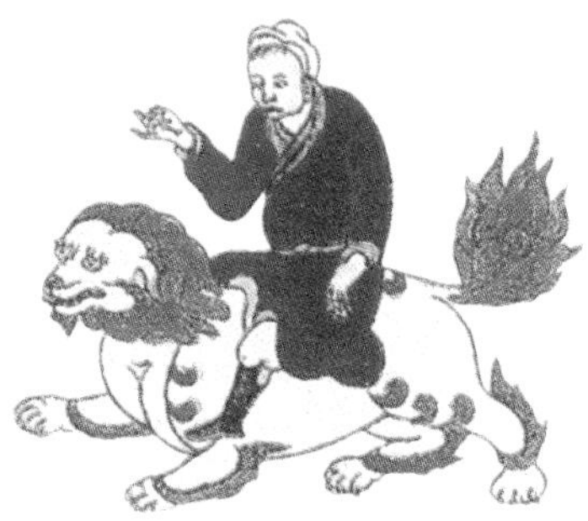

Riding on a lion.

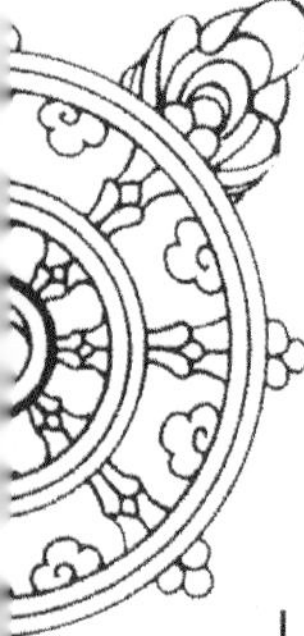

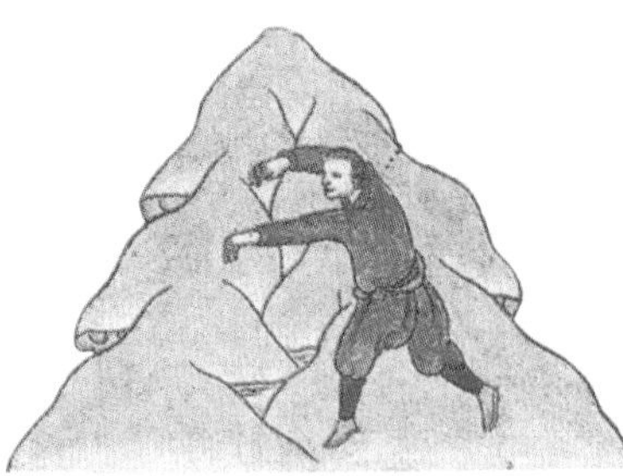

Climbing a mountain.

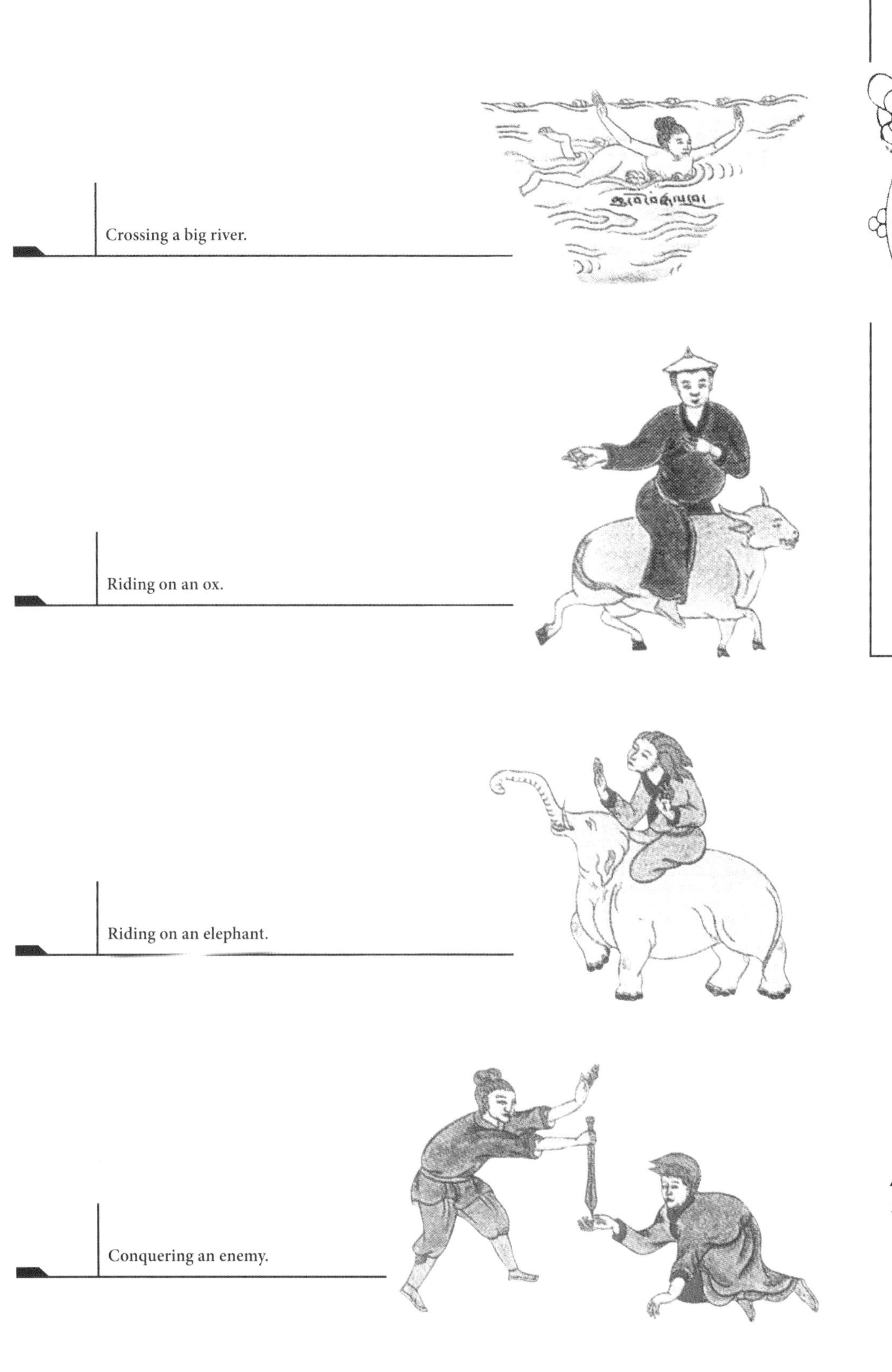

Crossing a big river.

Riding on an ox.

Riding on an elephant.

Conquering an enemy.

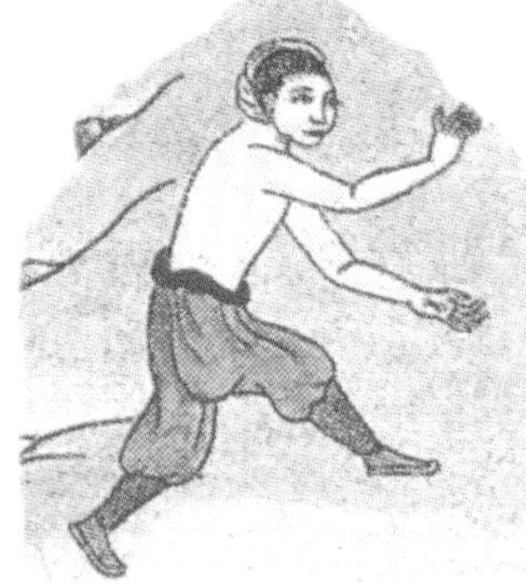

Walking toward the north or the east.

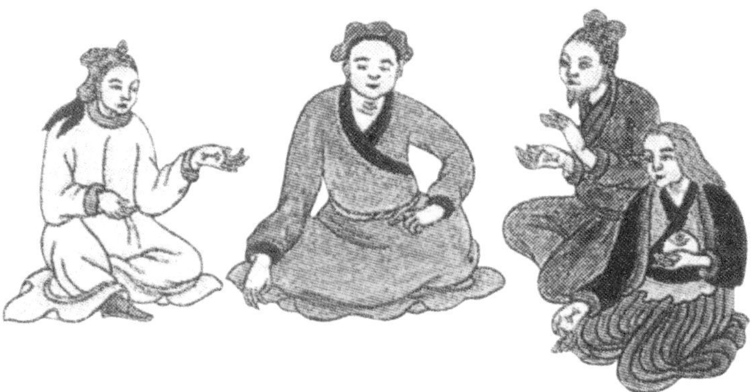

Taking care of one's parents.

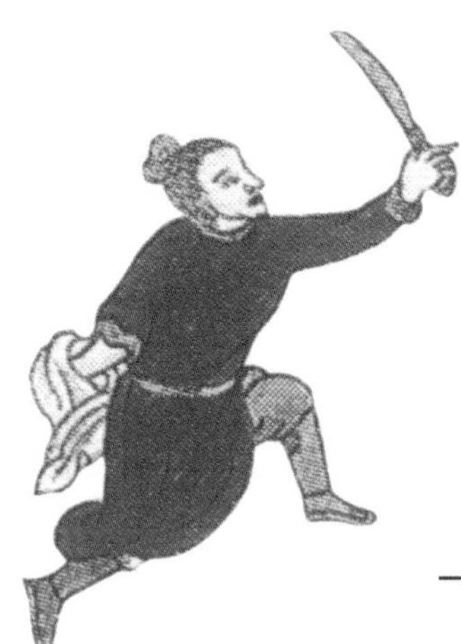

Escaping from a difficult predicament.

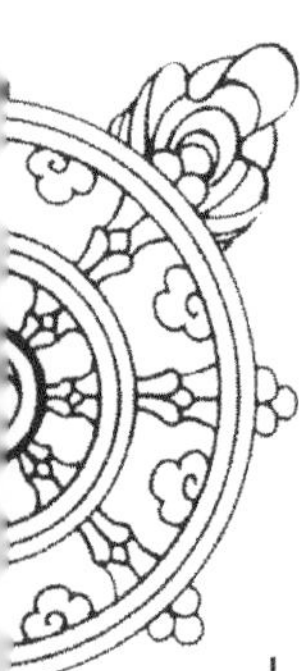

Auspicious signs in daily life

When a physician meets a man practicing Buddhism or a religious follower on his way to visit a patient, this is an auspicious sign.

When on the road and one encounters a basket full of grain, a barrel full of milk, a bottle full of wine, a Buddhist bell, burning flame, butter lamp with a soft and warm fire, flowers covering the ground, a Buddhist icon or streamer, khada (a white scarf that means respect or goodwill), a man wearing white clothes, someone giving a discourse on Buddha's teachings, performing rituals, or a horse giving birth to a foal, a sheep giving birth to a lamb, a cow giving birth to a calf, or people happily welcoming a new born child, all these are auspicious signs, signifying the patient will recover.

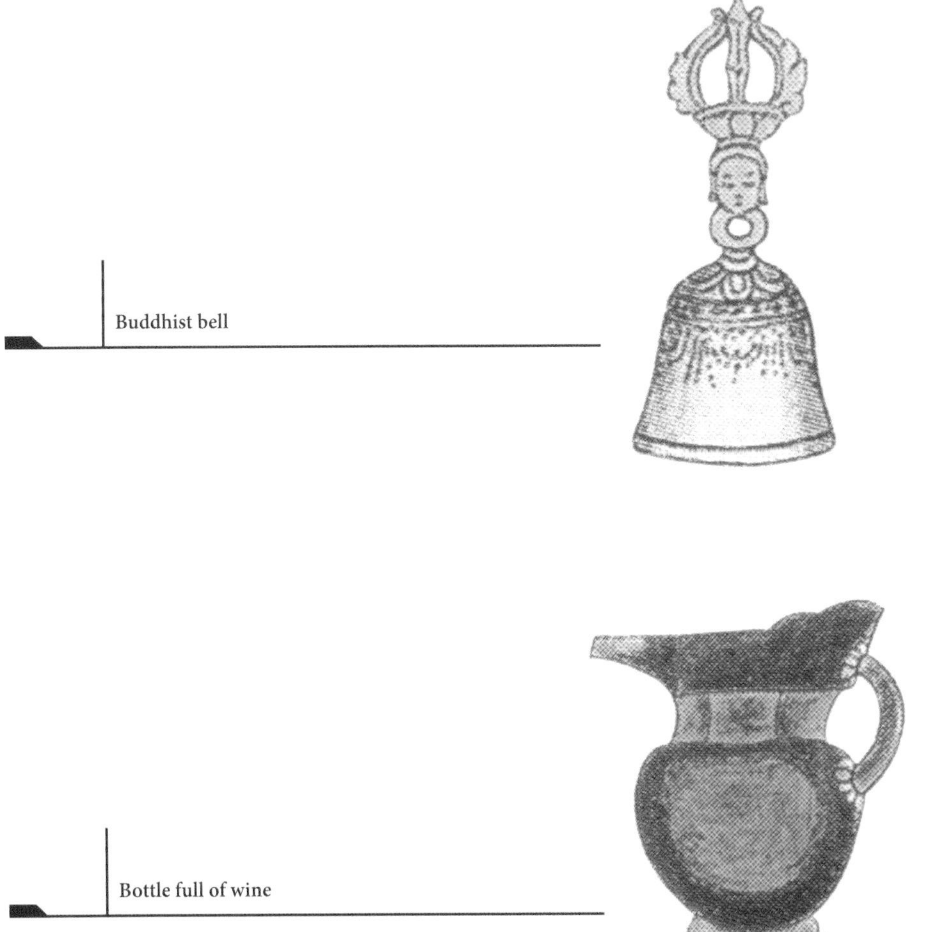

Buddhist bell

Bottle full of wine

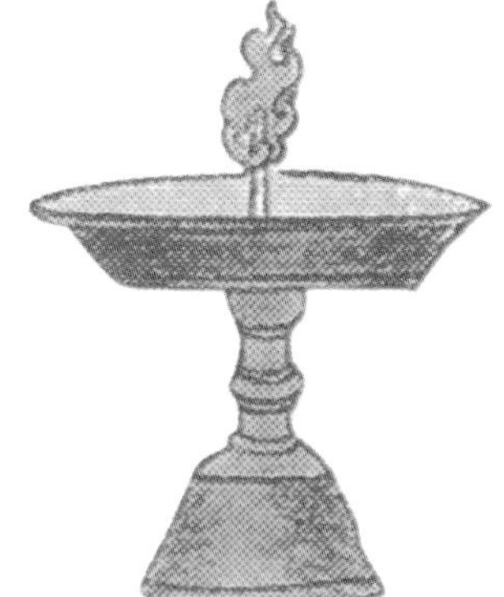

Butter lamp

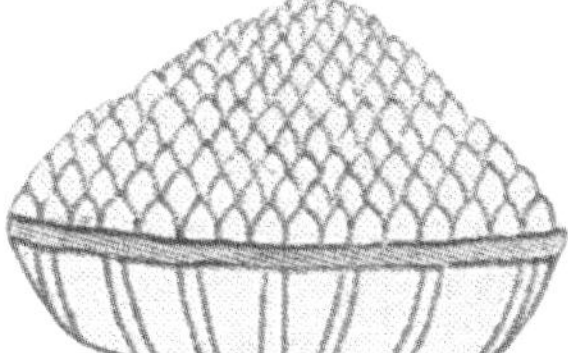

Basket full of grain

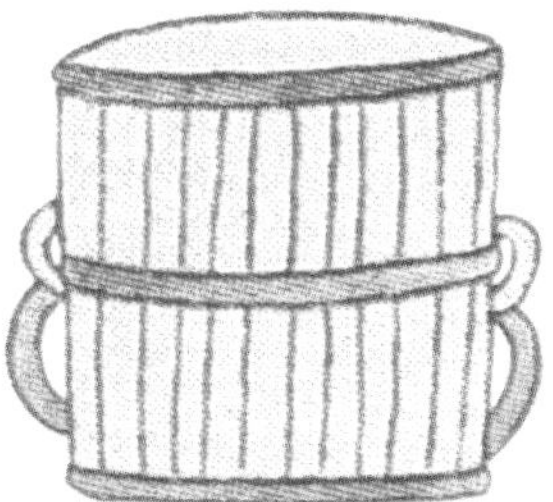

Barrel full of milk

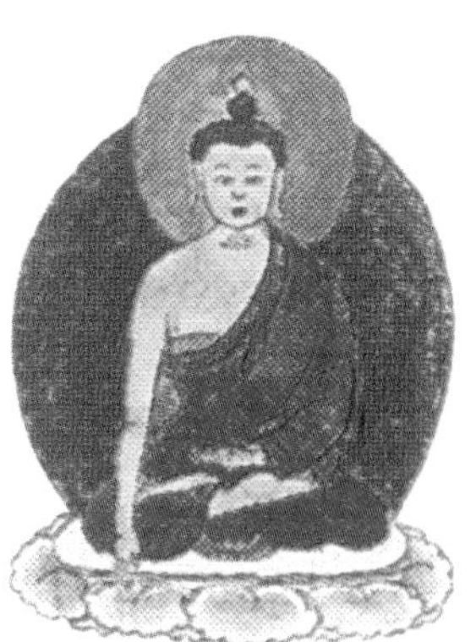

Bodhisattva

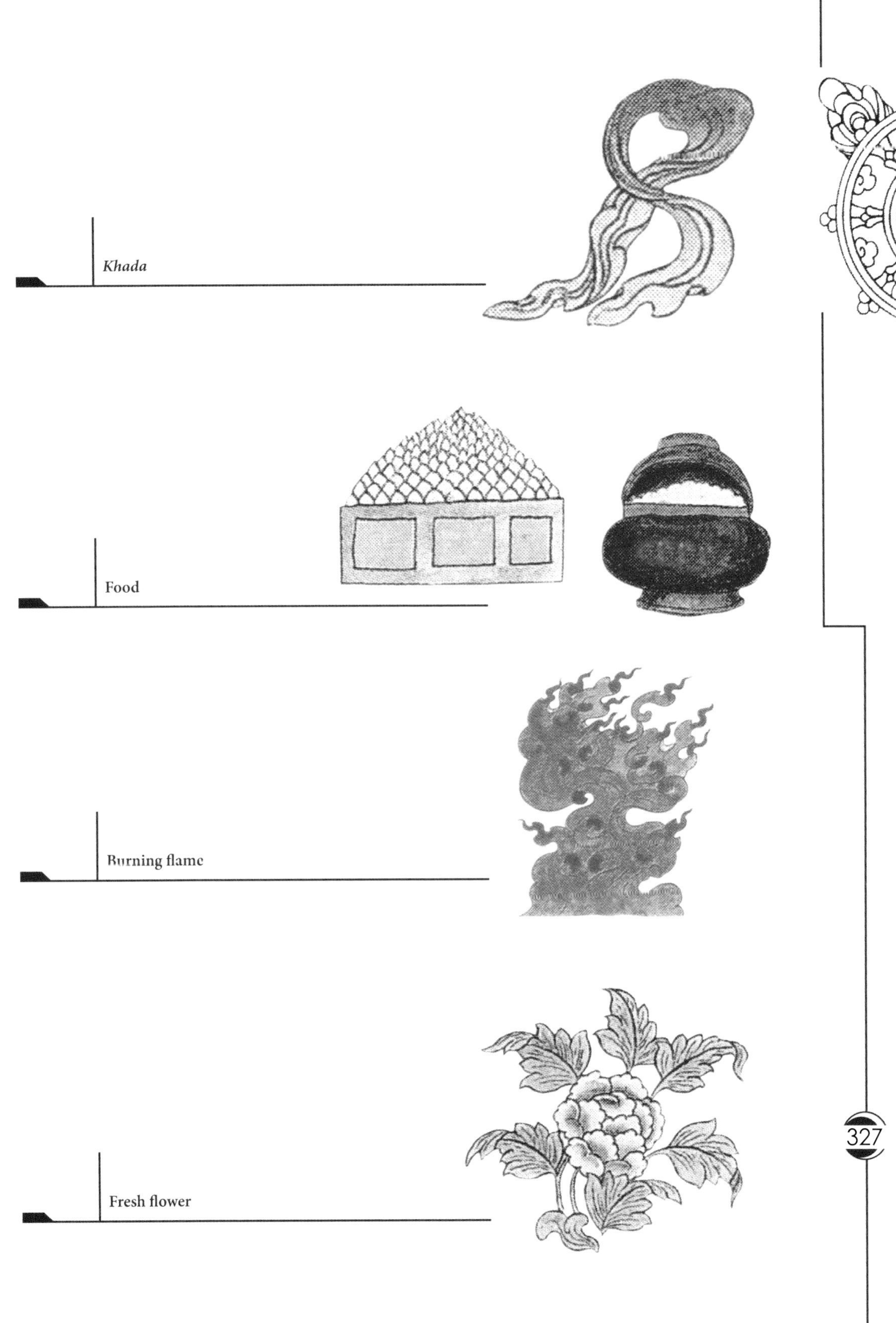
Khada
Food
Burning flame
Fresh flower

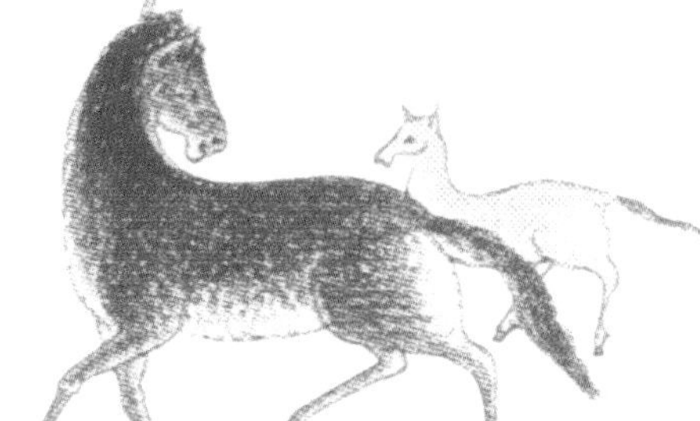

A horse giving birth to a foal.

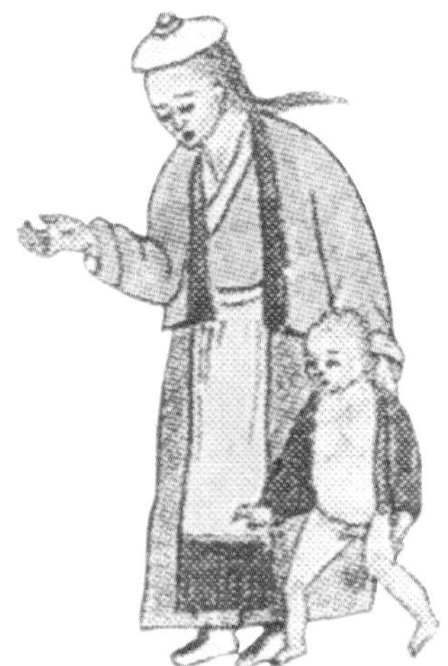

Mother giving birth to a child.

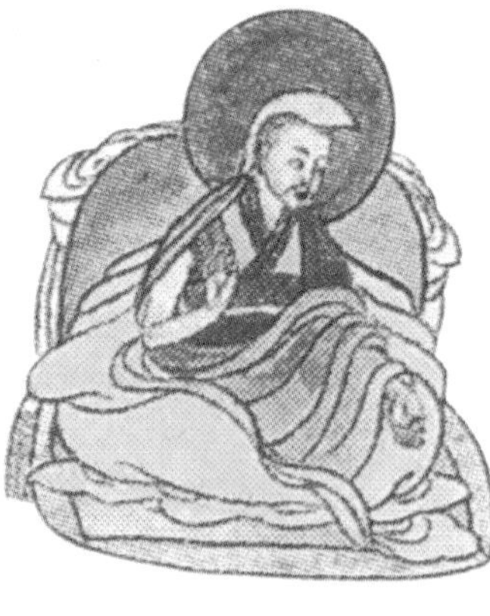

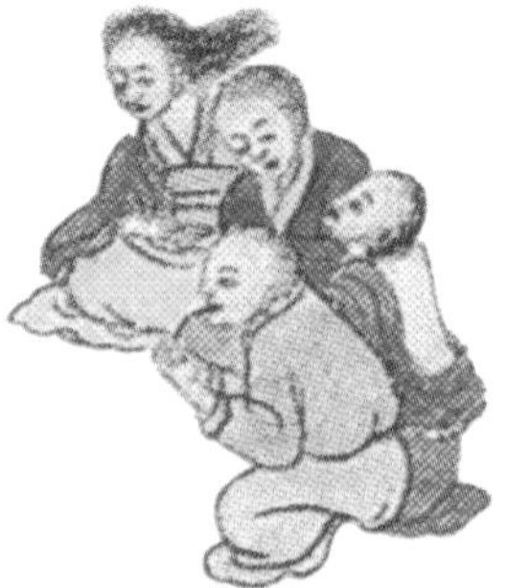

Someone reciting sutras and Buddhist teachings.

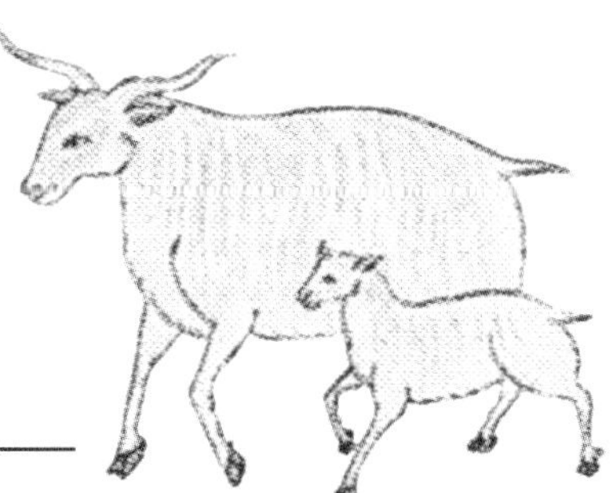

A sheep giving birth to a lamb.

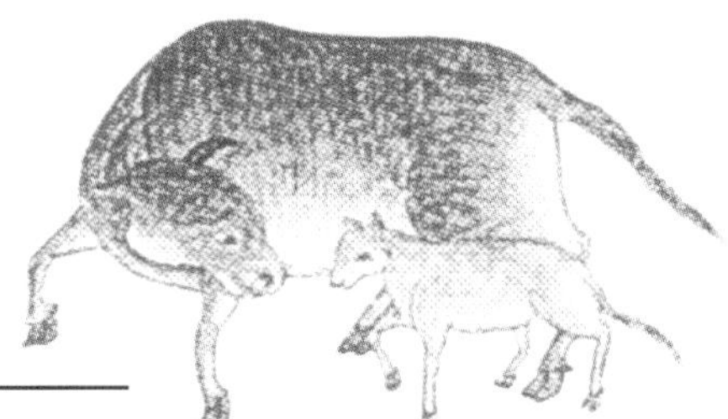

A cow giving birth to a calf.

Tibetan medicine divides signs into four groups: far, near, definite and indefinite signs. Distant signs are further subdivided into messenger, dream, and attitude signs.

Signs of Illness

There are numerous minute channels that run between the heart and the outside world. If these channels are blocked by diseased *rlung*, *mkhris pa*, or *badkan*, then people will dream. In the initial stage of a disease, even if one doesn't feel any uneasiness during the daytime, because the minute channels are already blocked, mild discomfort will be present but will very likely be overlooked. However, during the night the heart is vulnerable due to the blocked minute channels and dreaming will occur. The dreams alarm the body to changes that are happening, reminding them to prepare for disease or even death. Those who already suffer from disease and encounter inauspicious dreams become increasingly weak and unable to fight the disease. These dreams are death signs.

To learn how to decipher such dreams is an important part of health cultivation, and a necessary skill of an excellent physician.

Dreaming of riding on a cat, monkey, tiger, fox or dead body with an uneasy sensation, or when the animal is ferocious or frightening are signs that the death rope of the King of Hell is around a person's neck.

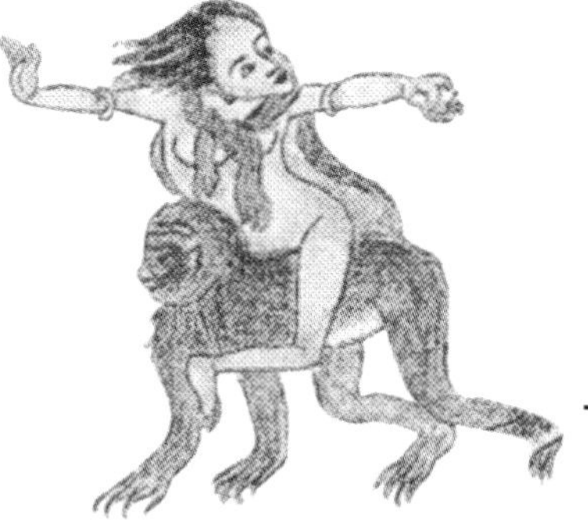

Riding on a monkey.

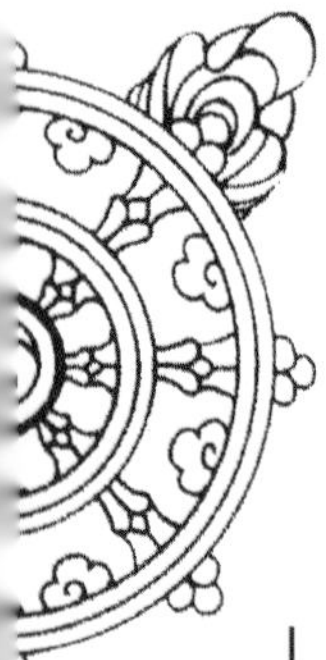

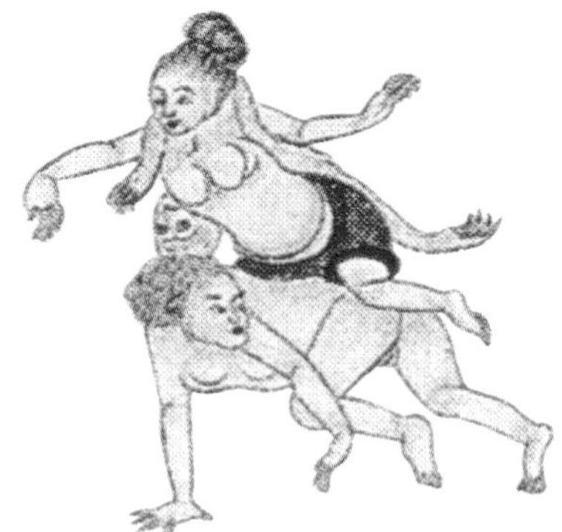

Riding on a dead body.

Riding on a cat.

Riding on a tiger.

Riding on a fox.

Dreaming of riding naked on an ox, horse, pig, camel and going southward are signs of death.

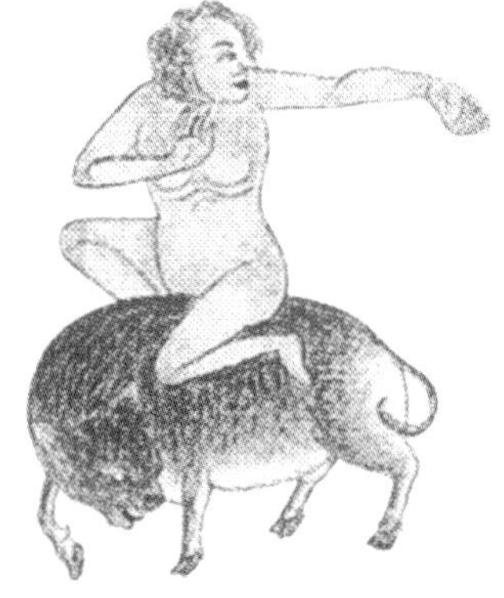

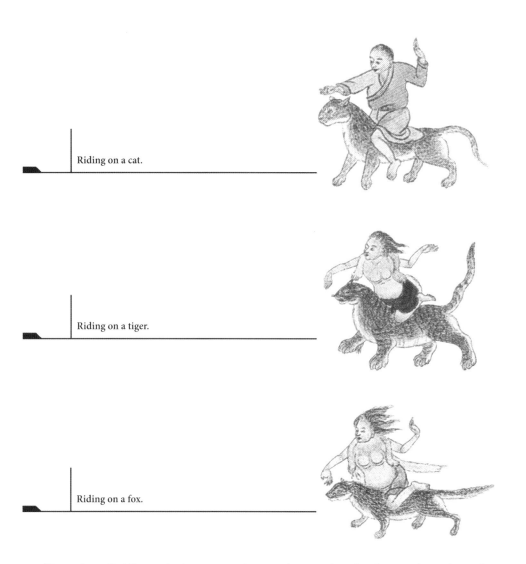

Riding naked on a pig.

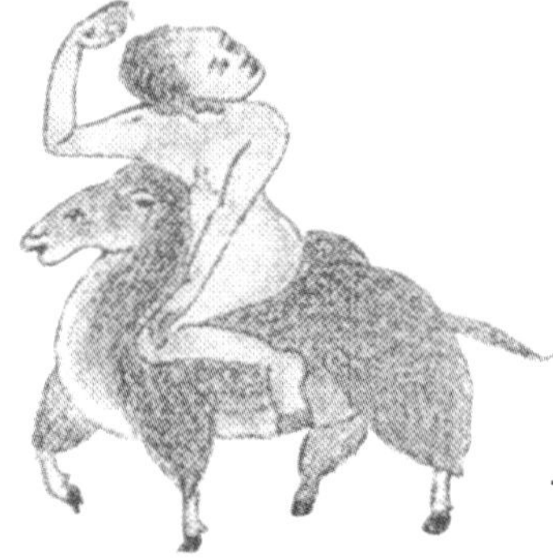

Riding naked on a camel.

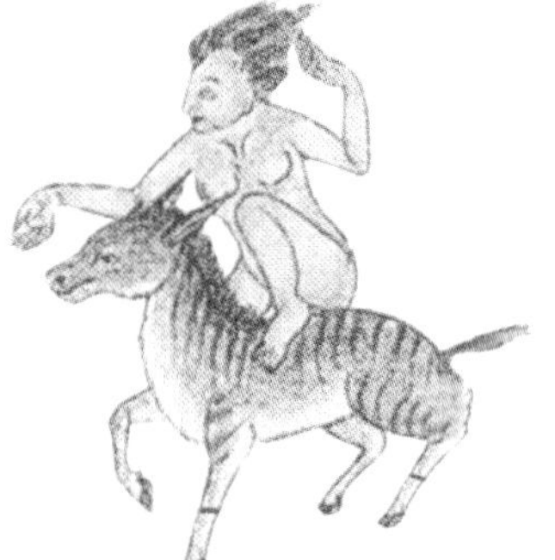

Riding naked on a donkey.

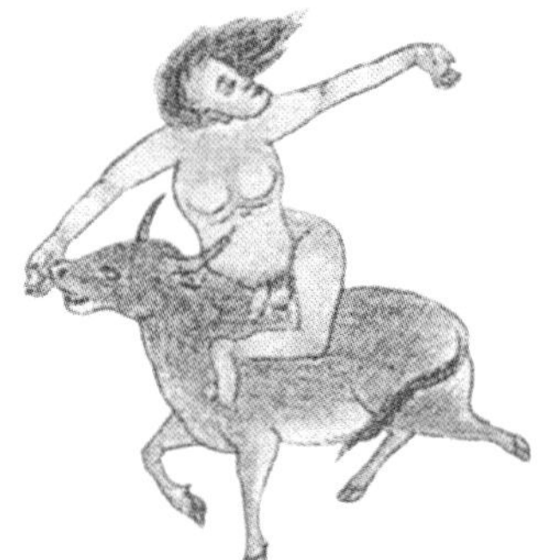

Riding naked on an ox.

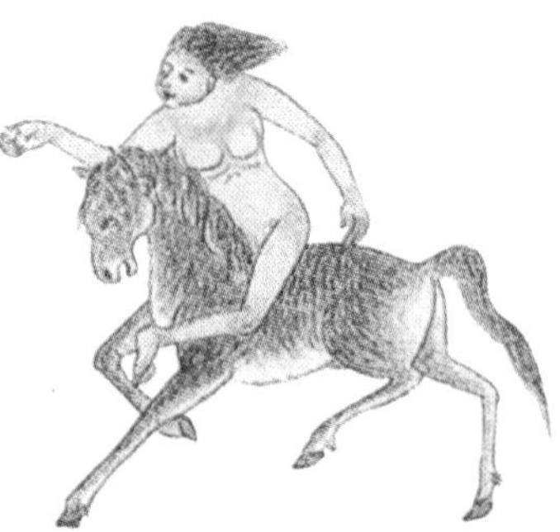

Riding naked on a horse.

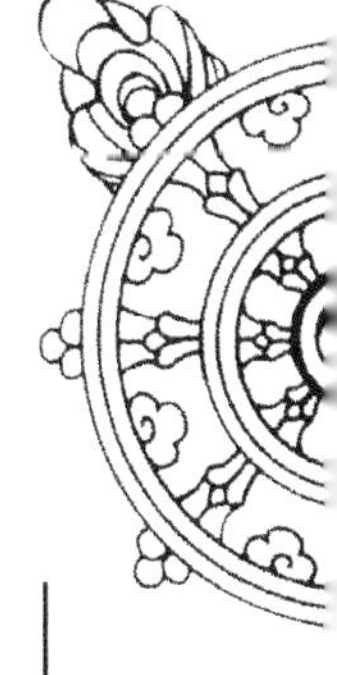

Dreaming of branches and leaves of a tree growing out of the head, or growing out of the chest, or trees with thorns, lotus flowers, trees with tender branches, green leaves and sharp thorns and flowers that are fresh and beautiful signifies that death is pending.

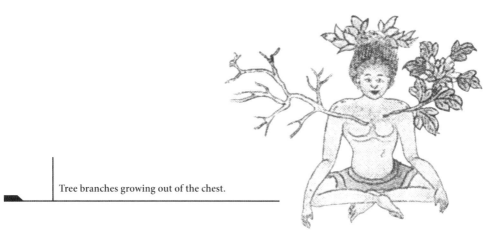

Tree branches growing out of the chest.

Dreaming of looking over the edge of a cliff or even falling over the edge, or sleeping in a cemetery, or the head being hit and broken, or being surrounded by crows, scorpions, and devils, or a low and terrible sound with no escape or help signifies a person has fallen ill.

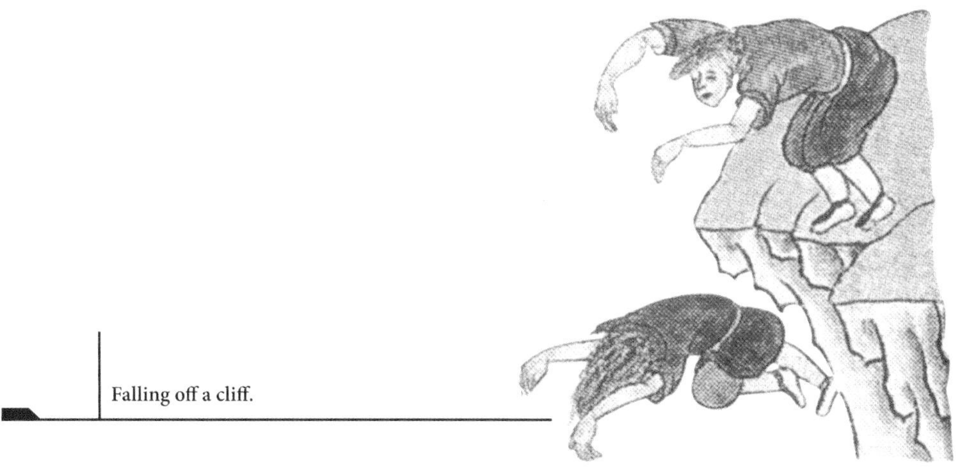

Falling off a cliff.

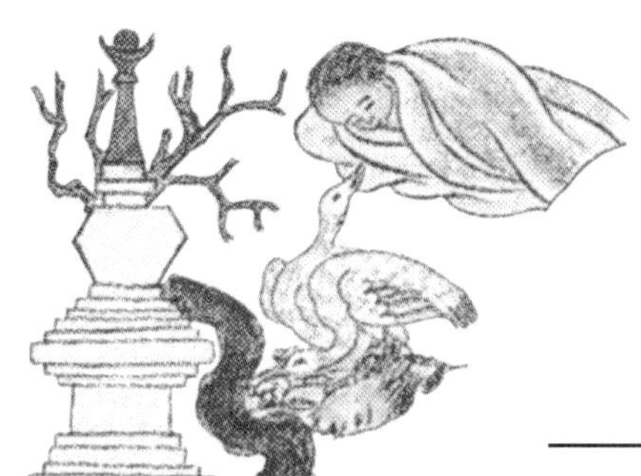

Sleeping in a cemetery.

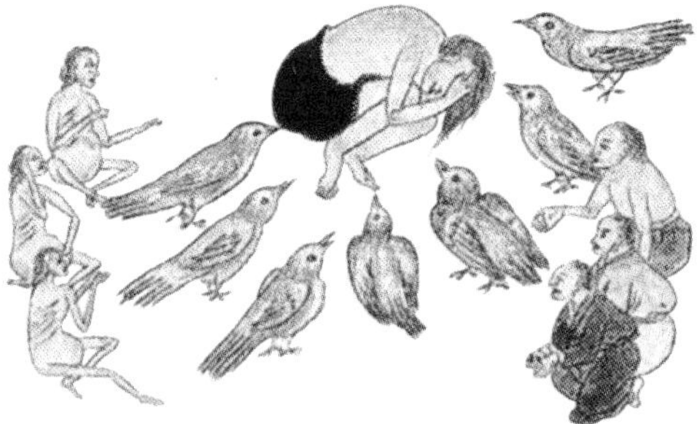

Surrounded by devils and crows.

Dreaming of harming oneself, cutting one's own skin with a knife and severe bleeding; or being in turbulent water and trying to swim but seeing no coastline, becoming exhausted and eventually floating away on the water, or dreaming of being swallowed by a big fish little by little signifies pending death.

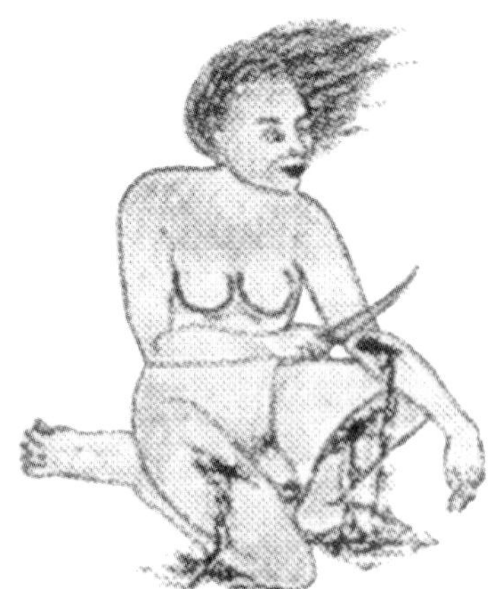

Harming oneself

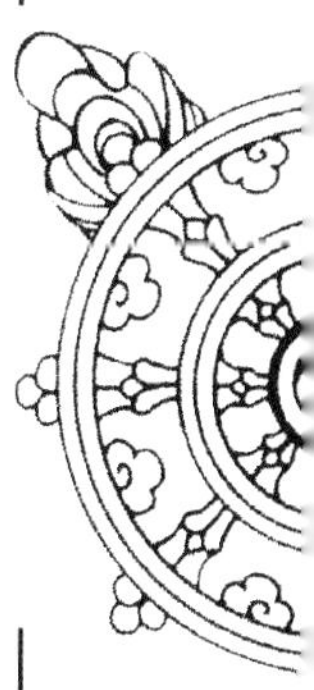

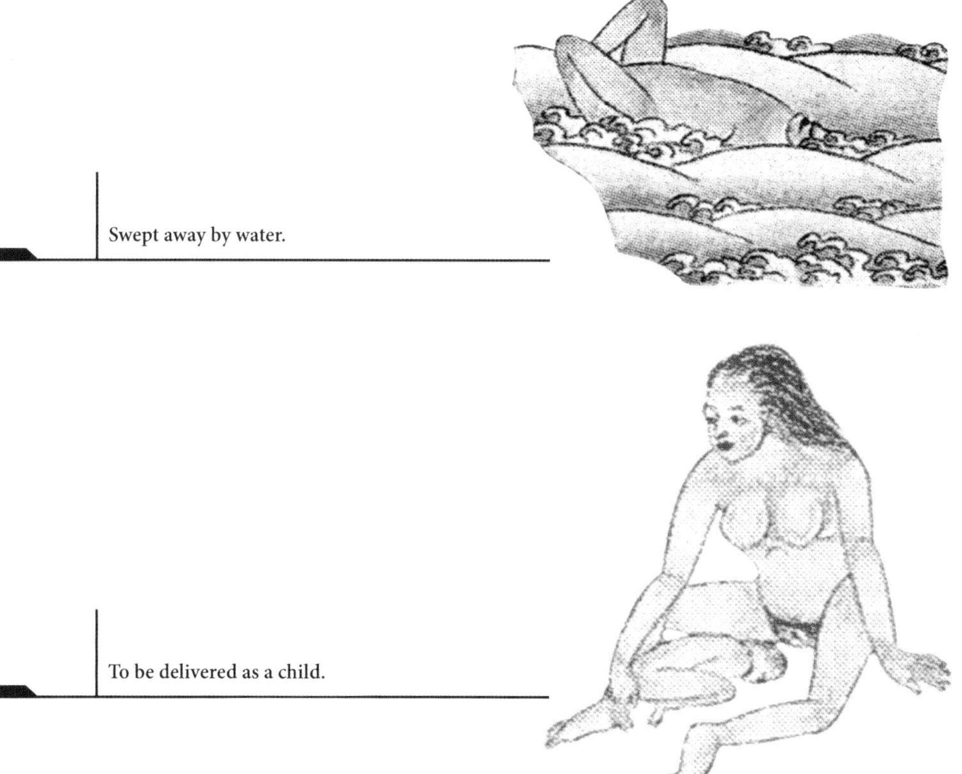

Falling into a swamp or being swallowed by a fish.

Swept away by water.

To be delivered as a child.

Dreaming of picking up metals such as steel and iron and piling them up like a hill, of fighting with an enemy, being hurt and surrendering, failing in business, making heavy debt and trying to avoid the creditors even when escape is impossible, or kneeling down to beg for more time to pay signifies that the body has succumbed to disease.

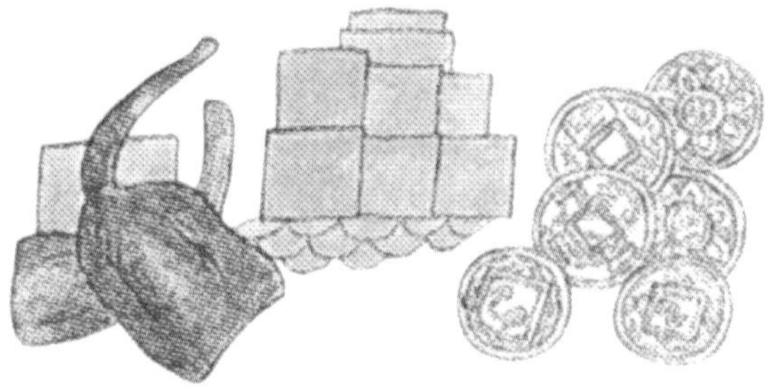

Piling up a large amount of metal.

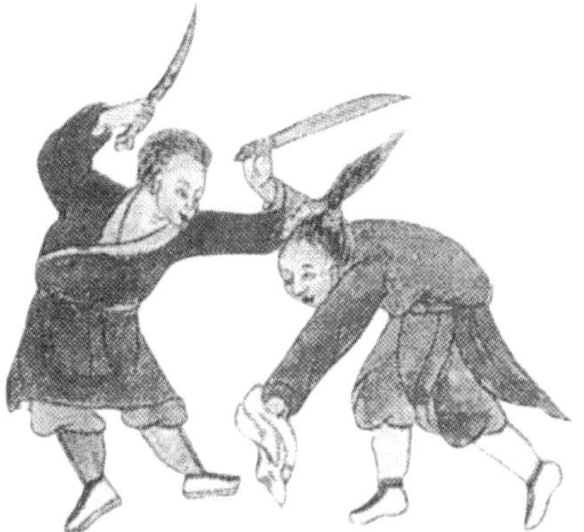

Fighting

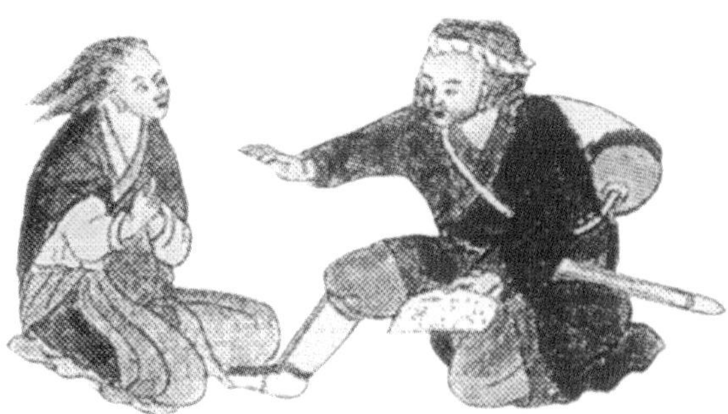

Failure in business.

Dreaming of getting engaged and marriage are not auspicious signs, but signify disease or even death.

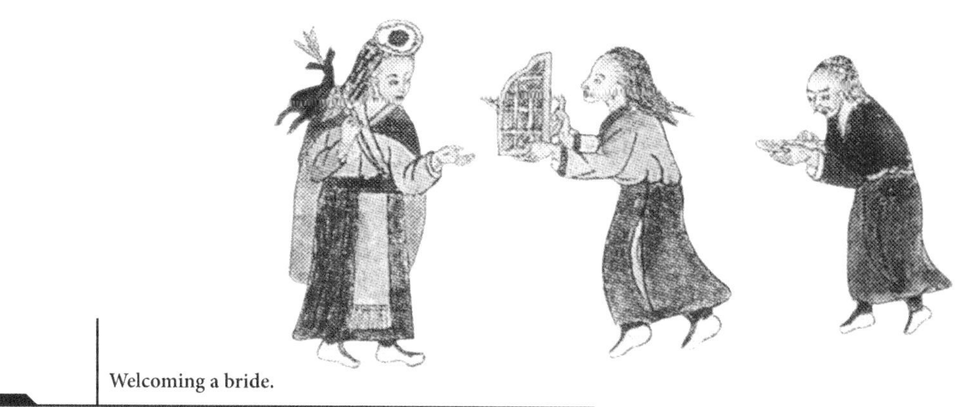

Welcoming a bride.

Dreaming of sitting naked, of hair being cut and the beard shaved, of drinking with dead relatives or friends, or being asked to stay and unable to leave, or dreaming of wearing a red robe and a red rosary, or dancing with dead relatives and friends signifies bad fortune and are mastered by the King of Hell.

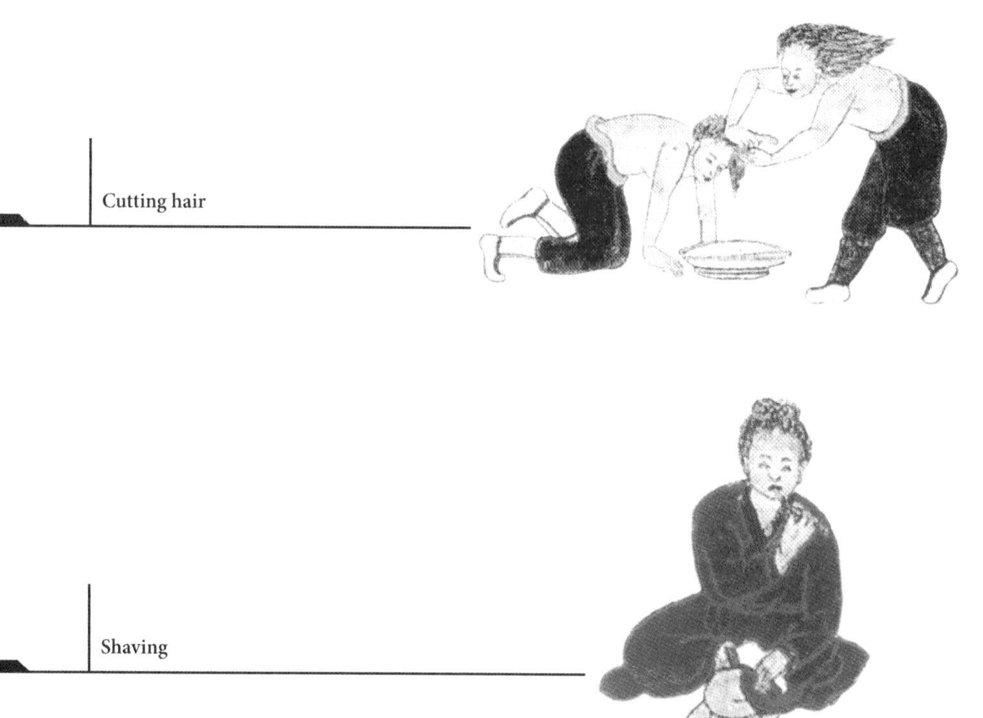

Cutting hair

Shaving

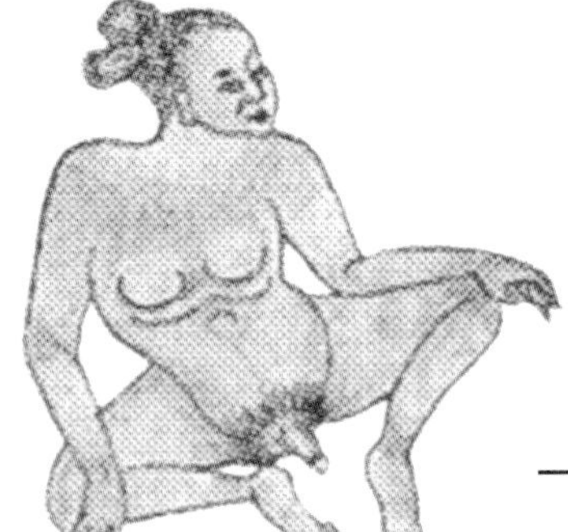

Sitting naked

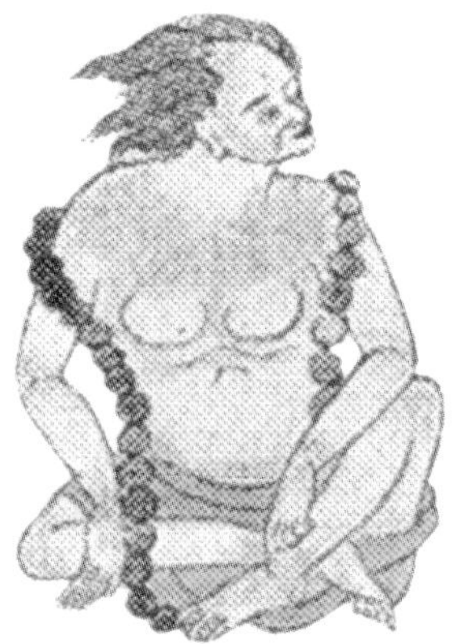

Wearing red clothes and a red rosary.

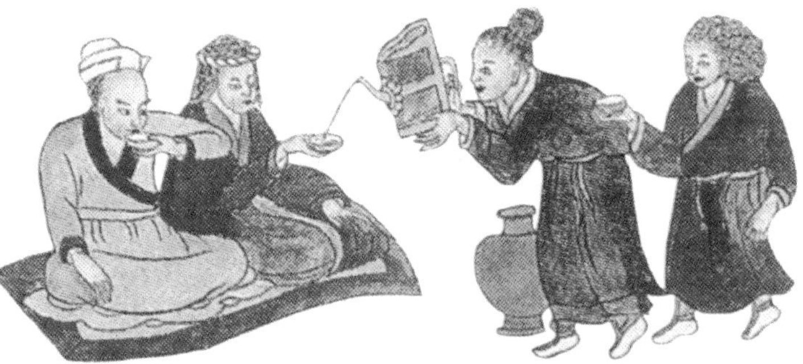

Drinking with dead relatives or friends.

Dreaming of a woman laughing for no reason or riding on a yellow cow that walks unsteadily signifies a poor prognosis or unavoidable death.

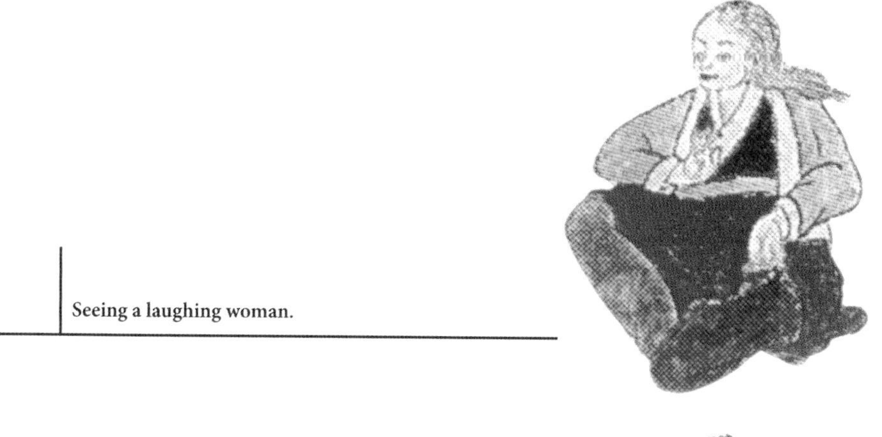

Seeing a laughing woman.

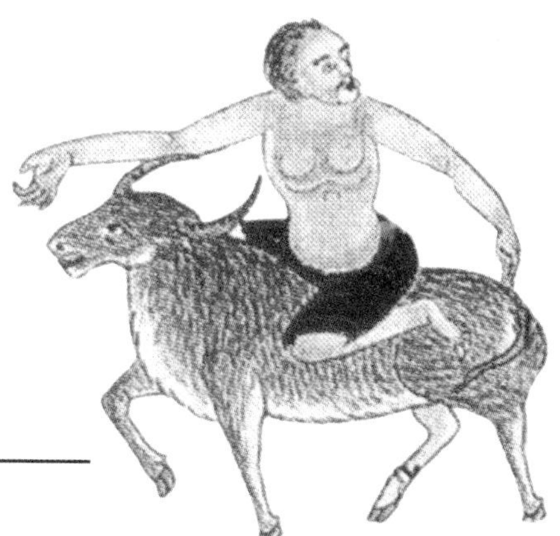

Riding on an ill yellow cow.

All the following dreams are death signs.

A tumor patient dreams of a tree growing from the chest, or even blooming and fruiting.

A person with leprosy dreams of a fire-offering, or someone rubbing oil over their body.

Dreaming of drinking vegetable oil with a criminal and feeling scared while doing so, a beautiful lotus flower blooming from the chest, or drowning in a rushing current.

A manic patient dreaming of dancing with a Yaksha.

An epileptic patient dreaming of dancing when drunk, or carrying a dead body.

A blind man dreaming of the sun or moon falling into the earth and not rising again.

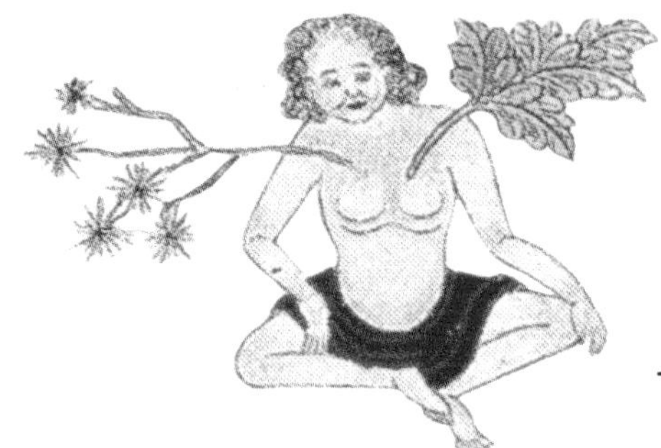

A tumor patient dreams of a tree growing from the chest.

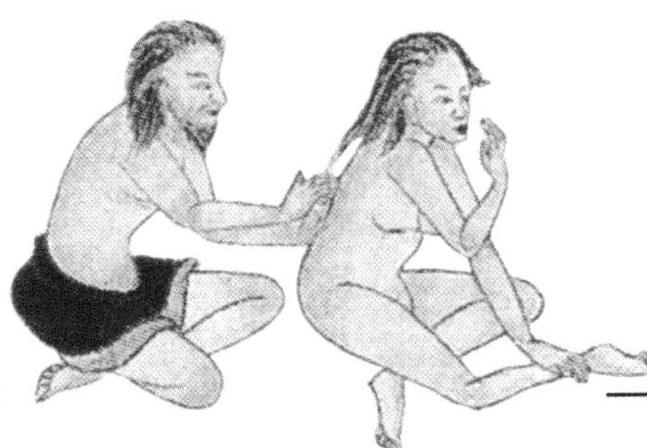

A leprosy patient dreams of rubbing oil over the body.

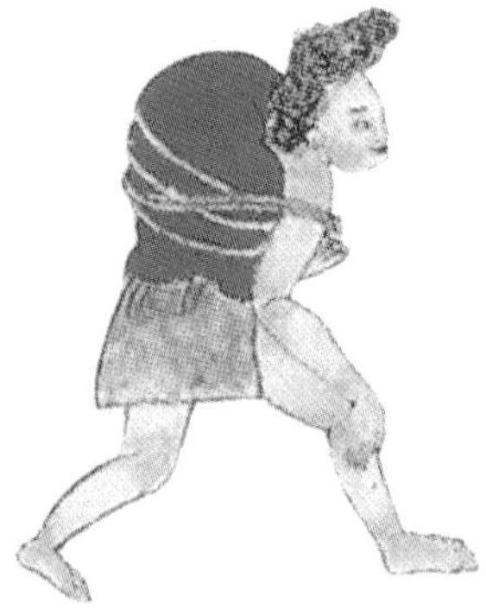

An epileptic patient dreams of carrying a corpse.

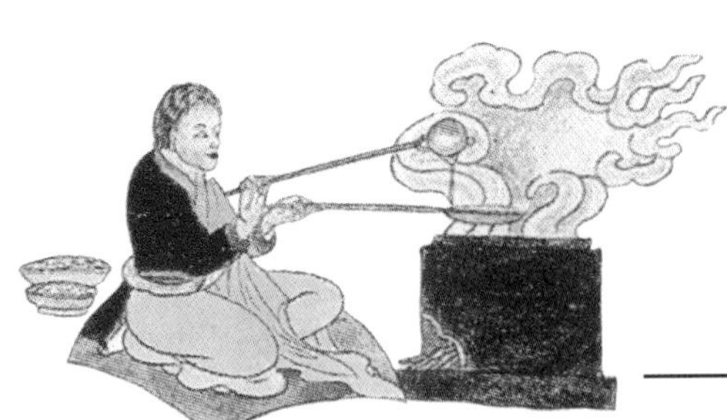

A leprosy patient dreams of a fire-offering.

Someone with urinary block dreams of a lotus flower growing from the chest.

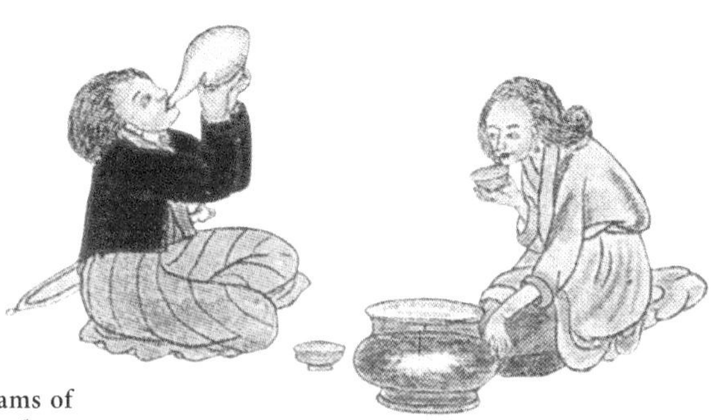

Someone with urinary block dreams of drinking vegetable oil with a criminal.

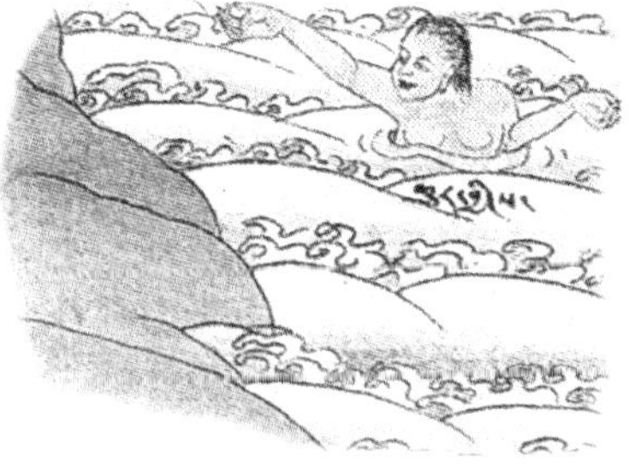

Someone with urinary block dreams of drowning.

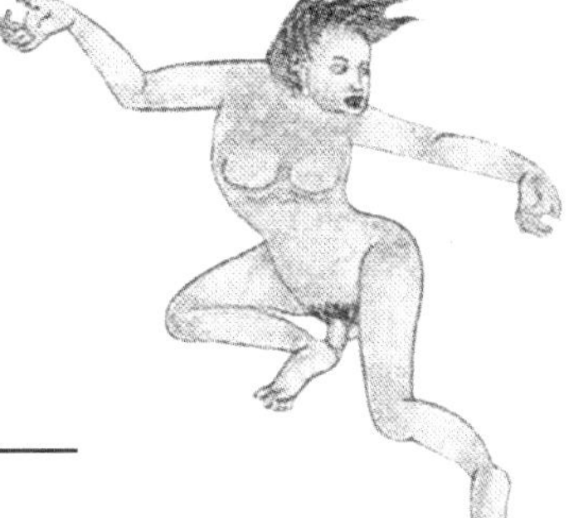

An epileptic patient dreams of dancing when drunk.

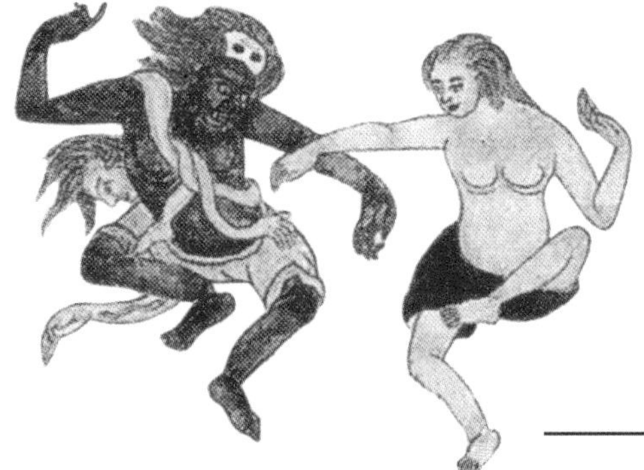

A manic patient dreams of dancing with a Yaksha.

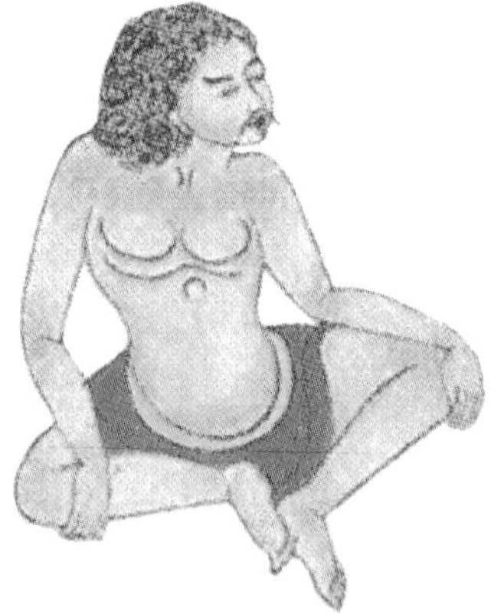

A blind patient dreams of the sun and moon falling onto the earth.

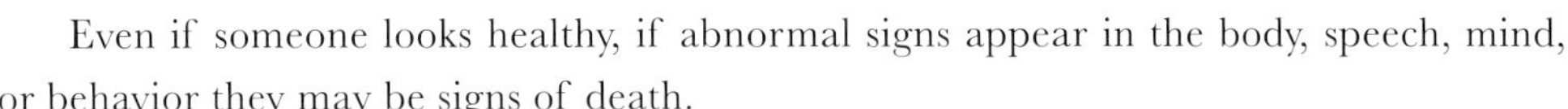

Signs of Death

Even if someone looks healthy, if abnormal signs appear in the body, speech, mind, or behavior they may be signs of death.

Signs of attitude

These are when someone begins to unreasonably hate their respected parents, teacher, relatives, or friends and is unwilling to communicate with them or avoids meeting them, hates the physician or medicine and refuses to accept treatment, hates the flavor or smell of medicine and throws away the bowl of medicine, or insults a physician with dirty language or throws him out of the home.

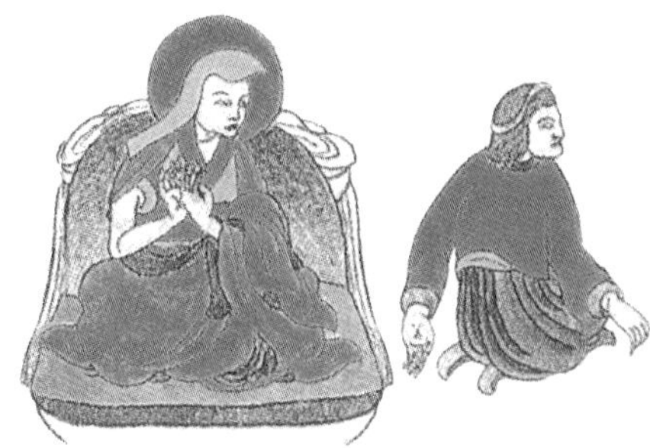

Hating Buddhist monks and relatives.

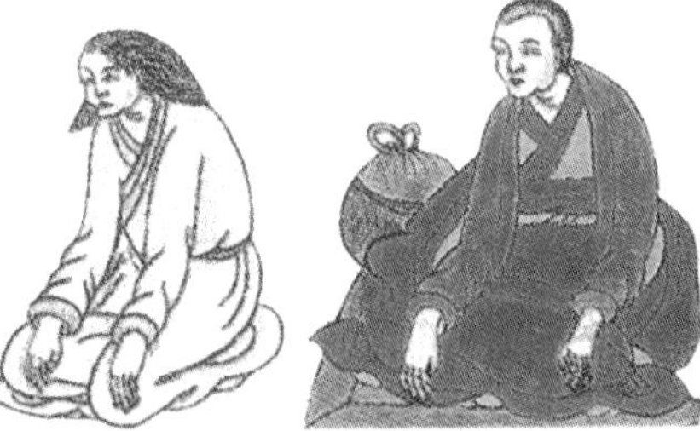

Unreasonable hate towards a physician or medicine.

When one's disposition and behavior changes from impatience to tenderness, and the body and facial appearance change from normal to unusual beauty, one becomes unusually irritable, estranged from one's relatives, but close to those he hates, a beautiful appearance becomes withered and dim, becomes uneasy, unreasonably enraged like a mad man, or willing to stay alone and refusing to communicate with others, these unusual behaviors are all signs of being on the verge of death.

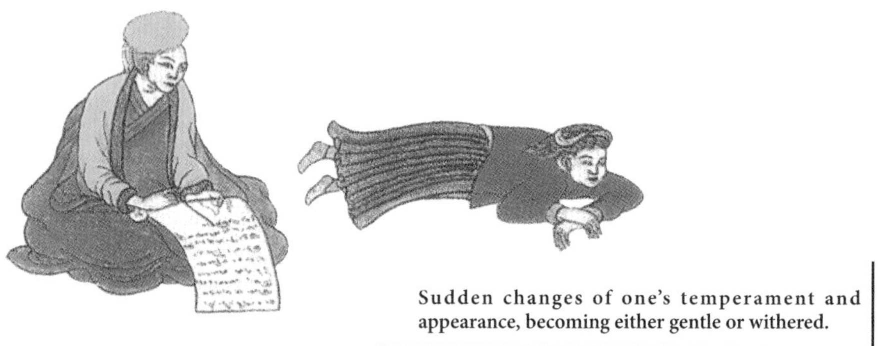

Sudden changes of one's temperament and appearance, becoming either gentle or withered.

All the following are signs of death.

A person is uneasy, always feels scared, or gives food that birds refuse to pick up.

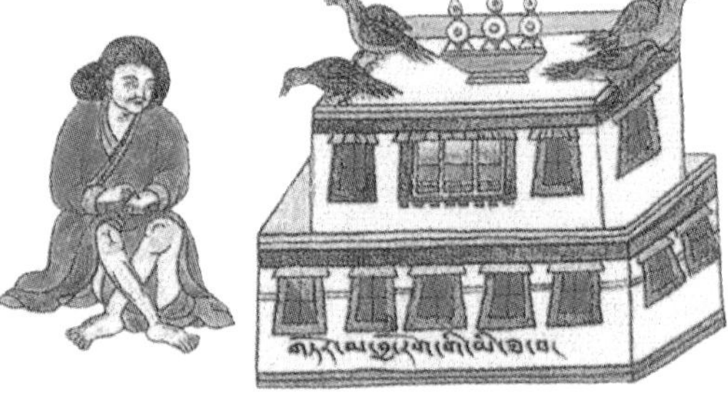

Crows refuse to take the food given.

When soaking in the bath, the area in front of the heart remains dry. Even when a drop of water is splashed on the area, it leaves no trace. When pressing the finger joints, no sounds can be heard.

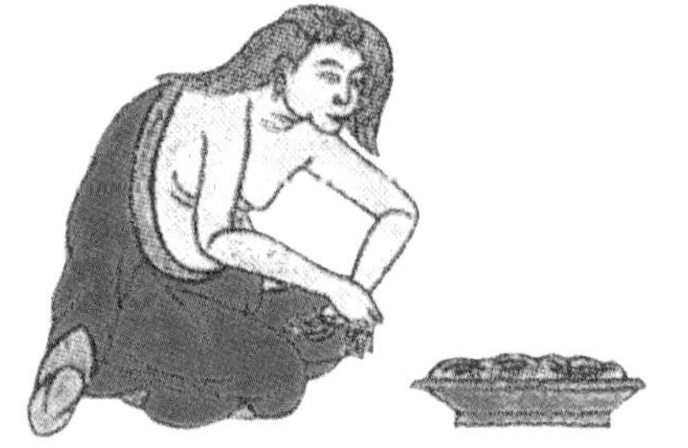

The chest stays dry while bathing.

The body gets weaker no matter how much nourishing food one eats. The body has a bad odor that can't be washed away even when rubbed with aromatics. Ticks, lice, and mites that originally lived off the body vanish suddenly or appear suddenly in large number in people who originally had none of such parasites.

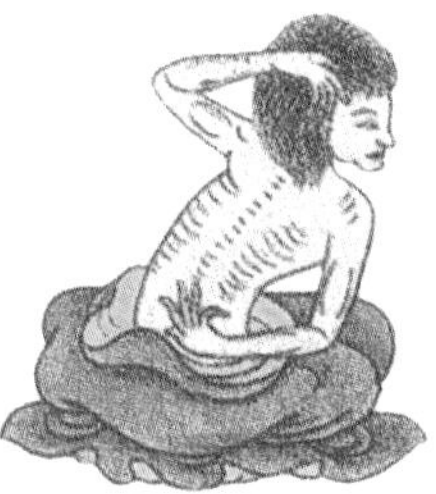

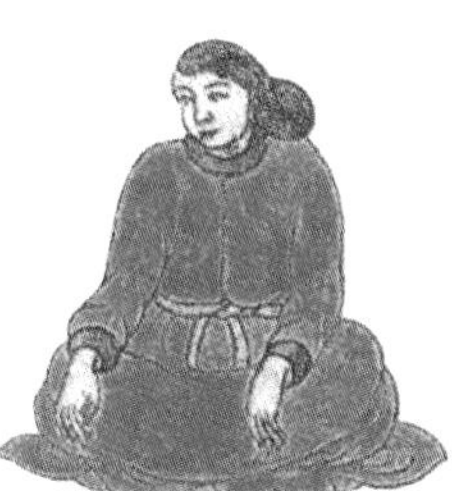

A sudden increase of body parasites
in great number or the sudden disappearance of parasites.

When under sunlight, no shadow can be seen. When looking into a mirror or water, no reflection appears, or only a blurred image like a thin gauze was covering the eyes. Double images may also appear, the image may seem like it is shaking even when the mirror or water is still, or the image may have defects such as a missing limb, deviated mouth, or white complexion. When there is strong sunlight a person stands with their back facing the sun so they can watch their shadow, and after a while they look at the sky and a vague image of themselves can be seen in the sky.

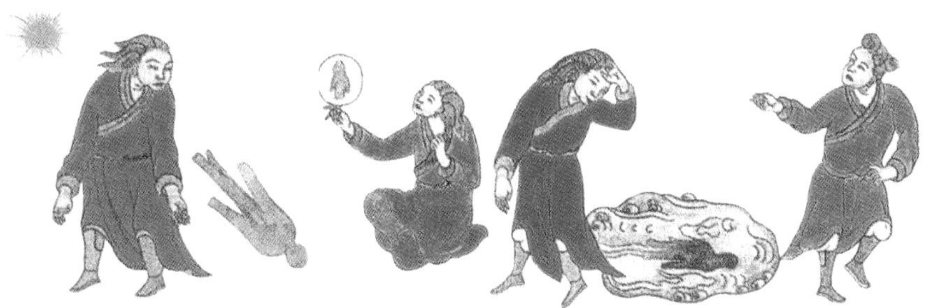

Incomplete shadows or reflections in water or mirrors.

In summary, if a person suddenly loses their ambition or hope, feels unreasonably tired of all things, is full of hatred, becomes worrisome, can't sleep even though they used to be lazy, becomes easily angered when originally they were kind or vice versa, or their image and shadow changes as explained above, they are going to die.

Near death signs

All the following signify a pending death.

Seeming like one has been poisoned despite not taking any poisonous substances, manifesting as foamy saliva or spontaneous bleeding from the orifices.

Forgetting what one said as soon as it is spoken, even if other people remind them.

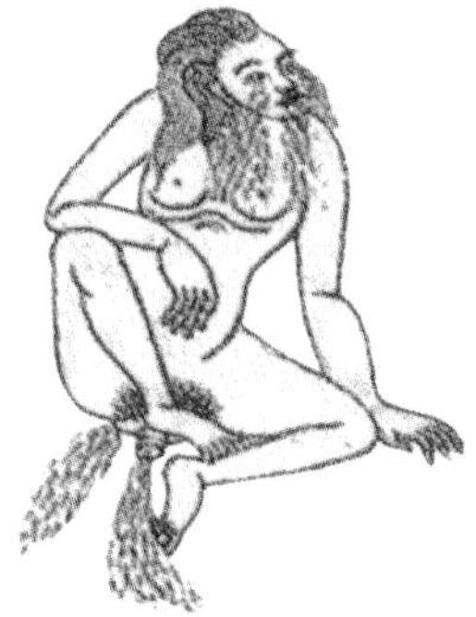

Spontaneous bleeding from the nine orifices.

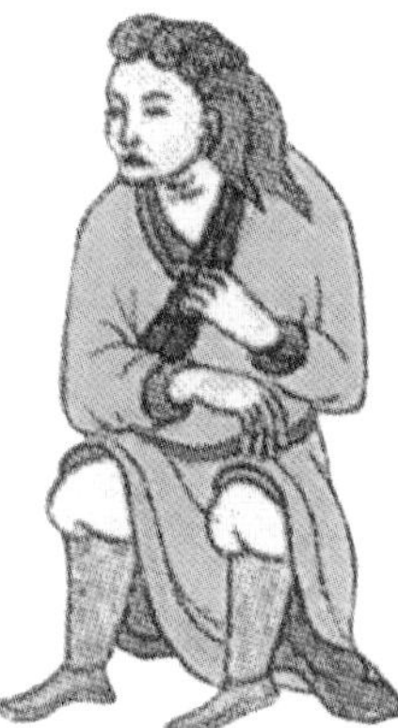

Forgetting what one has just said.

Retraction of the penis, prolapse of the scrotum or penis without any reason.

Retraction of the penis and prolapse of the scrotum.

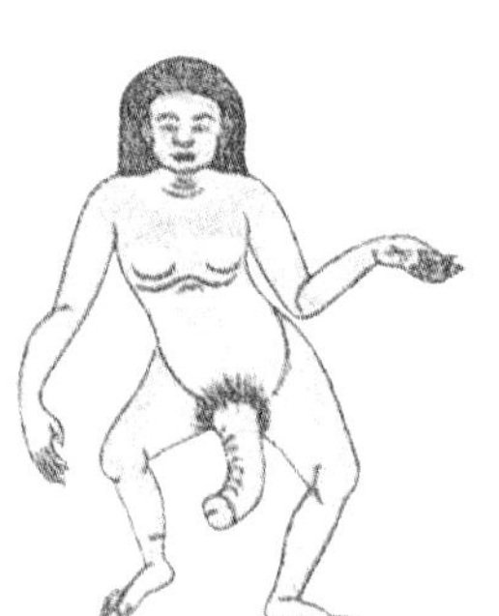

Prolapse of the penis and retraction of the scrotum.

Coughing or sneezing sounds very unusual, like a cock crowing.

Unable to smell an extinguished oil lamp even though the nose is not plugged and the lamp is just under one's nose.

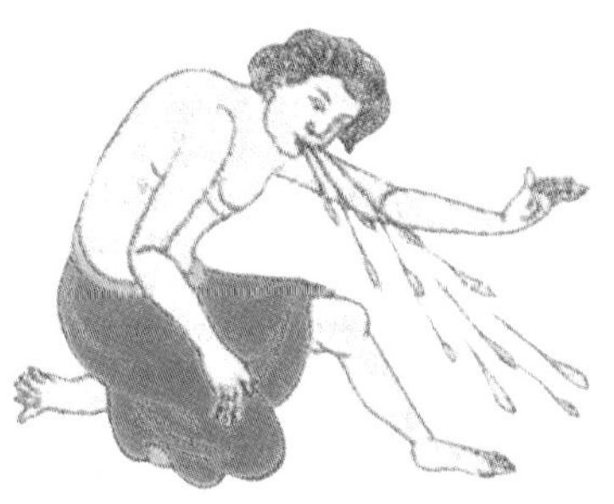

Unusual sound when sneezing or coughing.

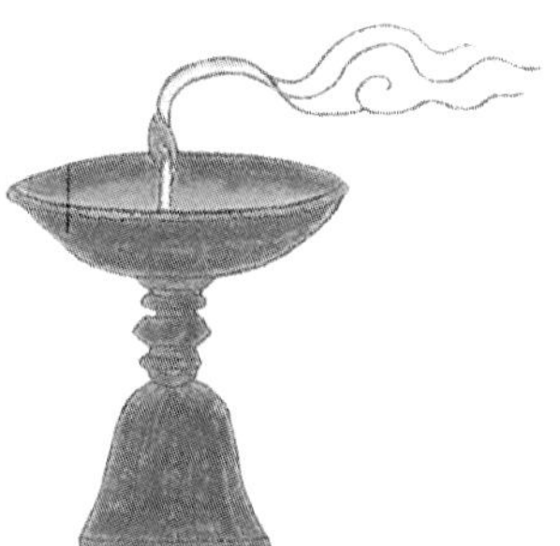

Unable to smell the smoke after an oil lamp is extinguished.

The top of the head is greasy even when no ointment is applied, or the hair has just been washed, dropping out of the eyebrows and hairs without realizing it, and the hair becoming very scanty, curly and rough. One feels nothing even when the head is touched by the hands.

Crescent patterns appear on the forehead or in the perineum, becoming more conspicuous day by day like an old person. During the day time heaven and hell are both visible, while during the night the Milky Way and the big dipper are invisible.

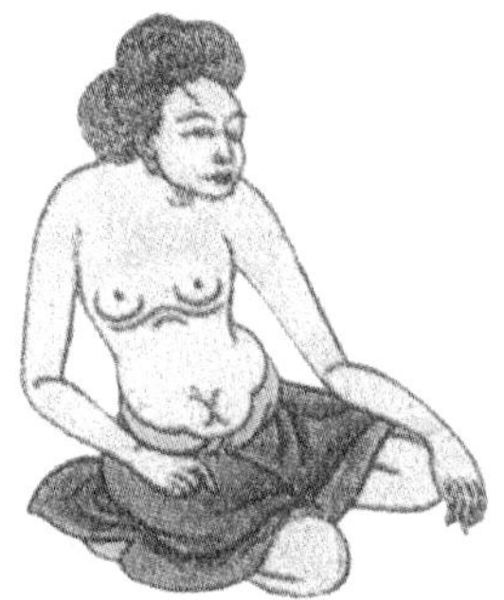

The top of the head is greasy.

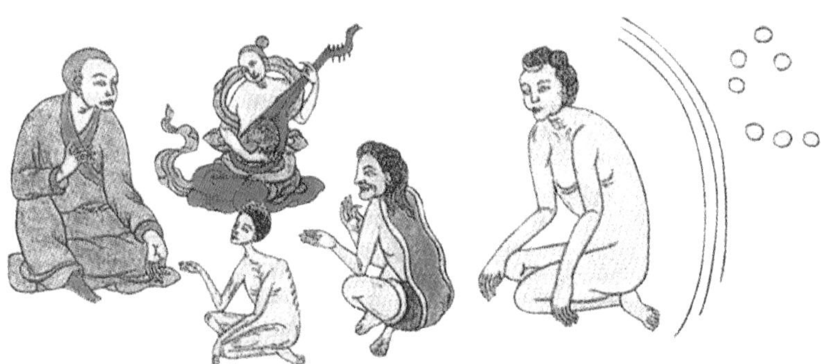

Crescent-shaped wrinkles on the forehead, appearance of heaven and hell in the daytime, and unable to see the Milky Way and the big dipper at night.

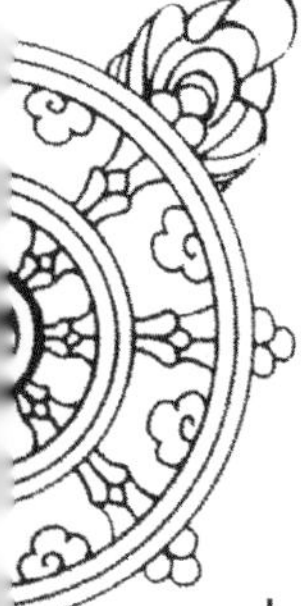

Dysfunction of the eyes, ears and body when they are not injured, with loss of the sense of hearing, smelling, tasting and touch. Sense disturbances like being unable to see a hand placed in the middle of the eyebrows, or the area between the eyes becoming deformed or broken. When the eyes are covered with the hand, no visual changes are noticed, and even when the eyes are opened no light can be seen. The eyes, like a scared rabbit, can't be closed. The eyes may be sunken with dim pupils, looking spiritless. The ears stick to the skull, and no sound can be heard after pressing on the ear.

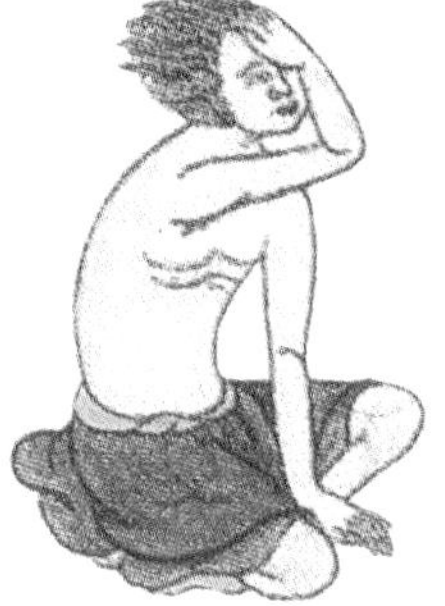

Nothing can be seen when putting the wrist on the space between the eyebrows.

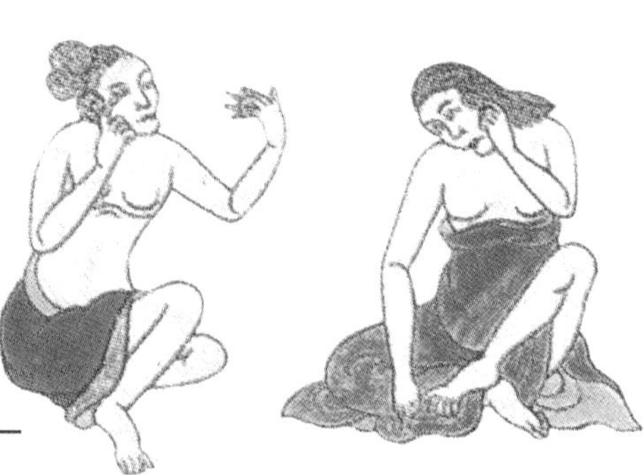

No sounds can be heard when pressing tightly against the ear.

After working hard or staying under the sun no sweat appears on the vertex, filth can be seen in the nose, the lower lip droops down and the upper lip turns upward with tartar-scum in between the teeth. The tongue becomes dark, dry and cracked, and the person will not want to drink even when they feels thirsty, the tongue can't move freely, causing unsmooth and incomprehensible speech, facial complexion looks like a layer of dust covers it that can't be washed away, and cool air is exhaled when panting.

The skin may be cool and rough, without luster, a hot sensation in the face with dizziness, or refusal to take warming medicines even when having contracted a cold disease, or vice versa. If the person can be convinced to take medicine, vomiting immediately follows. If the patient is treated with medication, manual treatments, dietary and lifestyle regulation, no effects are seen. However, treatment of reversed principles such as treating cold disease with cool drugs, and heat disease with warm drugs yields some effects and the condition can be ameliorated a little.

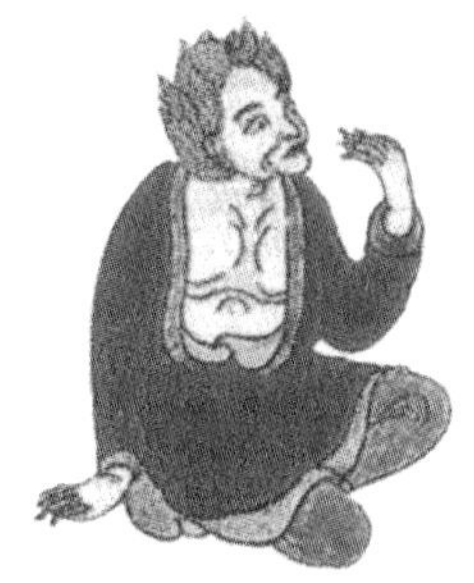

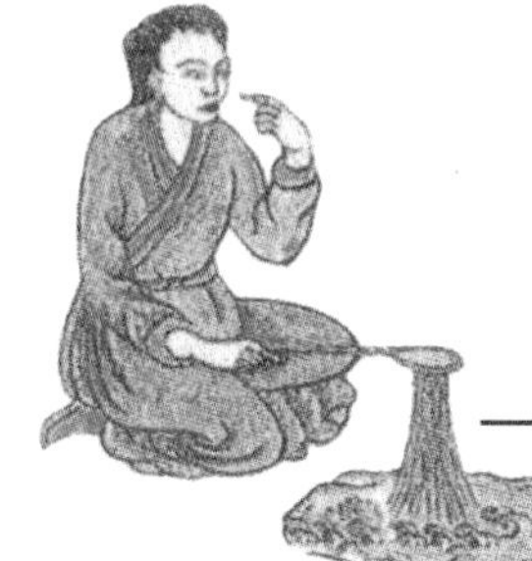

The nostrils are filthy inside and the tongue is dry and dark.

When all the above signs appear, death will come soon. However, some of the signs will not lead to death when treated correctly and the patient can even recover. This is because of all diseases caused by *rlung*, *mkhris pa*, and *badkan* there are many different manifestations. After the disease is cured the signs will also eventually disappear.

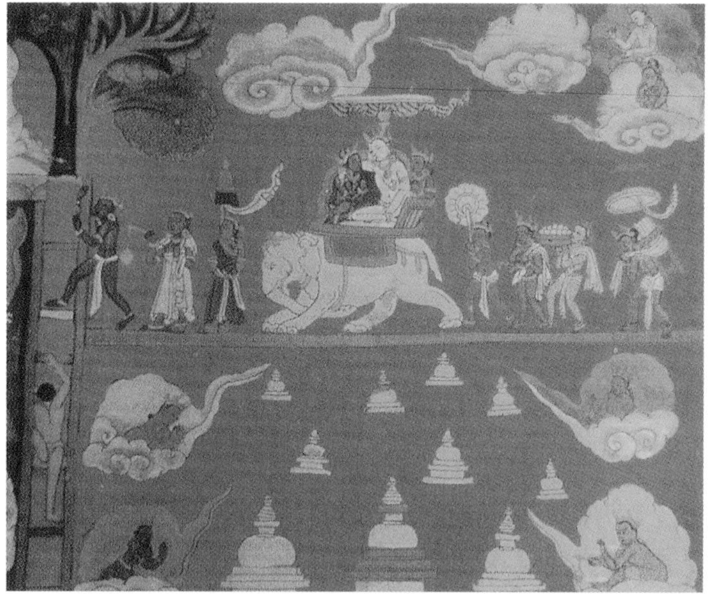

This picture is based on the legendary "celestial ladder," showing the image of an excellent life under Buddha's teachings. (part of a Tibetan mural).

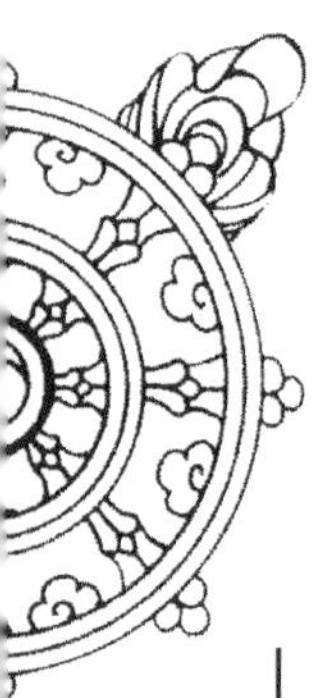

The End of Life

Generally speaking, after treatment when a patient is feeling better, all death signs should disappear. However, if a patient's condition improves, most of the symptoms vanish and the death signs still exist, the life is doomed. When the three vital sectors of energetic muscles, the ability to take food, and a beating pulse are withered and weak, death is pending.

Disappearance of the five sources

Blindness - when the function of earth is absorbed by water.

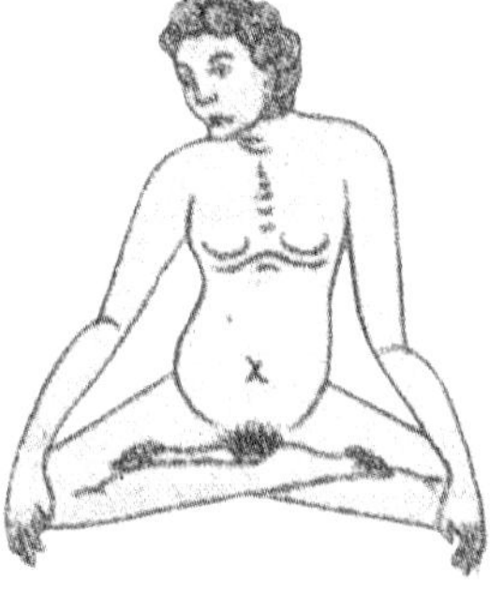

Withering of the nine orifices - when the function of water is absorbed by fire.

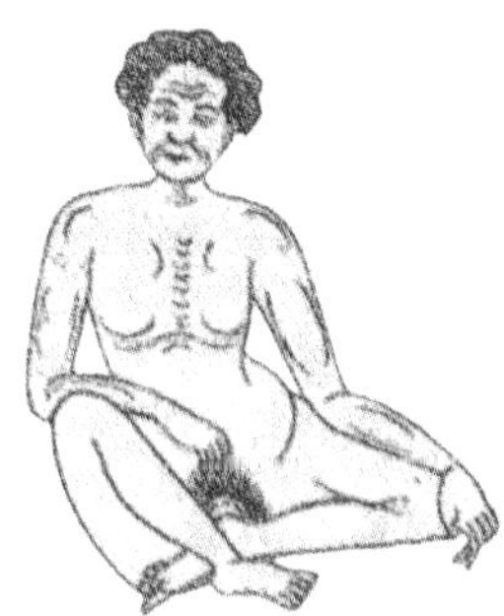

Lowering of body temperature - when the function of fire is absorbed by wind.

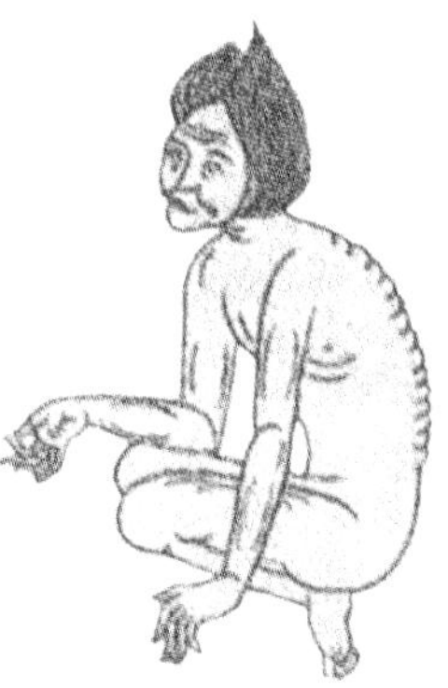

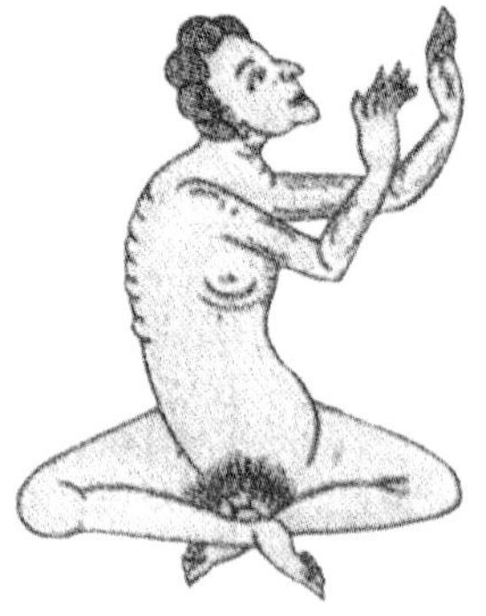

Interruption of breathing - when the function of wind is absorbed by space.

Life is built on the basis of the five sources: earth, water, fire, wind, and space. When the sources become gradually exhausted, the process of death begins.

When the function of earth is absorbed by water, there will be a loss of vision, from blurred vision to complete blindness.

When the function of water is absorbed by fire, manifestations are loss of moistening of the nine orifices, and their withering like trees in drought.

When the function of fire is absorbed by wind, manifestations include cool breathing and a lowering of body temperature.

When the function of wind is absorbed by space, there will be an interruption of breathing.

Disappearance of the five sense organs

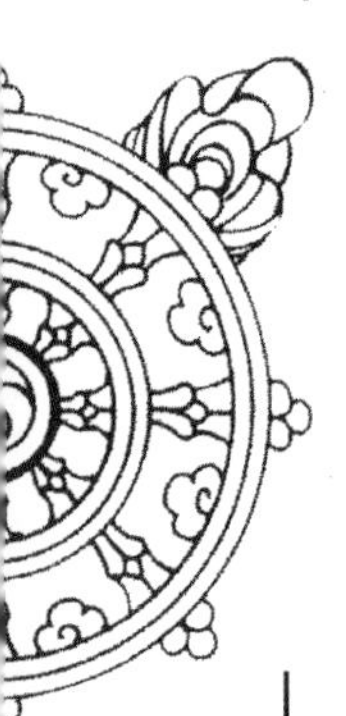

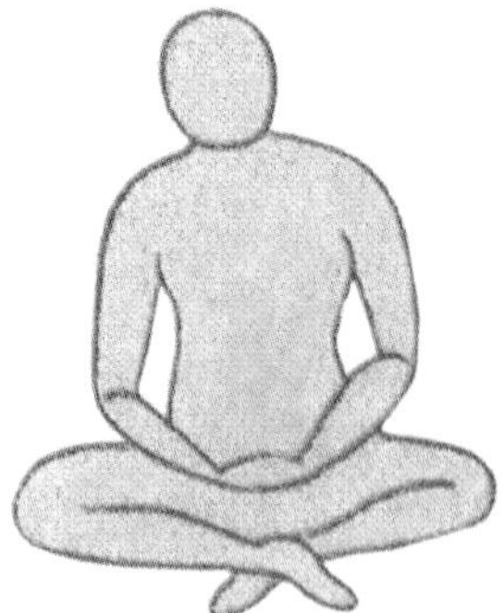

End of vision.

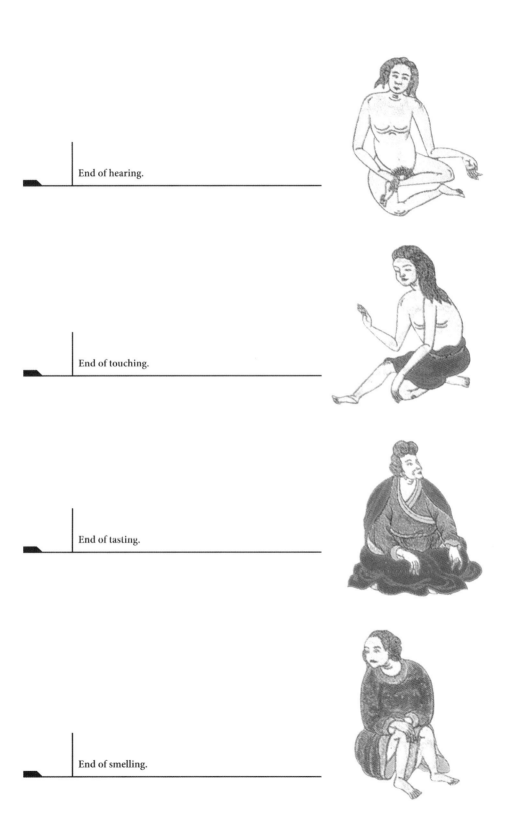

End of hearing.

End of touching.

End of tasting.

End of smelling.

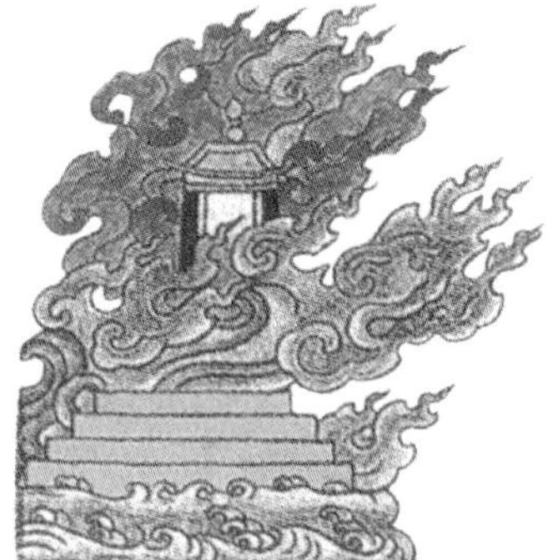

End of life.

The process of disappearance of the five sources is followed by the disappearance of the functions of the five sense organs.

When vision vanishes within hearing, the function of the eyes vanishes gradually from blurred vision to total blindness.

When hearing vanishes within smelling, the function of the ears vanishes gradually from vague hearing and inability to answer questions to a total loss of hearing.

When smelling vanishes within tasting, the function of the nose can't differentiate a foul stench from fragrance to a total loss of smell.

When tasting vanishes within touch, the function of the tongue vanishes gradually from unable to differentiate the various tastes until there is no more reaction to tastes.

Finally, when touch vanishes within the midst of life-preserving *rlung*, the sensation on the body surface also vanishes bit by bit until nothing can be perceived.

This is the end of life.

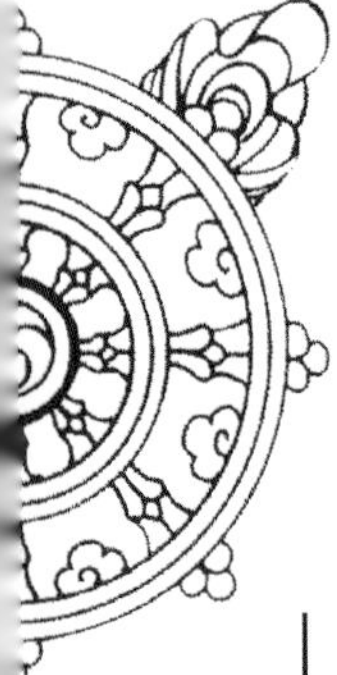

Birth, senility, disease, and death are natural processes quite similar to the transformation of four seasons of spring, summer, autumn and winter. Only when one cultivates their health and takes good care of their life can one live to the end of one's life without disease.

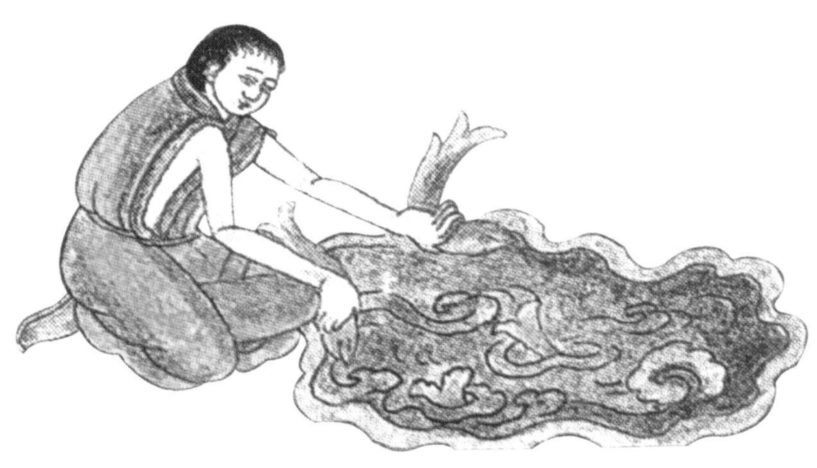

བཅུད་ལེན་གྱི་གཏམས་ངག

CHAPTER 9 HEALTH CULTIVATION ADVICE

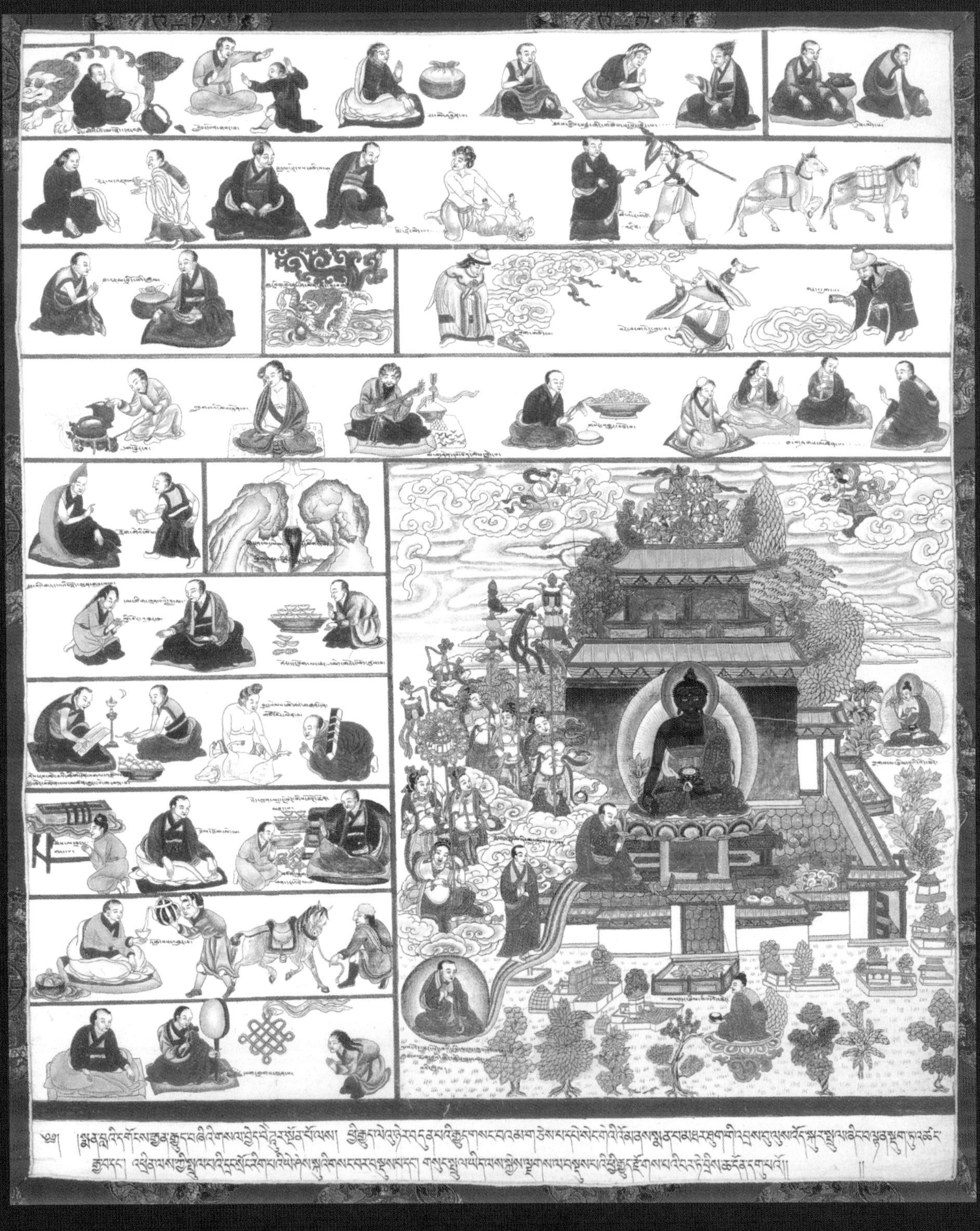

Thangka seventy-nine in the *Sman thang* series of *The Four Medical Tantras*: The Transmission and Heritage of *The Four Medical Tantras*

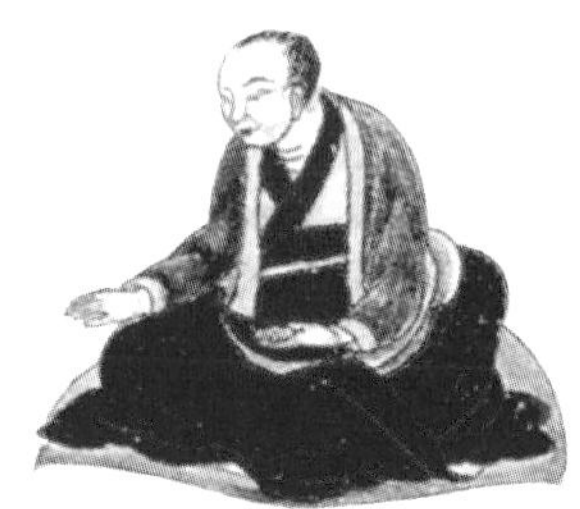

How can one assess the value of health cultivation during such a rapid thing as human life?

How can one summarize the true meaning of health cultivation within the constantly changing state between health and disease?

How can one reveal the secrets of health cultivation among the thousand threads between the universe and human life?

This is an ancient, eternal topic.

In the eighth century, *The Four Medical Tantras* was compiled. This great Tibetan medical work instructed the people on how to care for their lives. Its comments on the nature of health cultivation is a model for later generations. Like a bottle full of nectar, it gives health and wellbeing to the physical world.

The Development and History of *The Four Medical Tantras*

The history of Tibetan medicine is as long as the history of the Tibetan people.

Based on archeological findings, some 40,000 - 50,000 years ago humans began to live on the Qinghai-Tibet plateau. From this point, knowledge and experience about health cultivation gradually accumulated. By examining historical artifacts from about three thousand years ago, it can be seen that the ancestors of the Tibetan people already had knowledge of how to maintain health and prevent disease, creating a foundation for the maturity of Tibetan medicine in later generations.

Before the compilation of *The Four Medical Tantras*

During the second half of the 6th century AD, the powerful lord Darbu Nesie of the Southern Mountain region became strong. His son and successor, Namri Srongtsan, was well respected by several clans as a *tsanpo*, meaning a powerful king. Also during this period medical arts and astrology was imported from China.

Srongtsan Gampo, the son of Namri Srongtsan, later unified Tibet and showed extraordinary ability and wisdom in ruling the territory. He reformed and unified the written Tibetan language and supported the spread of Buddhism and its related culture. The spread of medicine was also a part of the spread of Buddhism.

In 641 AD, Srongtsan Gampo proposed a marriage between his kingdom and the Tang emperor of China. The Tang emperor approved and Princess Wencheng was sent to Tibet to be the king's wife. She carried with her many treasures and knowledge from the advanced Tang culture, including many medical books. As recorded in the *Mani Instructions*, Princess Wencheng carried with her, "Information and medicinal materials for the treatment of the four hundred and four kinds of diseases, the eight kinds of observations, the fifteen kinds of diagnostics, and another four medical works." The texts were translated and compiled as the medical work that now goes by the name *Sman dpyad chen mo (A Complete Book of Medicine)*, which is the earliest known medical classic in Tibetan medicine. This work is, unfortunately, lost.

Srongtsan Gampo also invited many physicians from neighboring regions and nations to educate Tibetan doctors on advanced medical techniques. Of them, three notable physicians came from India, Tazig, and China. A comprehensive seven-volume work called *Mi 'jigs pa*

mtshon cha (The Fearless Weapon) was compiled under the cooperation of these three physicians. This second medical classic of Tibetan medicine has also been lost.

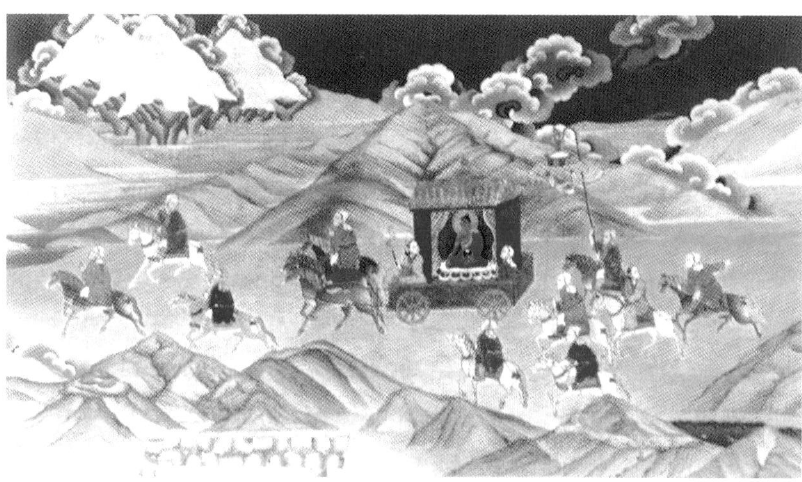

It is said that when Princess Wencheng entered Tibet she brought information and medicinal substances on four hundred and four kinds of diseases, eight observation methods, and fifteen kinds of diagnostics (a part of an illustration showing Princess Wencheng entering Tibet for marriage).

In the 8th century, King Khride Tsugtan again requested marriage with a member of the Tang imperial family. In 710 AD, Princess Jincheng entered Tibet and also brought with her a large number of medical works, techniques, and doctors. Under the common effort of Chinese Buddhist monk-physicians and Tibetan translators, another comprehensive medical work was compiled, the *Sman dpyad zla ba'i rgyal po (The Medical Investigation of the Lunar King)*. This is presently the earliest extant medical work of Tibet.

The birth of *The Four Medical Tantras*

The eight century saw a great leap forward for Tibetan medicine. In 755, Khrisrong Sdetsan, the son of Khride Tsugtan, became a *tsanpo* who gave great importance to medicine and invited many physicians to Tibet, including the Chinese physician Dongsum Gangwa, the Indian physician Sendi Garpa, Haracendi from Tazig, and Darmashila from Nepal. In addition, the Buddhist monks Jingxu and Sengneng also came to contribute. These physicians, scholars, and monks worked together to translate and write many medical works that were compiled together as *The Purple Book of Royal*

Healthcare. After their work, all the foreign physicians returned home safely, which was not easy in those days. Not long later, King Khrisrong Detsan became ill and again invited physicians from many different countries to come and treat him. This time, only Dongsum Gangwa of China accepted the invitation. Dongsum not only cured the King's disease, but also presented the King with a medical book called *The Purple Beacon Light for Therapy*. The King was overjoyed and granted the physician the title Tazi Dongsum Gangwa, indicating that the physician was a model physician for the four directions. The doctor was also granted two manors and chose to remain in Tibet for the rest of his life.

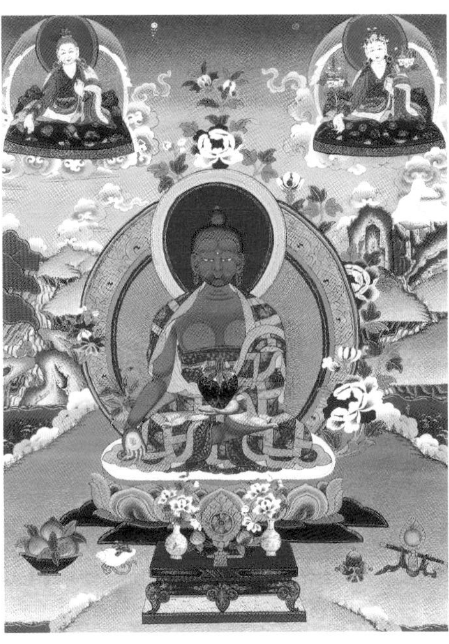

On the upper right of the image is Gyuthog Sningma Yontan Ganpo, author of *The Four Medical Tantras* (also known as old Gyuthog). On the upper left is the 13th generation descendant of old Gyuthog, Gyuthog Gsarma Yontan Ganpo (known as new Gyuthog). In the center is the Medicine Buddha.

The King decided to spread Dongsum's healing techniques throughout his kingdom and summoned nine excellent young men to follow Dongsum as his disciples. Under the instructions of Dongsum, the disciples became famous physicians. Among them, Gyuthog Yontan Gonpo became the most well known.

Gyuthog was born in a family whose members had been physicians for generations. The influence of his family, his natural talent, hard work, and bold style of practice all contributed to his great skill. Under the instructions of his famous mentor, he learned from all the medical works and traveled to neighboring countries and regions to study. To record his great knowledge, he wrote *The Four Medical Tantras* at the end of the 8th century. This work has become the most influential medical classic of Tibetan medicine and lays the foundation of medical practice.

The dissemination and development of *The Four Medical Tantras*

In the 9th century, the native religion of Tibet, Bon, struggled against the increasing influence of Buddhism. Eventually, during the reign of Darma Tsanpo (838-842 AD), a large scale campaign against Buddhism was carried out and many books and artifacts were destroyed. Since the content in *The Four Medical Tantras* was strongly linked to the teachings of Buddha, monks and lay Buddhists secretly kept it and other Buddhist sutras safely hidden. Because of this time of unrest, *The Four Medical Tantras* was not circulated immediately after it was compiled. It remained buried under ground for a considerable amount of time before it was safe enough to distribute publicly.

As soon as Buddhism was safely established in the Ngari region during the Guge dynasty, the buried sutras were unearthed and distributed. *The Four Medical Tantras* was also recovered during this period. Eventually, it was given to new Gyuthog (Gyuthog Gsarma, 1126-1202 AD), who made substantial revisions and supplements. The presently used version of *The Four Medical Tantras* is, in fact, the version that was revised by him and many later physicians. For this reason he is now knows as "The secular medical king."

In the 14th century, some important scholars appeared in Tibet, the most influential ones from the Northern Byang School and the Southern Zur School. They interpreted *The Four Medical Tantras* from different angles. The Southern School criticized the hypothesis that the text came from Buddhist teachings as was advocated by the Northern School, claiming that *The Four Medical Tantras* is a medical work written by Tibetan physicians themselves through long-term practice and study. This viewpoint was very influential and was especially respected by later scholars of Tibetan medicine.

In the 16th century the fifth Dalai Lama of the Gadan dynasty strongly encouraged the development of science and culture. His Regent Sde srid Sanggyas Gyatsho (1653-1705) paid special attention to the heritage of *The Four Medical Tantras*. By this time, the text of this classic had received many commentaries, some of which were archaic, some that were secret, and many that were contradictory. He collected various versions and checked them very carefully. He also summoned many doctors from different areas to discuss the text and finally reached an agreement on a thorough revision, supplementation, and annotation. At last, they rewrote the classic and included many popular texts. The published version was titled *Baidurya sngon po (Blue Lapis Lazuli).*

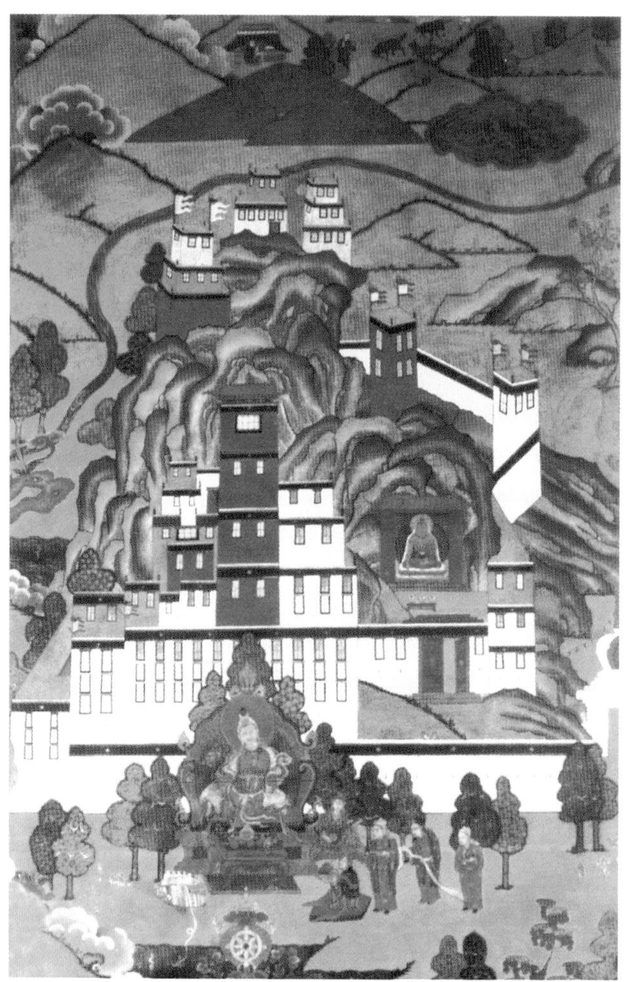

The Lcag-po-ri near Potala Palace is the academic center of modern Tibetan medicine (illustration of the ancient Lcag-po-ri).

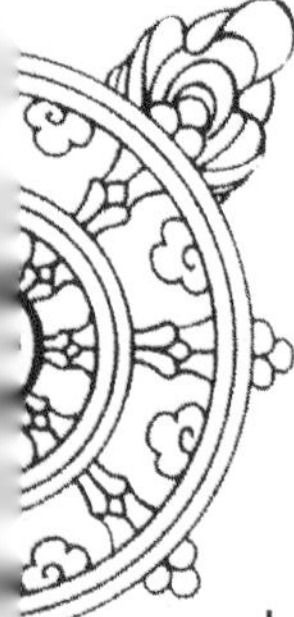

Not long later after the death of Sanggyas Gyatsho, an important Tibetan pharmacological book appeared called *Shel gong shel phreng (Crystal Materia Medica)*, which discussed 2,294 kinds of medicines and is both based on and develops the medicinal knowledge in *The Four Medical Tantras*. It became the most influential pharmacological text in Tibetan medicine. It preserves the essence of ancient Tibetan medicine so that medical experience can be preserved, and offers the broad arena for later physicians to improve their practice. It can be said that the history of Tibetan medicine is the history of the development of *The Four Medical Tantras*.

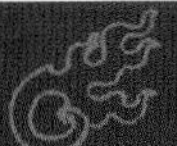

A Summary of Health Cultivation

In the *Phyi ma rgyud* (*Conclusion Tantra*), the Wise Sage (Vidyajnana) summarizes the root problems of health and disease, and answers the question of Sage Manasija by saying, "Oh! Sage Manasija! A popular saying goes that a fully drawn bow attempts to hit the target, and the planting of crops is for daily food. Although there are various professions, all workers expect good results. Similarly, *The Four Medical Tantras*, though very extensive, can be summarized as addressing only two conditions, health and disease".

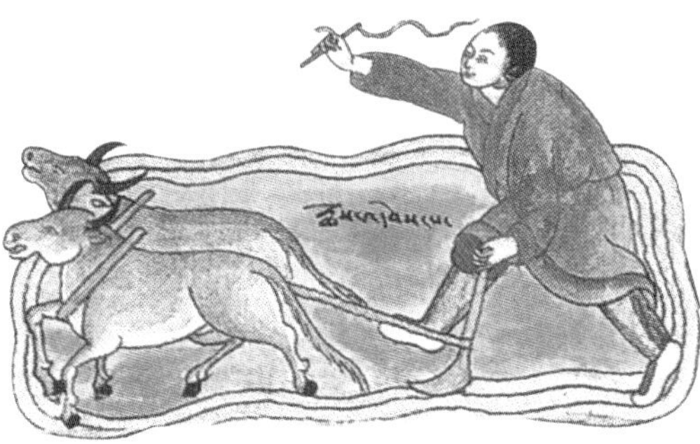

Farmers work for a living throughout the four seasons.

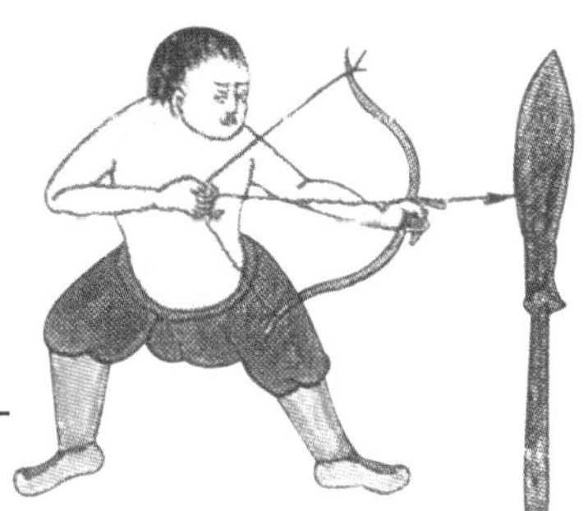

An arrow shot by fully drawn bow is bound to hit the target.

The two conditions of life

Sage Vidyajnana's answer is clear and simple. It explains not only the basic purpose of writing *The Four Medical Tantras*, and introduces the two conditions of health and disease, towards which all medical activities and health cultivation habits are directed. This makes the starting point clear and definite.

The first problem is how to protect health when one has it. Even when the body is healthy, one must pay attention to daily habits, including regular living, adequate work, and adequate nutrition with frequent bathing.

If one falls ill, then it is important to know how to treat the disease and how to recover. Diseases are many and so are their manifestations, but they can also be classified into two categories, hot and cold. No matter the conditions, timely diagnosis and comprehensive therapy is necessary. There are 1,200 different methods of diagnosis, but they can be categorized into only three methods: inspection, questioning and palpation. Life or death can be determined by palpation; hot and cold by inspection; and the cause by questioning.

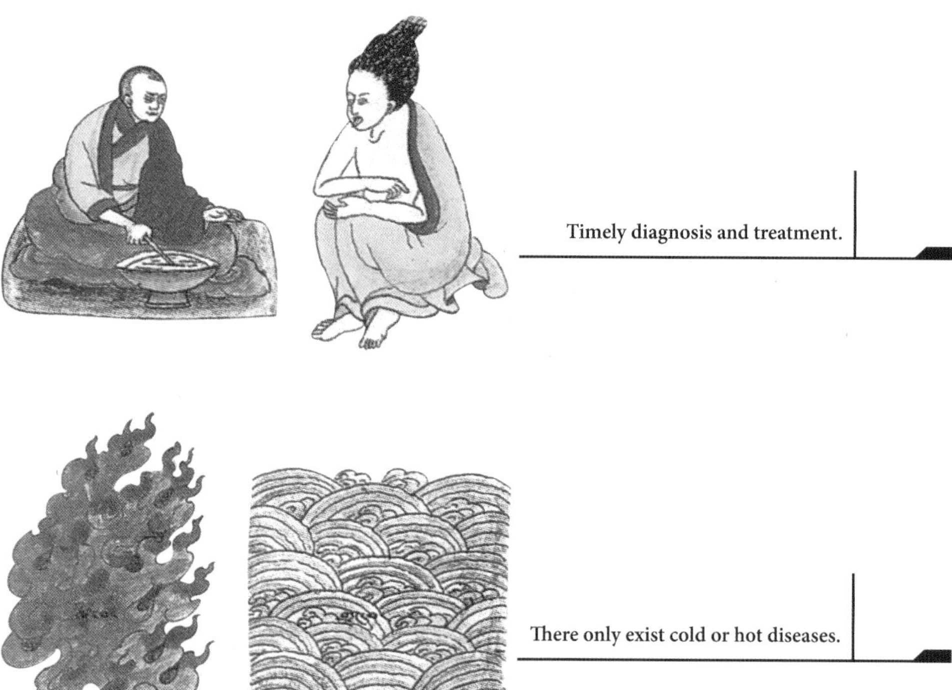

Timely diagnosis and treatment.

There only exist cold or hot diseases.

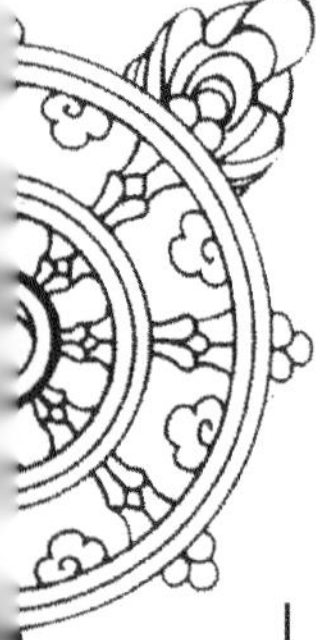

There are 1,003 approaches in the treatment of disease. But all of these methods fall under four basic methods: medication, external therapies, diet, and lifestyle. Medicine can be divided into two groups, calming and clearing. The former group has two kinds, hot and cold; the latter group also has two kinds, mild and drastic. For external therapies there are rough and moist types; for diet there are beneficial and harmful practices. For lifestyle, one must pay attention to strong and gentle habits. "There are 360 methods, which include diagnostic, therapeutic and treatment methods."

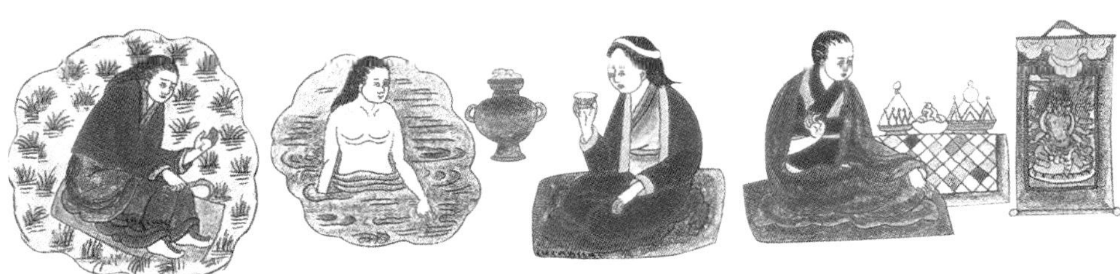

Adequate labor, bathing, nourishment and draining.

The connection between health and disease

Tibetan medicine claims that the five sources (earth, water, fire, wind and space) are the most important factors that form the body. *The Four Medical Tantras* say, "If the five sources are incomplete, there will be no fertility. A lack of earth and water will lead to the body being unable to be formed. In the absence of fire, the body won't mature; in the absence of wind, the body won't develop, and in the absence of space, there will be no room for development." "By the nature of earth, the muscles, bones, nose and smell of the fetus are developed. By the nature of water, the blood, tongue and taste of the fetus can be developed. By the nature of fire, the body temperature, complexion, and eyes of the fetus are developed. By the nature of wind, breathing and the sense of touch of the fetus can be developed. By the nature of space, the ear and voice of the fetus are developed".

Similarly, what harms the body is also derived from the five sources. *The Four Medical Tantras* says, "All creatures have the ability to live happily. But due to unclear reasons, they can't be separated from disease. These unclear reasons lead to greed, anger and ignorance, which, in turn, produce disasters of *rlung*, *mkhris pa* and *badkan*." "When the five sources are used up and disappear, it is a sign of death. When the action of earth is absorbed by water, one can't see; when that of water is absorbed by fire, the nine orifices are exhausted; when that of fire is absorbed by wind, the body temperature will drop; when that of wind is absorbed by space, the breathing will be interrupted." In summary, life comes from five sources, and so does disease.

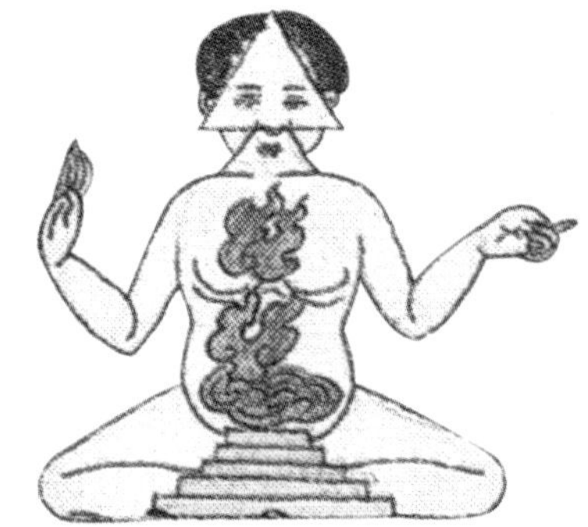

Life comes from the five sources.

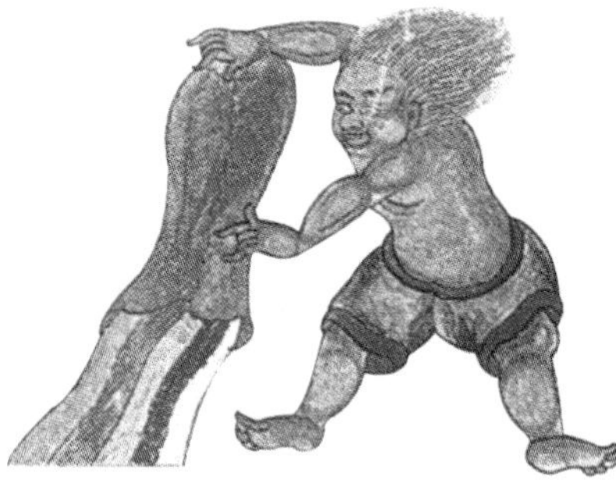

Diseases come from the five sources.

All medicine also comes from the five sources. Earth is the root of medicinal growth; water's moisture is also necessary for growth; the heat of fire supports growth; wind's activity makes medicine move; and space provides room for growth and movement. Also, the tastes of medicine come from different combinations of the five sources. In *The Four Medical Tantras* it says, "When earth and water predominate, the sweet taste is born; when fire and earth predominate, the sour taste is born; when water and fire predominate, the salty taste is born; when water and wind predominate, the bitter taste is born; when fire and wind predominate, the spicy taste is born; when earth and wind predominate, the astringent taste is born."

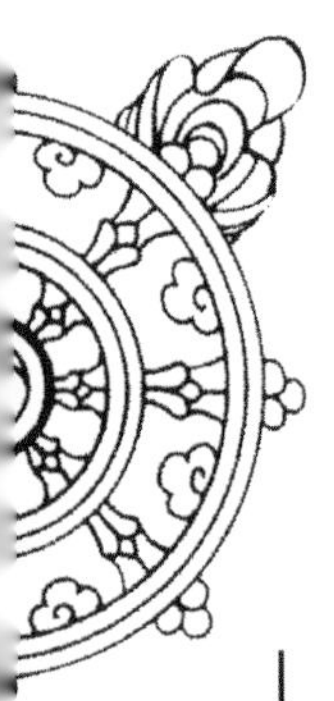

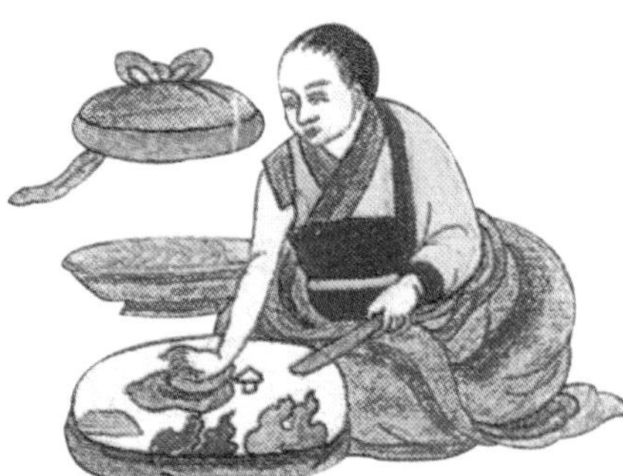

Medicine comes from the five sources.

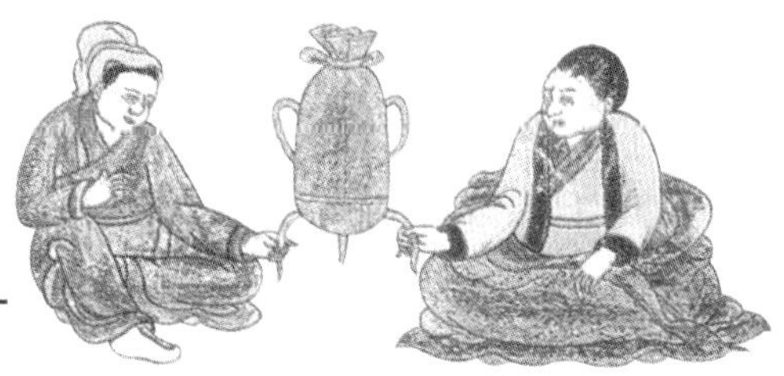

Coexistence of human beings and medicine.

Since life, disease, and medicine all come from the five sources, by the various natures, actions and tastes of different medicines, disharmonies among the three factors (i.e. disease) can be rectified to treat disease.

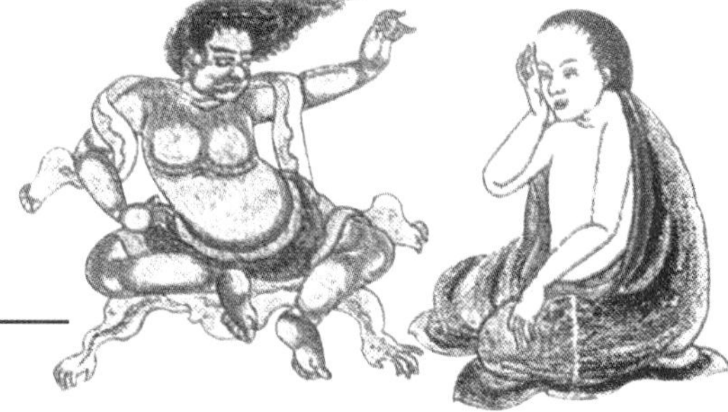

Coexistence of health and disease.

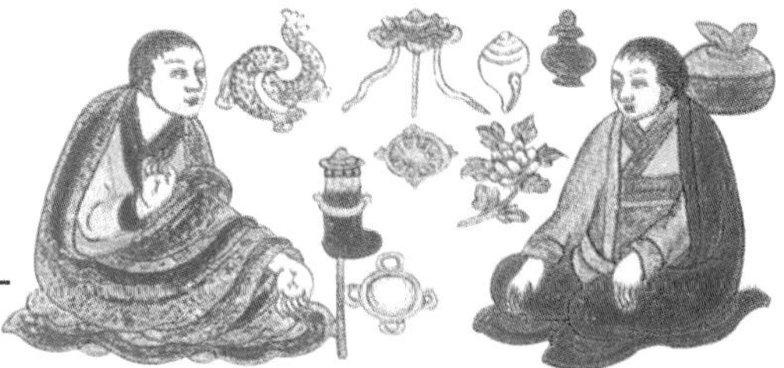

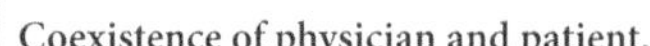

Coexistence of physician and patient.

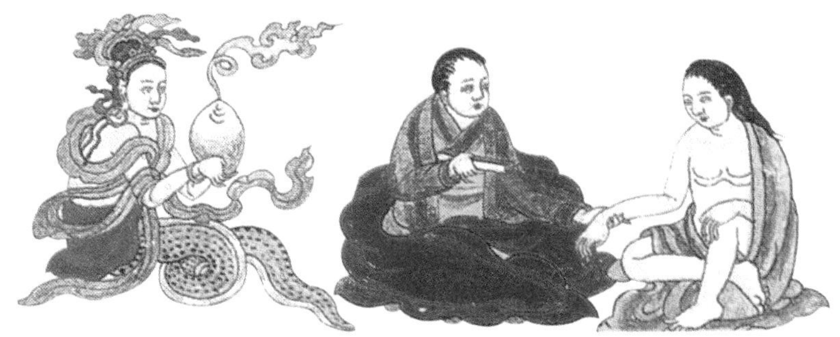

Coexistence of fate and fortune.

In summary, medicine and the body are mutually connected and health and disease also coexist. Based on the recognition of the above, if the communication between the physician and the patient and the selection of medicine are both appropriate, medicine can restore harmony among the three factors. It is by this approach that auspicious fate and wellbeing are achieved, and hope is acquired.

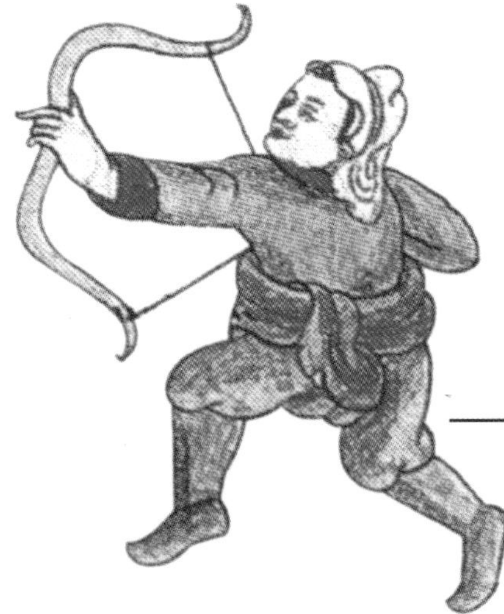

The recovery of harmony among the three factors leads to a healthy body.

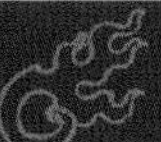 The Four Medical Tantras

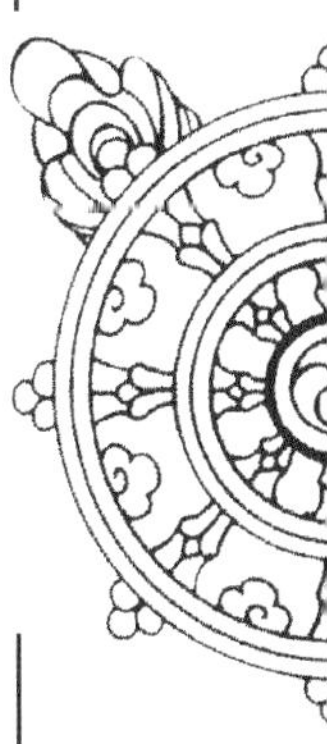

As the most important work in Tibetan medicine, *The Four Medical Tantras* creates the foundation for the academic system of Tibetan medicine. Since the 8th century, physicians have annotated and developed this medical classic, pushing Tibetan medicine to new frontiers. Numerous other classic works were created in later times, but physicians of these later generations view *The Four Medical Tantras* as the sun and anything that came afterward as the stars.

In the 17th century, based on *Baidurya sngon po (Blue Lapis Lazuli)*, the teaching scrolls of *Sman thang* were born. These scrolls annotate the rich contents of *The Four Medical Tantras* in a unique way, and perfectly combine Tibetan medicine and the painting. They are still regarded as a glory in the history of world medicine.

What do *The Four Medical Tantras* say?

The Four Medical Tantras consist of four parts: the *Root Tantras*, *Description Tantras*, *Secrecy Tantras*, and *Conclusion Tantras*.

There are six chapters in the *Root Tantras*, which is the general introduction that introduces the fundamental system of Tibetan medicine. It uses an allegorical tree to introduce physiology, pathology, treatment, health cultivation and an introduction to diagnosis and treatment.

The *Description Tantras* deal with the development of the embryo, internal organs, internal and external causes of disease, daily life, the nature, taste and effects of medicinals, surgical instruments, and a chapter dealing with the proper conduct of a physician.

The *Secrecy Tantras* introduce the etiology, symptoms, and treatment of diseases of the heart, liver, spleen, lung, kidney, large intestine, small intestine, male and female genital organs, diseases of the five sense organs, miscellaneous internal diseases, skin diseases, surgical diseases, children's diseases, and gynecological diseases. This is the encyclopedia of clinical medicine.

The *Conclusion Tantras* introduce all therapeutic and diagnostic approaches, including pulse examination, urinalysis, and the different forms of giving medicinals, such as boiling, powders and all other therapeutic methods, such as emesis and purging.

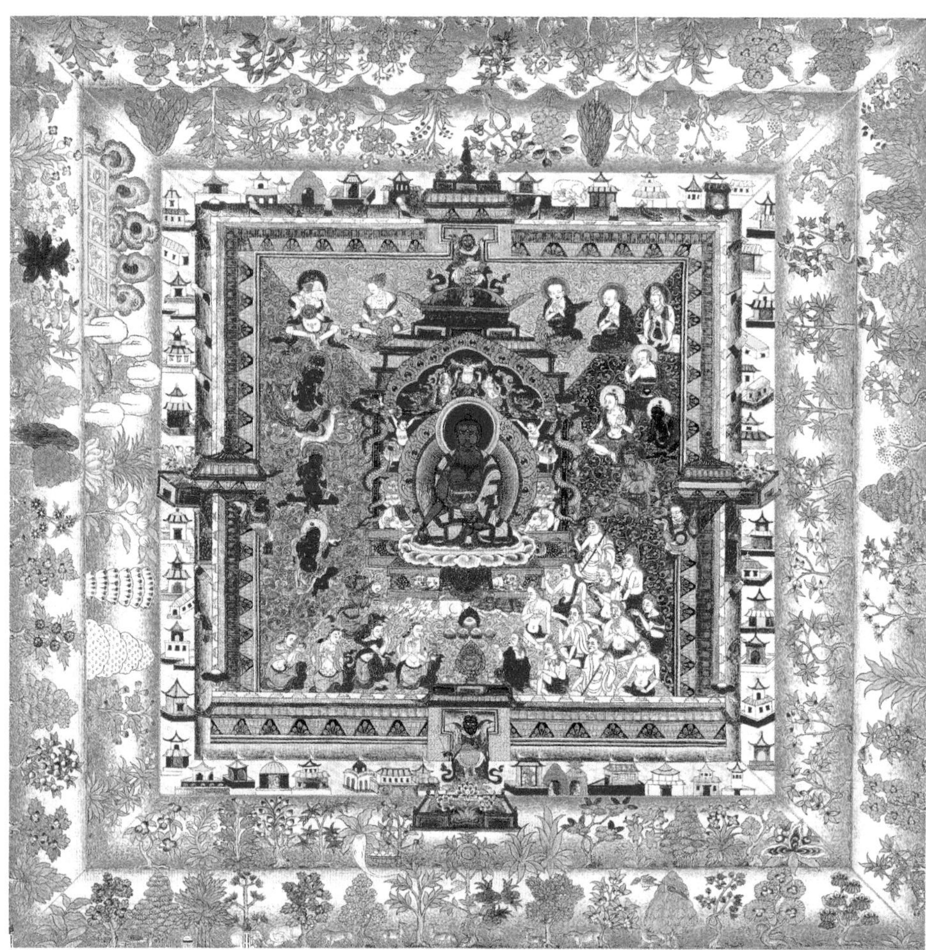

A picture of the Lta-na-sdugs painted on the basis of *Root Tantras* of *The Four Medical Tantras* (*Thangkha* one in the *Sman thang* series of the *The Four Medical Tantras*).

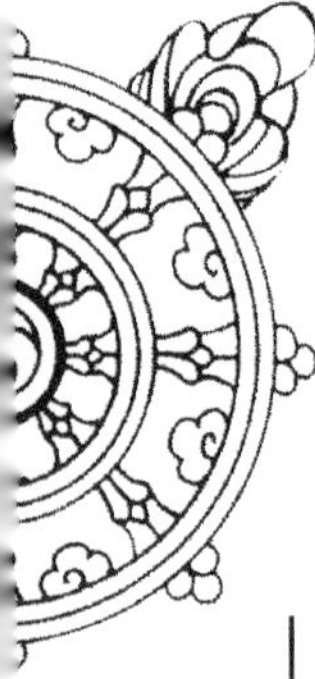

Based on the above description, it is clear that *The Four Medical Tantras* is a fundamental work that embraces all aspects of Tibetan medicine. After its compilation, Khrisrong Detsan treated it as a treasure and buried it in the Samye Monastery until Tsaba Ngonshe found it in the 12th century. Physicians of later ages respected it as a classic. Tsaba Ngonshe gave it to the 13th generation grandson of old Gyuthog, the Gyuthog Gsarma who made a thorough revision and supplement with detailed annotations. After that the classic was finalized into the present version of *The Four Medical Tantras*.

The treasure of Tibetan medicine, the *Sman thang*

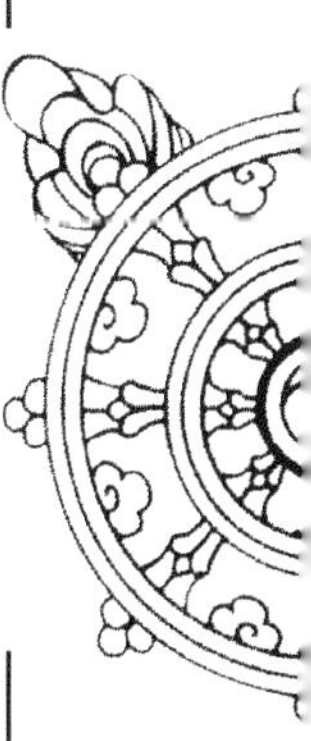

Sman thang is a transliteration from Tibetan language in which *sman* refers to medicine, while *thang*, or *thangkha*, means a "hanging painted scroll." In other words, *Sman thang* is a medical painting.

The whole series of *Sman thang* is based on the text of *Baidurya sngon po* (*Blue Lapis Lazuli*), supplemented with some contents from *Sman dpyad zla ba'i rgyal po* (*The Medical Investigation of the Lunar King*). All the paintings in this series are basically the same size, roughly 30-43 cm × 90-100 cm. There are altogether eighty paintings in the series.

Thangkha one is the legendary city of the Medicine Buddha (Lta-na-sdugs). *Thangkha* two to four are based on the *Root Tantras* and deal with the physiology, anatomy, pathology, diagnostics and basic principles of treatment; *Thangkha* five is about the development of the embryo; *Thangkha* six to eighteen deal with the vessels, organs, blood letting points, vital points and physiological characteristics based on the *Description Tantras; Thangkha* nineteen to twenty deal with the signs of death; *Thangkha* twenty-one to twenty-four deal with the causes of disease and good and bad habits in daily life and diet; *Thangkha* twenty-five to thirty-five all deal with medicinal substances; *Thangkha* thirty-six to thirty-eight deal with the methods and principles of treatment; *Thangkha* thirty-nine deals exclusively with the proper conduct of a physician; *Thangkha* forty to forty-one deal with the points for moxibustion, acupuncture and blood letting; *Thangkha* forty-two to forty-eight deal with the cause of diseases; Thangkha forty-nine to fifty-two deal with the body structure in a more detailed way; *Thangkha* fifty three deals with the source of toxins; *Thangkha* fifty-four to fifty-five deal with the methods of health cultivation; *Thangkha* fifty-six to sixty-nine deal with diagnostics in detail; Thangkha seventy to seventy-six deal with all sorts of therapeutic methods; *Thangkha* seventy-seven to seventy-nine deal with Tibetan medicine in general and the significance of *The Four Medical Tantras*. The last *thangkha* deals with important figures throughout the history of Tibetan medicine.

As mentioned by Sanggyas Gyatsho, his goal in painting the *Sman thang* series is, "To render the *The Four Medical Tantras* popular and easily understood, for both the academic circle and the young novices that learn Tibetan medicine, we have prepared this series of medical wall hangings. Through this series, the text of *The Four Medical Tantras* can be clearly seen like a transparent chebule flower on one's palm."

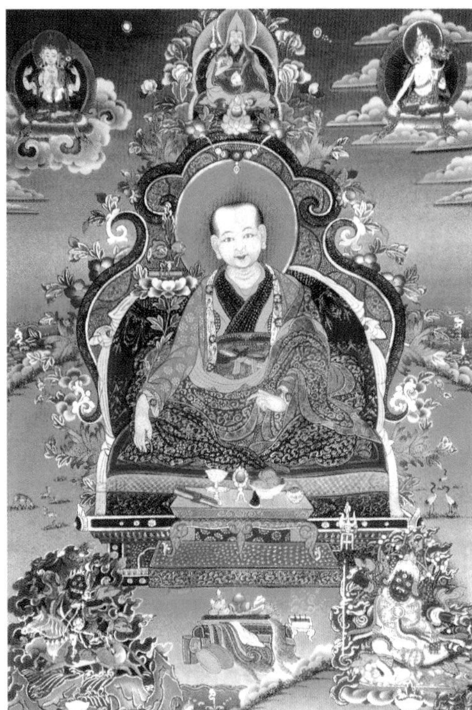

Sanggyas Gyatsho (1653-1705).

Presently, the use of hanging scroll paintings in medical teaching is very common and may not seem special. However, the *Sman thang* series is different, because it is also a rare treasure of one of the ancient medical systems in the world. Not only is it several hundred years old, but it possesses very rich contents and includes almost all aspects of Tibetan medicine. It also has strong ethnic features, as the paintings in the whole series manifests the unique Tibetan flavor, including figures, architecture, habits, customs, language, and painting techniques. The *Sman thang* series is a unique teaching tool and is the only one of its kind in the world.

Eulogy on the classic

Because of the great value of *The Four Medical Tantras* to life and health, in the style of our predecessors, here we have composed a poem to this classic.

The *Root Tantras* are the seed of medicine from which all medical techniques are derived;

The *Description Tantras* are the sun and the moon in the sky by which all darkness and ignorance are eliminated;

The *Secrecy Tantras* are a treasure in which everything is included;

The *Conclusion Tantras* are a diamond dagger, by which all diseases are overcome without any obstacles;

Like the pleasing song of the cuckoo, *The Four Medical Tantras* make all creatures relaxed and happy;

Like the glory of the Sun, *The Four Medical Tantras* overshadows the light of the stars.

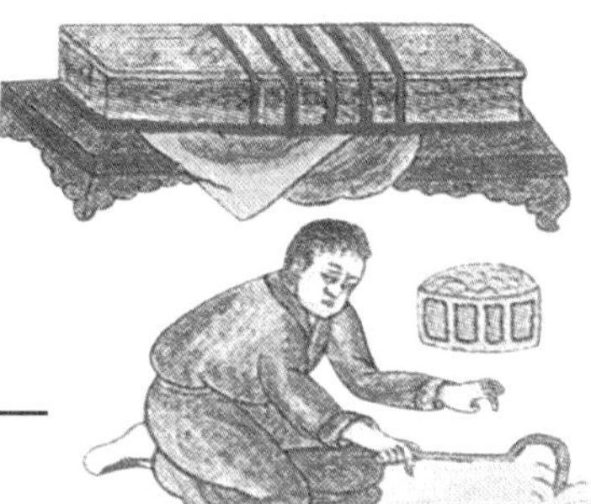

Like a fertile seed, all medical techniques are derived from it.

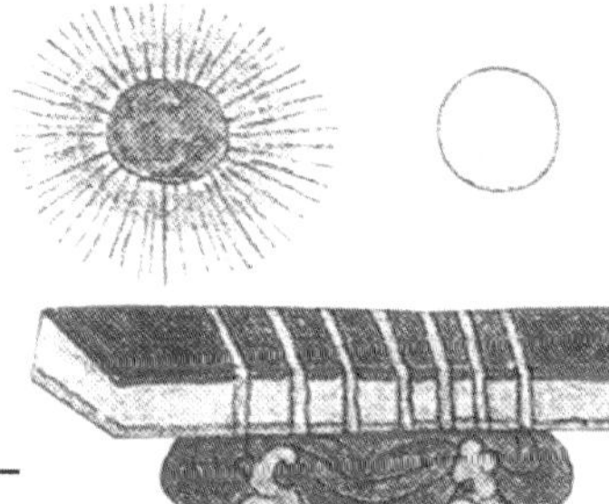

Like the sun and moon in the sky, it eliminates all ignorance.

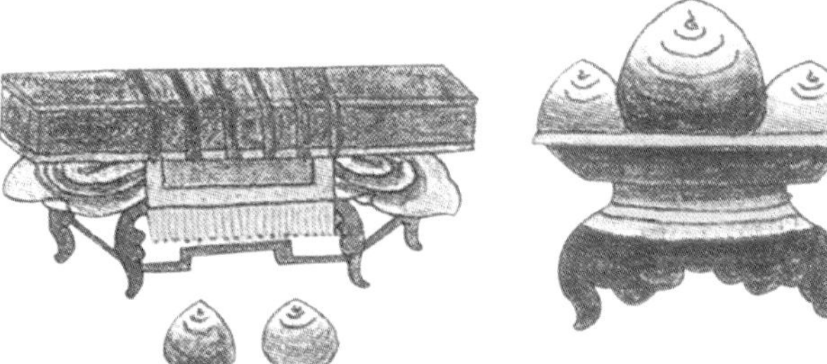

Like a diamond dagger, all diseases are eliminated without obstacle.

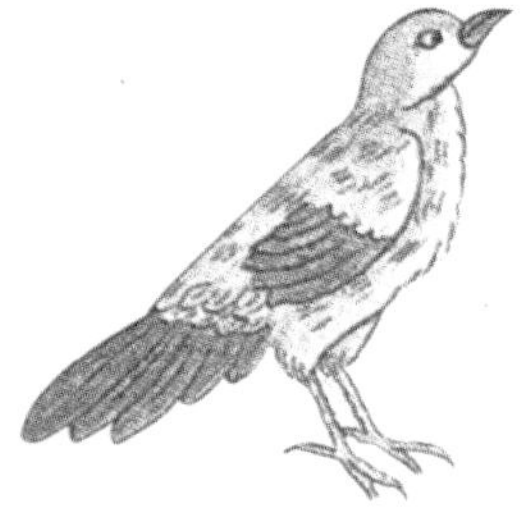

Like the pleasing song of a cuckoo, it makes all creatures relaxed and happy.

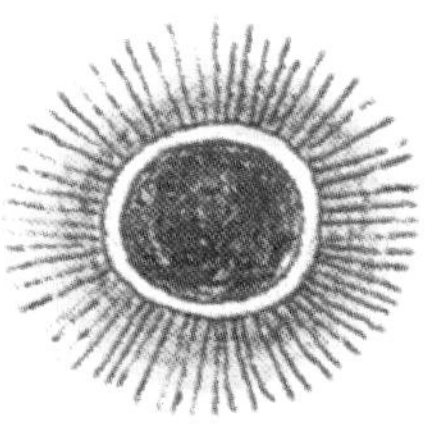

Like the pleasing song of the cuckoo, it makes all creatures relaxed and happy.

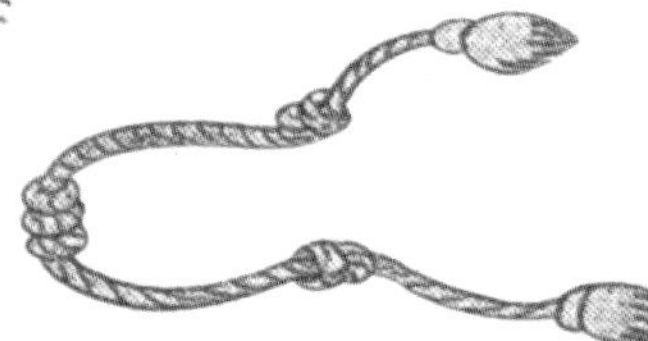

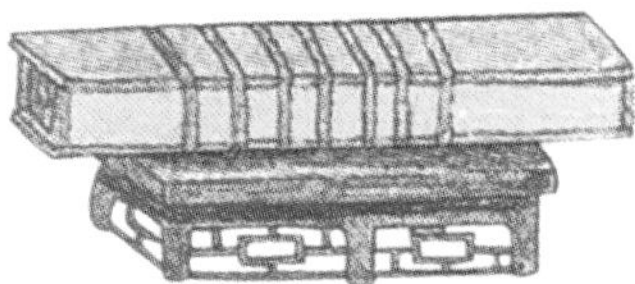

Like a vulture flying high, seeing all small diseases in a deep valley.

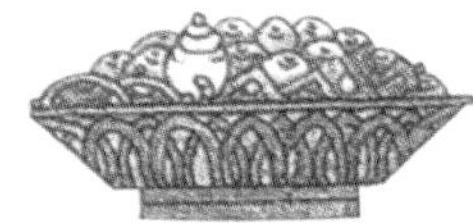

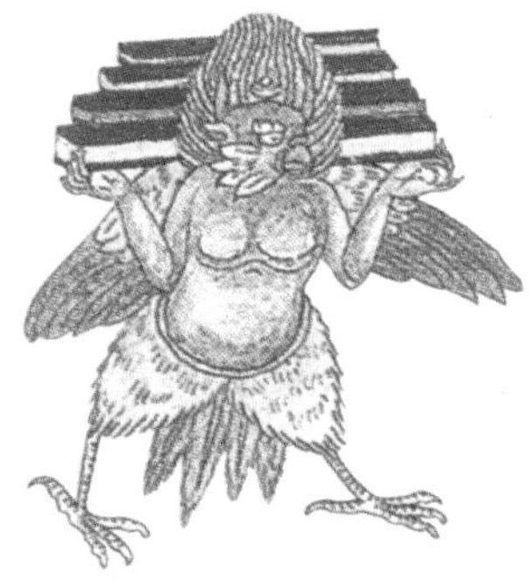

Like the glory of the Sun, it overshadows the star.

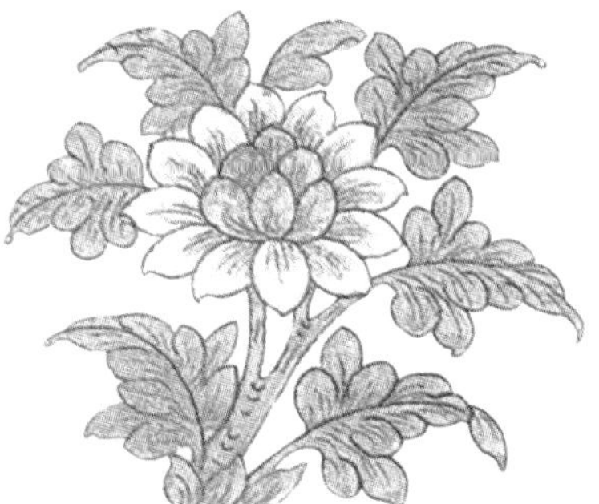

Like the reappearance of the broad leafed epiphyllum, it is rare and pure.

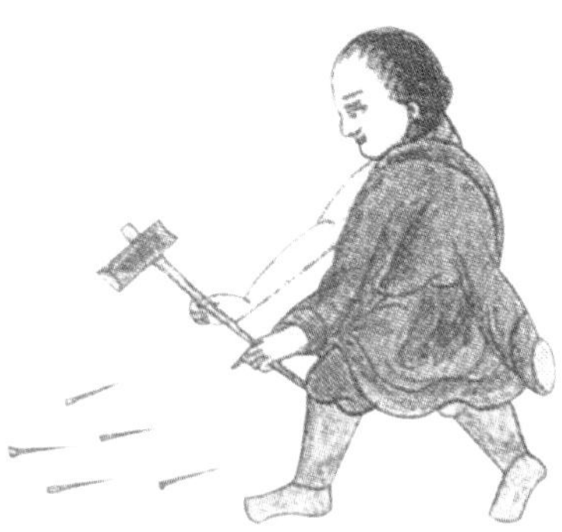

It is the hammer that smashes all diseases.

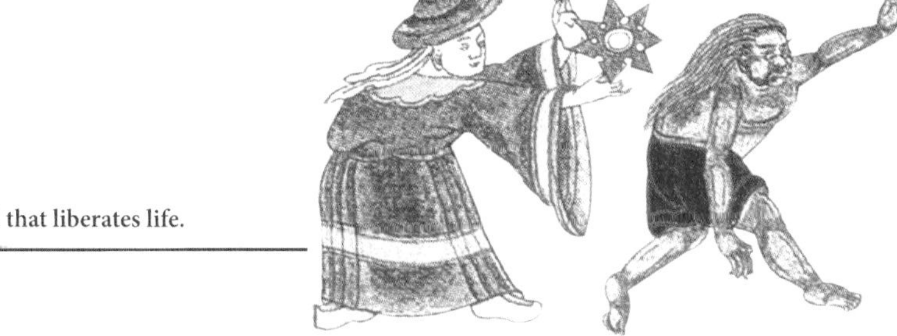

It is the gift that liberates life.

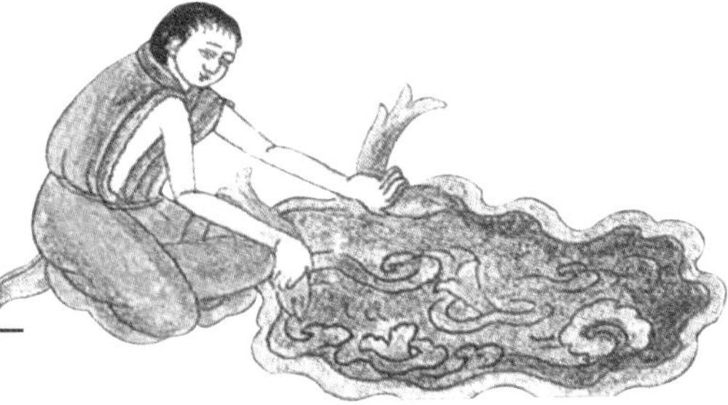

It is the diamond wheel expelling all disease devils.

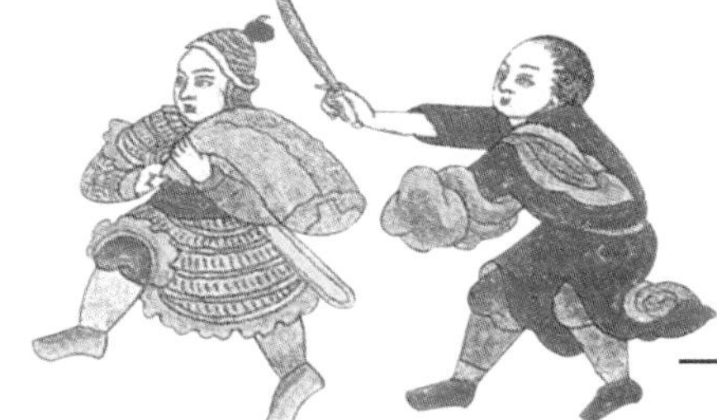

It is a warrior destroying all diseases.

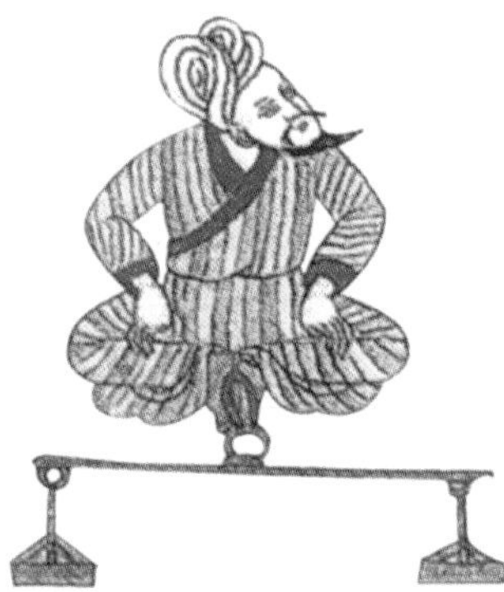

It is a balance that adjusts the three factors.

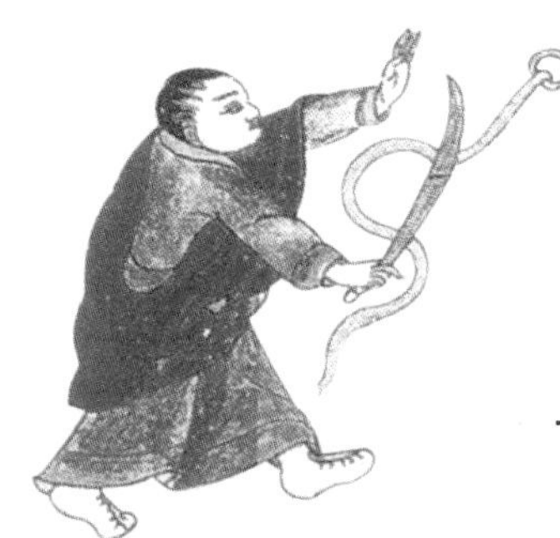

It is a sword severing the path to death.

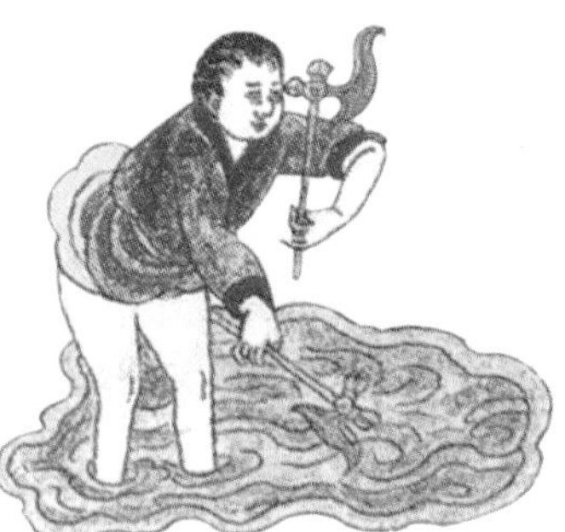

It is a blessed ladder leading all creatures to escape from the sea of bitterness.

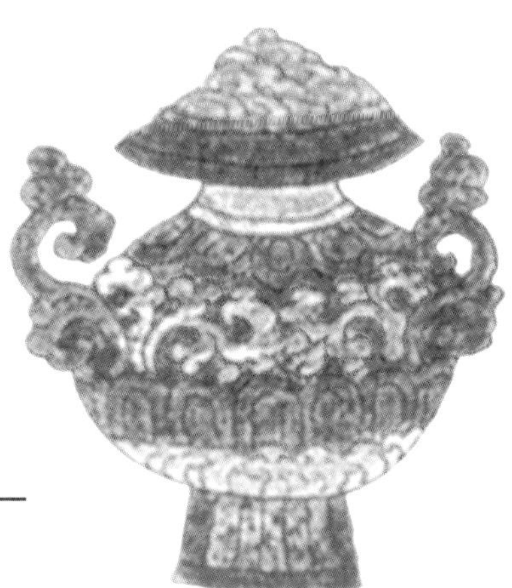

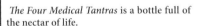

The Four Medical Tantras is a bottle full of the nectar of life.

Like the reappearance of a broad leafed epiphyllum, *The Four Medical Tantras* is very rare and pure.

The Four Medical Tantras collects all prescriptions to reach the peak of medicine, just like a vulture flying high, seeing all small diseases in a deep valley.

The Four Medical Tantras is a spiritual treasure destroying the devils of death, a hero conquering all disease evils, a scale adjusting harmony; a sharp dagger severing the rope that kills life, a hammer smashing the causes of pain, and a benefactor saving lives.

The Four Medical Tantras is the crown of medical theories, the protection of the lives of humans, the diamond wheel destroying diseases, the warrior eliminating disease, the sword severing the path to death, the blessed ladder that saves lives from the pool of misery, the gift that protects lives, and the precious bottle of nectar that saves lives from death.

The Four Medical Tantras makes great contributions to the health of all human beings. Tibetan physicians of later ages composed numerous poems in praise of it. The *Conclusion Tantras* summarizes all these poems as eleven kinds of metaphor. Let's use these poems to spread the seeds of fortune and health the world over.

This is the peak of all medical theories, the king governing all medical instruments, the key explaining all therapies, the foundation of all medical systems, the source of all medical thought, the precious mirror observing all diseases, the sea collecting all medical essence, the nectar eliminating all misery, the donation saving all lives, the item satisfying all wishes, and the valuable treasure preserving health and longevity.

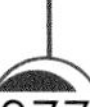

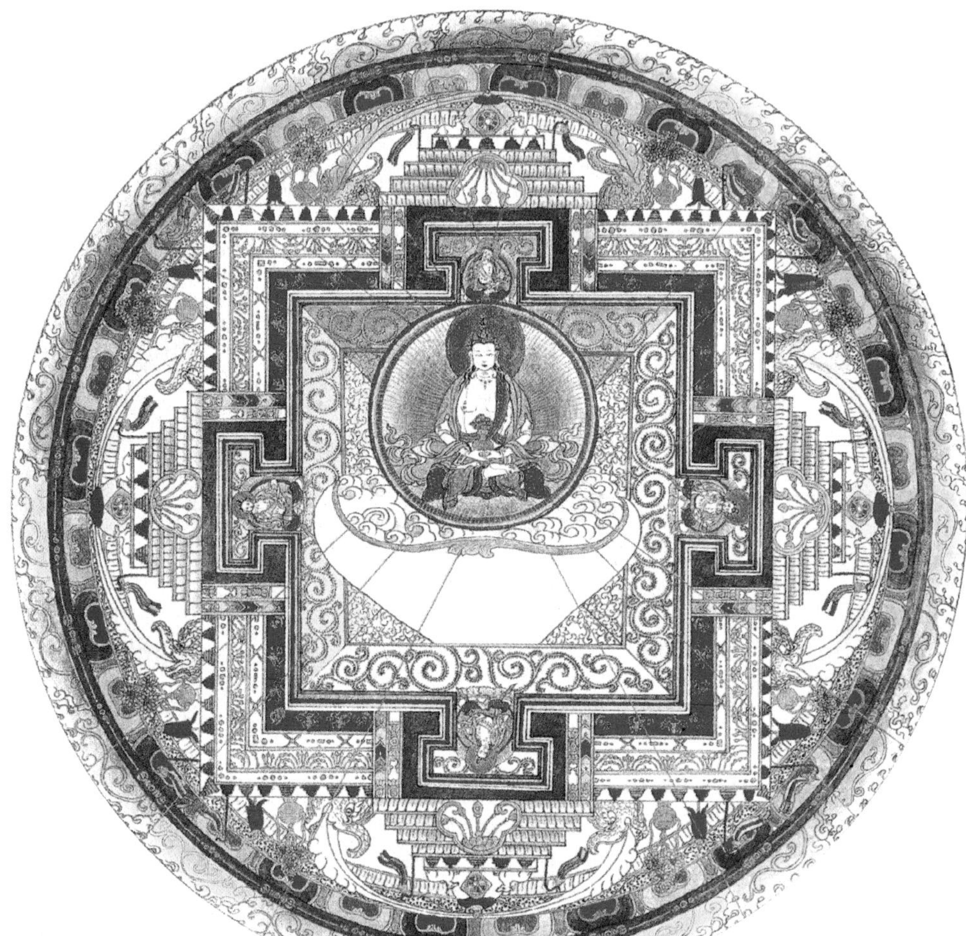

After the incarnation of the Medicine Buddha, the wise immortal instructs the world about health cultivation in the *Secrecy Tantras* of *The Four Medical Tantras*, he then returns to the City of Medicine Buddha (Lta-na-sdugs). (From *Thangkha* fifty-five in the *Sman thang* series, the life preservation II of *The Four Medical Tantras*)

INDEX BY BOOKS, TERMS AND PERSON'S NAME

Books

Terms

Persons' Names

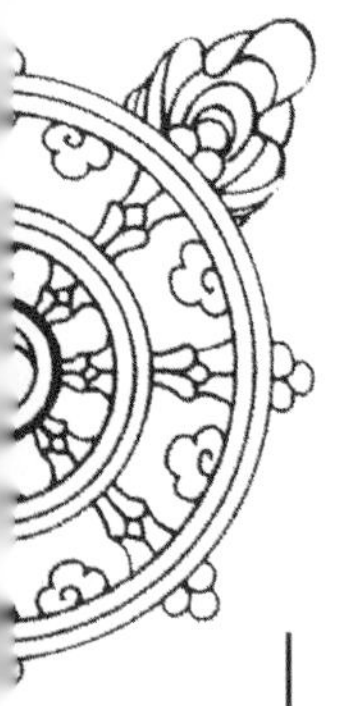

GENERAL INDEX

A

B

C

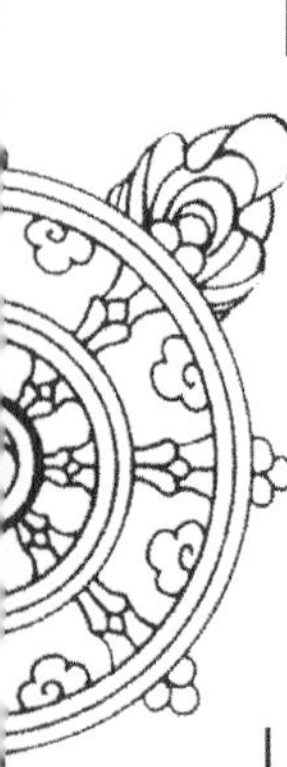

D

E

F

G

N

O

P

Q

R

S

T

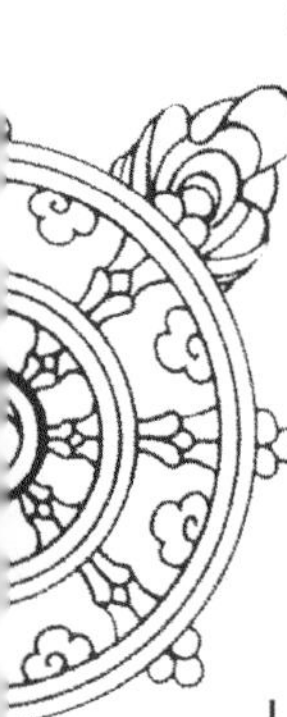

U

V

W

X

Y

Z

图书在版编目（CIP）数据

图说藏医养生（英文）/黄福开主编.—北京：人民卫生出版社，2008.4

ISBN 978-7-117-09101-5

Ⅰ.图… Ⅱ.黄… Ⅲ.藏医－养生（中医）－普及读物－英文 Ⅳ.R291.4-49

中国版本图书馆CIP数据核字（2007）第121359号

图说藏医养生 (英文)

主　　编：黄福开

出版发行：人民卫生出版社（中继线+8610-6761-6688）

地　　址：中国北京市丰台区方庄芳群园三区3号楼

邮　　编：100078

网　　址：http://www.pmph.com

E - mail：pmphsales@gmail.com

发　　行：zzg@pmph.com.cn

购书热线：+8610-6769-1034（电话及传真）

开　　本：787×1092　1/16

版　　次：2008年4月第1版　　2008年4月第1版第1次印刷

标准书号：ISBN 978-7-117-09101-5/R·9102